ATLAS OF THE EAR

by Scanning Electron Microscopy

ATLAS OF THE EAR

by Scanning Electron Microscopy

Yasuo Harada

Hiroshima University Medical School
Hiroshima, Japan

Published, in association with
Nishimura Co., Ltd., Japan, by

MTP PRESS LIMITED
International Medical Publishers
LANCASTER · BOSTON · THE HAGUE

Published by
MTP Press Limited
Falcon House
Lancaster, England

British Library Cataloguing in Publication Data
Harada, Yasuo
Atlas of the ear by scanning electron microscopy.
1. Ear
I. Title
611'.85 QM507

ISBN-13: 978-94-009-6600-0 e-ISBN-13:978-94-009-6598-0
DOI: 10.1007/978-94-009-6598-0

Originally published in Japanese by Nishimura Co., Ltd.,
1-754-39 Asahimachi-dori, Niigata-shi 951, Japan.

Softcover reprint of the hardcover 1st edition 1983

Contents

Foreword

The physiology of the semicircular canals was my main research interest before I began to study their morphology. In 1966, by utilizing the isolated semicircular canal of the frog, I was able to show that cell activity in the horizontal semicircular canal has the opposite polarity to that in the vertical canals, which was the first physiological proof of Ewald's law. Several transmitting electron microscope (TEM) studies had already reported on the morphology of the semicircular canal cristae; however, my morphological work was motivated by a strong desire to see whether the morphological polarity accorded to the physiological polarity.

In 1968 I happened to see the paper written by Dr David Lim, one of my close friends. His findings concerning the vestibular morphology, when examined by scanning electron microscopy (SEM), fascinated me a great deal because of the three-dimensional quality of the micrographs. This stimulated me to become involved in vestibular morphology. In the beginning, however, I faced many problems with specimen preparation for SEM, and the first few years were spent simply solving technical problems, especially those of artifacts.

Many of the figures in this book have been photographed with a JEOL JSM U-3 scanning electron microscope over a decade. The sharpness of these pictures still, I think, bears comparison to the definition of those taken by the more sophisticated SEM scopes currently available.

My work on the morphology and physiology of the vestibular organ led me to research into the whole inner and middle ear system. This has been intensively investigated with a JEOL JSM T200 and a JEOL JSM F15 which were recently introduced to my department. Here, these micrographs from the inner and middle ear are compiled for publication together with brief captions. What is presented in the text is generally aimed at the level of the otolaryngologist, but would also be of interest to medical students. The structure of the inner ear is complicated, as is indicated by its alternative name of 'labyrinth', and it used to be a research field not easily accessible. In this atlas emphasis is placed on the surface structure, thus enabling better understanding of the anatomy. Furthermore, this book covers almost every aspect of the inner and middle ear, such as morphology beneath the surface, the nervous system and even clinical pathology.

It is my great pleasure that this publication may contribute to the work of those concerned with the ultrastructure of the ear.

Yasuo Harada, MD

Acknowledgements

Many thanks to Prof M. Cherubino at Pavia University, Italy, who invited me to conduct research on the physiology of the inner ear. Physiological work under guidance of Prof C. Casela and Prof G. Rapuzzi at the Istituto di Fisiologia Generale dell'a Università di Pavia, was further developed in Japan and stimulated my interest in vestibular morphology.

Prof S. Kurozumi's support for this study is acknowledged.

Dr N. Tagashira, Mr M. Murao, Ms Y. Ohki and Ms M. Hayashi have been extremely helpful in preparing pictures and the manuscript. Thanks are also due to Dr I. Hunter-Duvar and Dr M. Suzuki who have contributed to this English compilation. This work was supported by Grant-in-Aid for Scientific Research C 157399, B 248309 and A 440162.

The Middle Ear

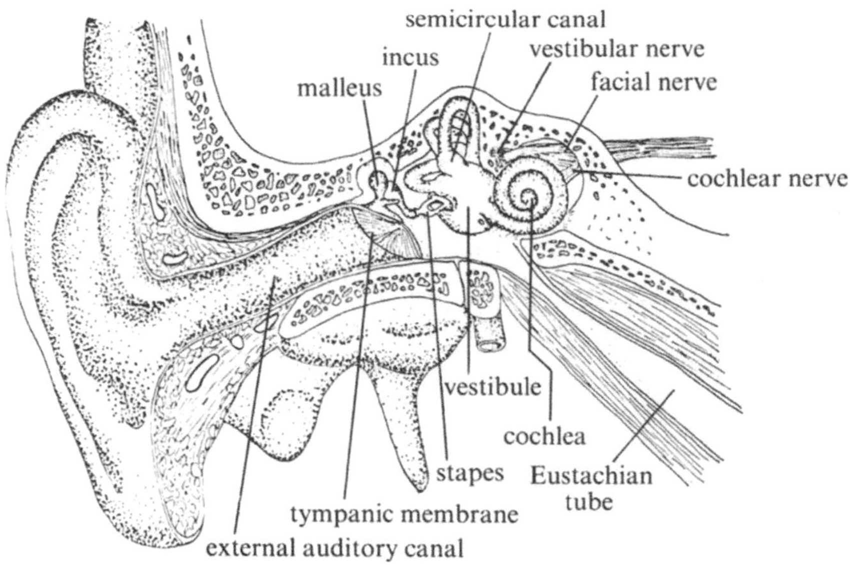

The tympanic membrane

The tympanic membrane of a human adult is oval or elliptical in shape, with its major axis 9.0–10.2 mm in length and minor axis 8.5–9.0 mm. The tympanic membrane is divided into tense and flaccid portions and histologically consists of three layers, epidermis, lamina propria and mucosa. The flaccid portion lacks the lamina propria. The annular ligament surrounds the tense portion, but it is interrupted at the flaccid portion.

(1) *Epidermis*

This is especially thick in the flaccid portion and is divided into the stratum corneum, stratum spinosum and stratum basale.

(2) *Lamina propria*

There are two layers; the radiate fibrous layer on the outside and the circular fibrous layer inside. These layers include collagen fibrils and other fine fibrils. Studies by SEM showed the radiate fibrous layer starts from the lower $\frac{4}{5}$ of the malleus manubrium (Shimada *et al.*, 1971) and ends at the annulus. The circular fibrous layer arises from the short process of the malleus, partly from the manubrium and is dense in the peripheral area of the tympanic membrane. A similar structure is seen in the guinea pig (Lim, 1970, Kawabata, 1971, Harada, 1972, Nomura, 1978).

(3) *Mucosa*

This layer consists of a single layer of squamous cells in the flaccid portion which partially includes multiple stratified cylindrical cells (Hentzer, 1969). There are microvilli in the cell surfaces and also some cells with a centriole.

References

1. Harada, Y. (1972). Scanning electron microscopic observation of the lamina propria of the tympanic membrane in guinea pig. *Practica Otologia (Kyoto)*, **65,** 995
2. Hentzer, E. (1969). Ultrastructure of the human tympanic membrane. *Acta Otolaryngol. (Stockholm)*, **68,** 576
3. Kawabata, I. and Ishii, H. (1971). Fiber arrangement in the tympanic membrane. *Acta Otolaryngol. (Stockholm)*, **72,** 243
4. Lim, D. J. (1970). Human tympanic membrane. Electron microscopic observation. *Acta Otolaryngol. (Stockholm)*, **70,** 197
5. Shimada, T., *et al.* (1971). The fiber arrangement of the human tympanic membrane. A scanning electron microscopic observation. *Ann Otol. Rhinol. Laryngol.*, **80,** 210

Figure 1 Epidermis (human). (**a**) There are some concave portions possibly due to the nucleus of the cell (× 400), (**b**) the surface is generally smooth, but partially desquamated (× 1300)

a

b

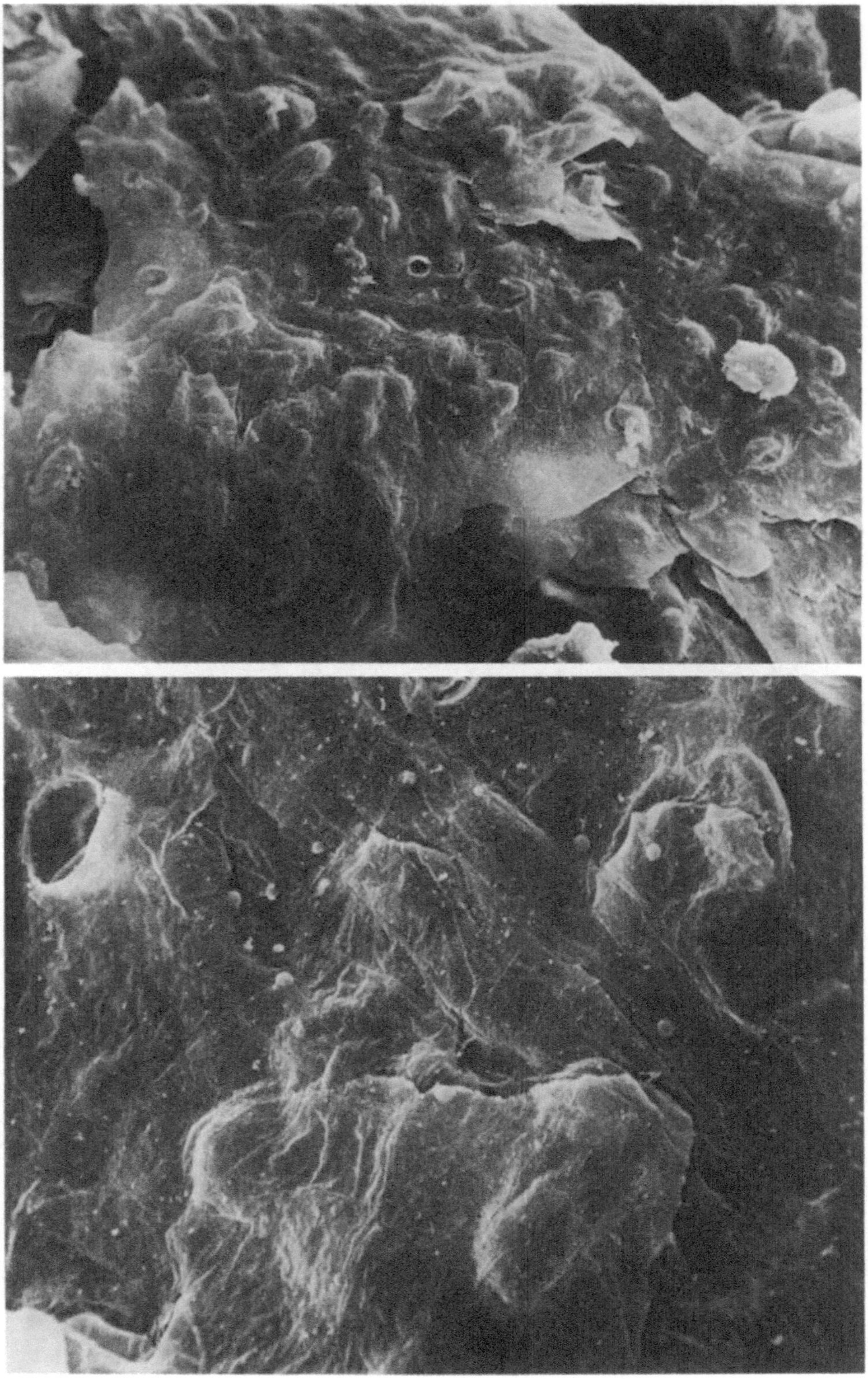

Figure 1

a

b

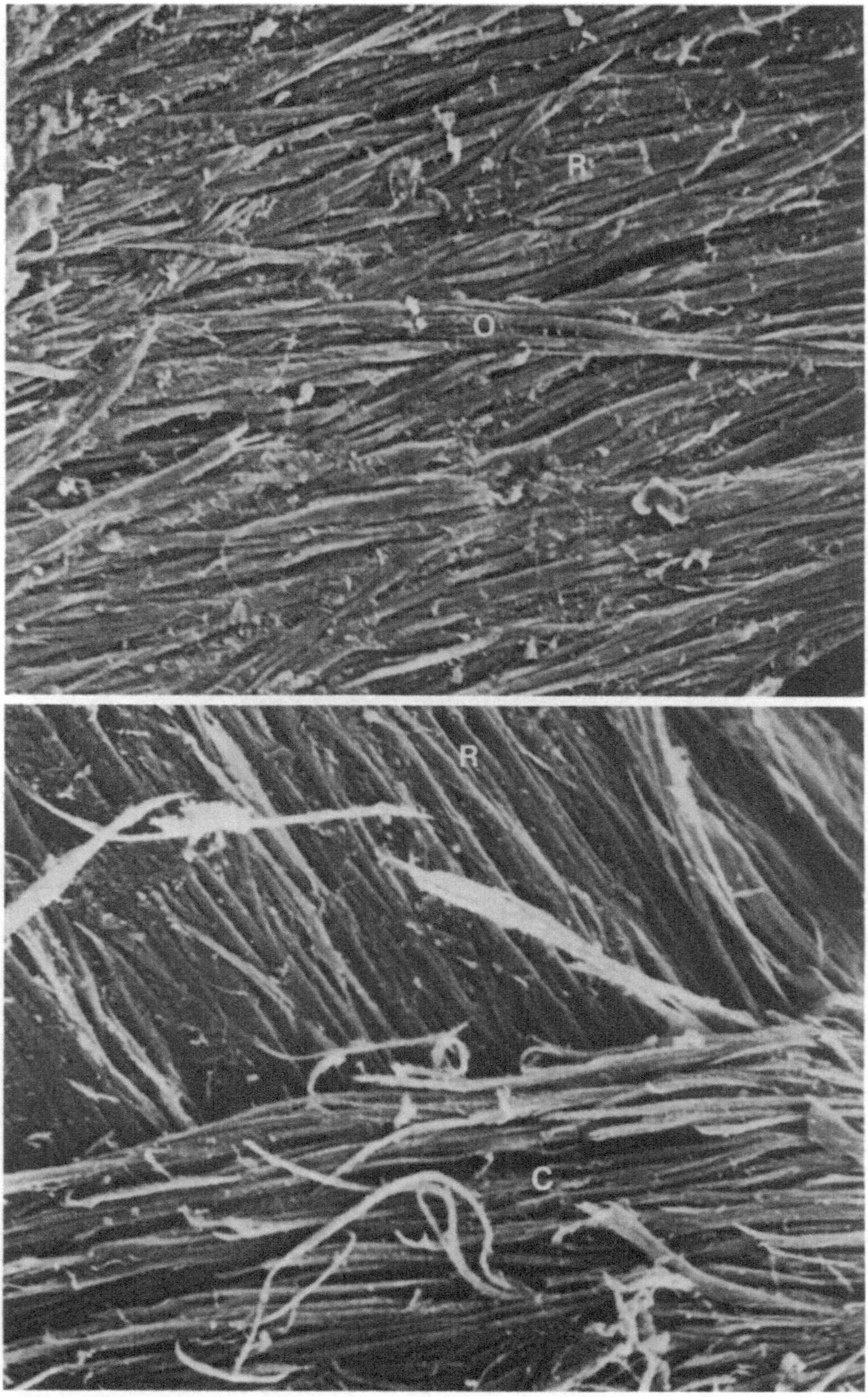

Figure 2 Lamina propria (human). C: circular fibre, R: radiate fibre, O: oblique fibre. (**a**) × 400, (**b**) × 400

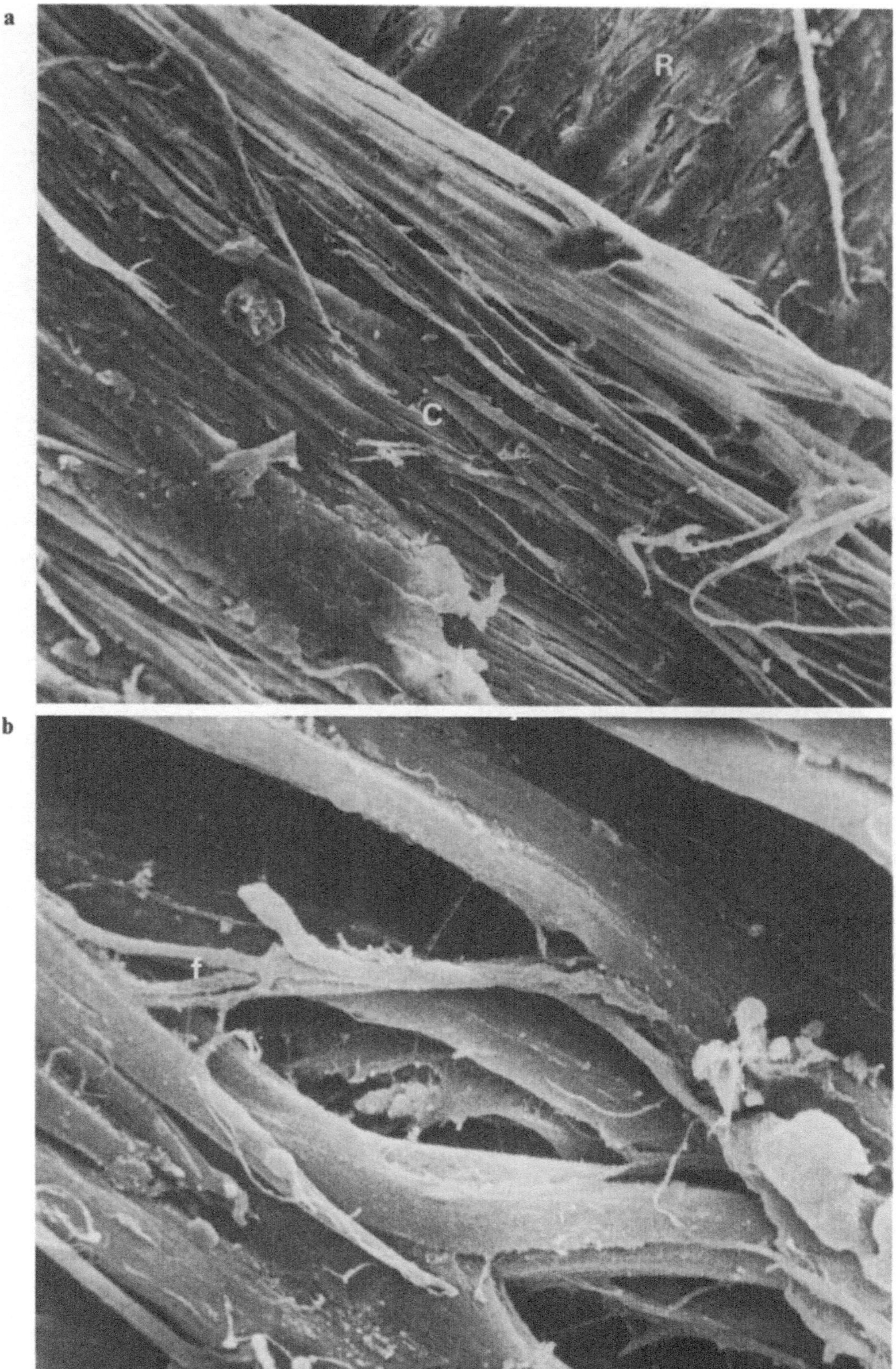

Figure 3 The circular (C) and the radiate (R) fibrous layers (human) (**a**) × 400, (**b**) × 4000

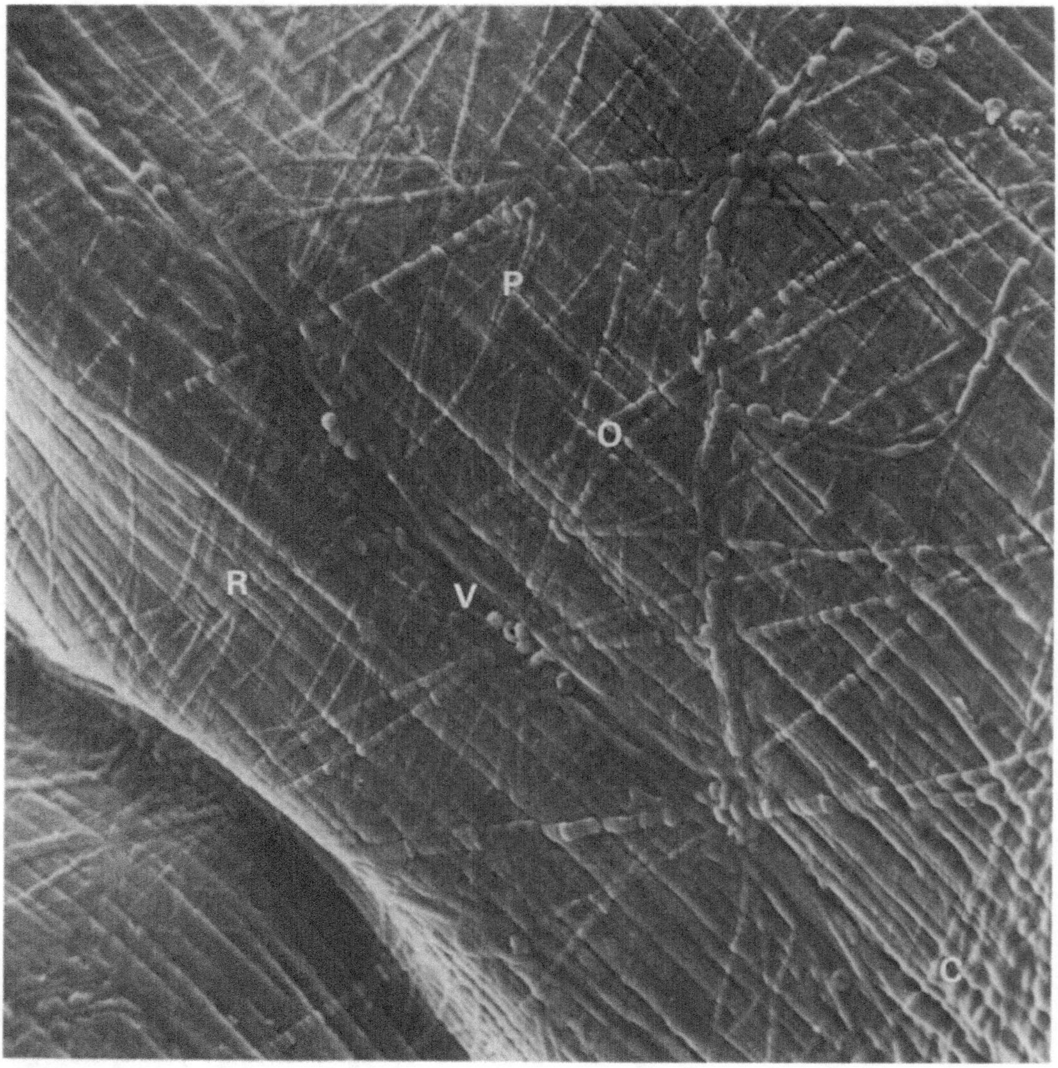

Figure 4 Lamina propria (guinea pig). The lamina propria of guinea pig is thinner than that of human. The oblique (O) and the circular fibres (C) are observed on the radiate fibres (R). Small vessels (V), which contain blood cells, are also seen (× 500)

Figure 5 Mucosa (human). The mucosa is covered by flat cells with a few microvilli. Since each cell body is relatively thin, the nucleus sometimes causes bulging on the cell surface. (**a**) Polygonal large cells are seen together with smaller cells (× 1400), (**b**) a cell with a centriole (× 4200)

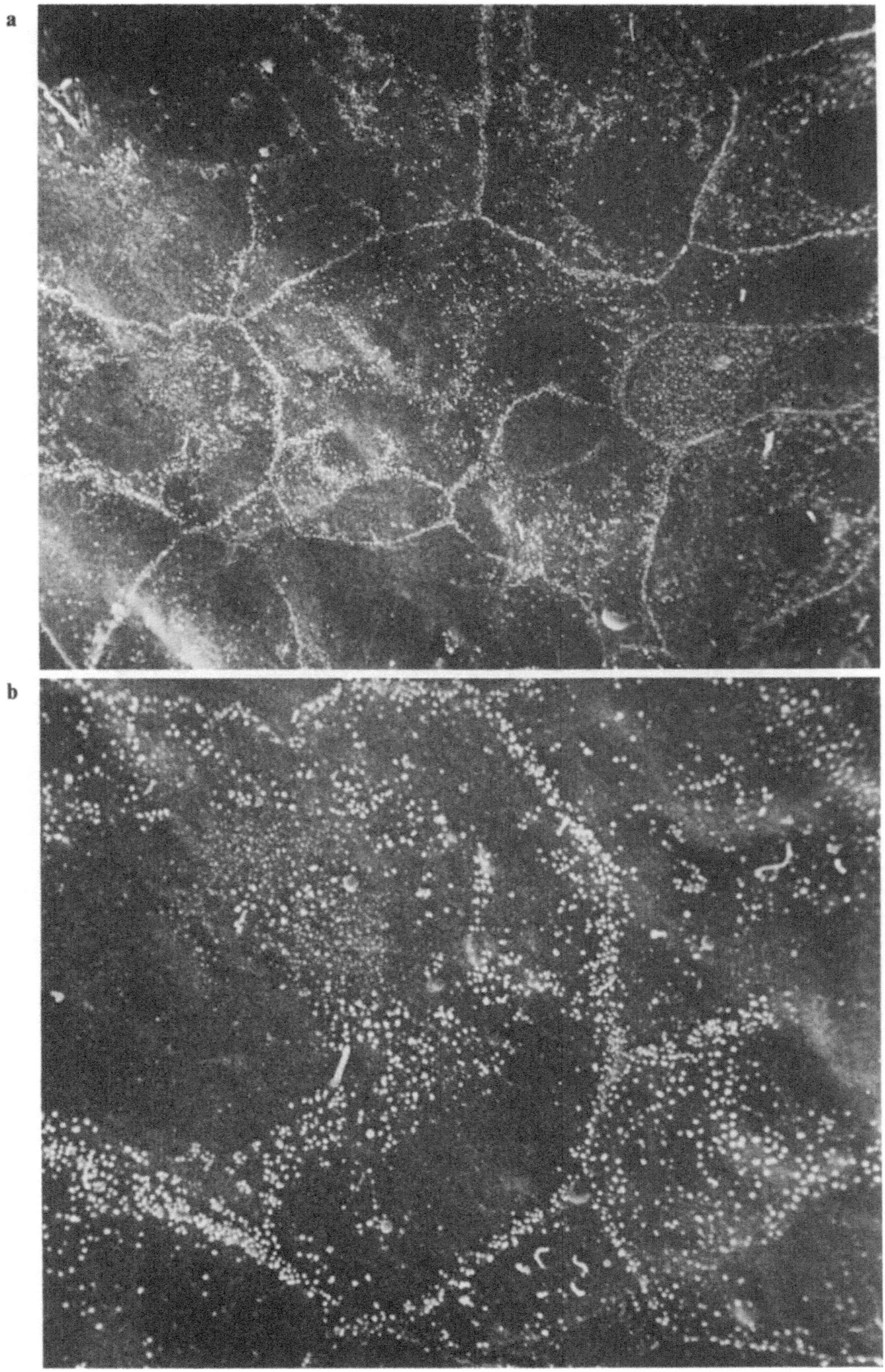

Figure 5

The auditory ossicles

The auditory ossicles are composed of three small bones in the upper tympanic cavity. Ossicles are bound to each other by joints, thus creating an ossicular chain. They connect the tympanic membrane with the oval window to conduct the sound from the air to the fluid of the cochlea.

(1) *Malleus, hammer*

The malleus is the largest of all ossicles and weighs 24.91 ± 0.61 mg. The upper portion is called the head of the malleus.

Anteriorly below the head of the malleus is the anterior process. Other portions are the neck, lateral process and handle of the malleus. The head of the malleus forms the incudomallear joint with the incus. The tip of the handle (manubrium) adheres to the tympanic membrane.

(2) *Incus*

This ossicle is located in the recessus epitympanicus and weighs 27.39 ± 1.03 mg. There is a saddle-shaped surface in the body which forms an articulation with the head of the malleus. The body continues to a short leg (short process, crus breve) and a long leg (crus longum). The short process attaches to the fossa incudis and the long leg has the lenticular process at its end which forms the incudostapedial joint with the stapes.

(3) *Stapes*

This is the most medially located and the lightest of all the ossicles, weighing 3.38 ± 0.48 mg. There are four portions, the foot plate, anterior crus, posterior crus and head. The foot plate is flat and covers the oval window. Anterior and posterior crura are the same length and continue to the head. The lateral side of the head articulates with the lenticular process of incus (incudostapedial joint).

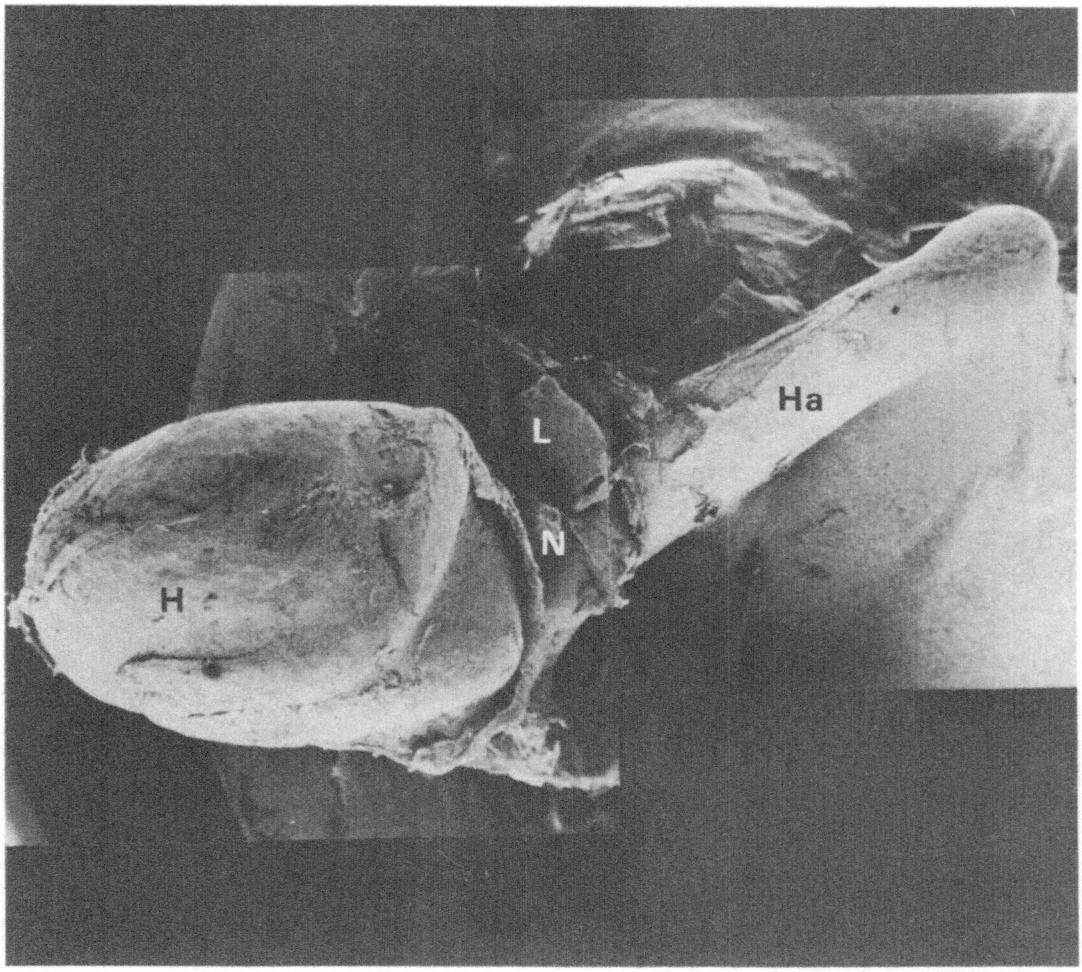

Figure 6 Malleus (human). H: head, capitulum mallei; N: neck, collum mallei; Ha: handle of malleus, manubrium mallei; L: lateral process, short process, processus lateralis (× 20)

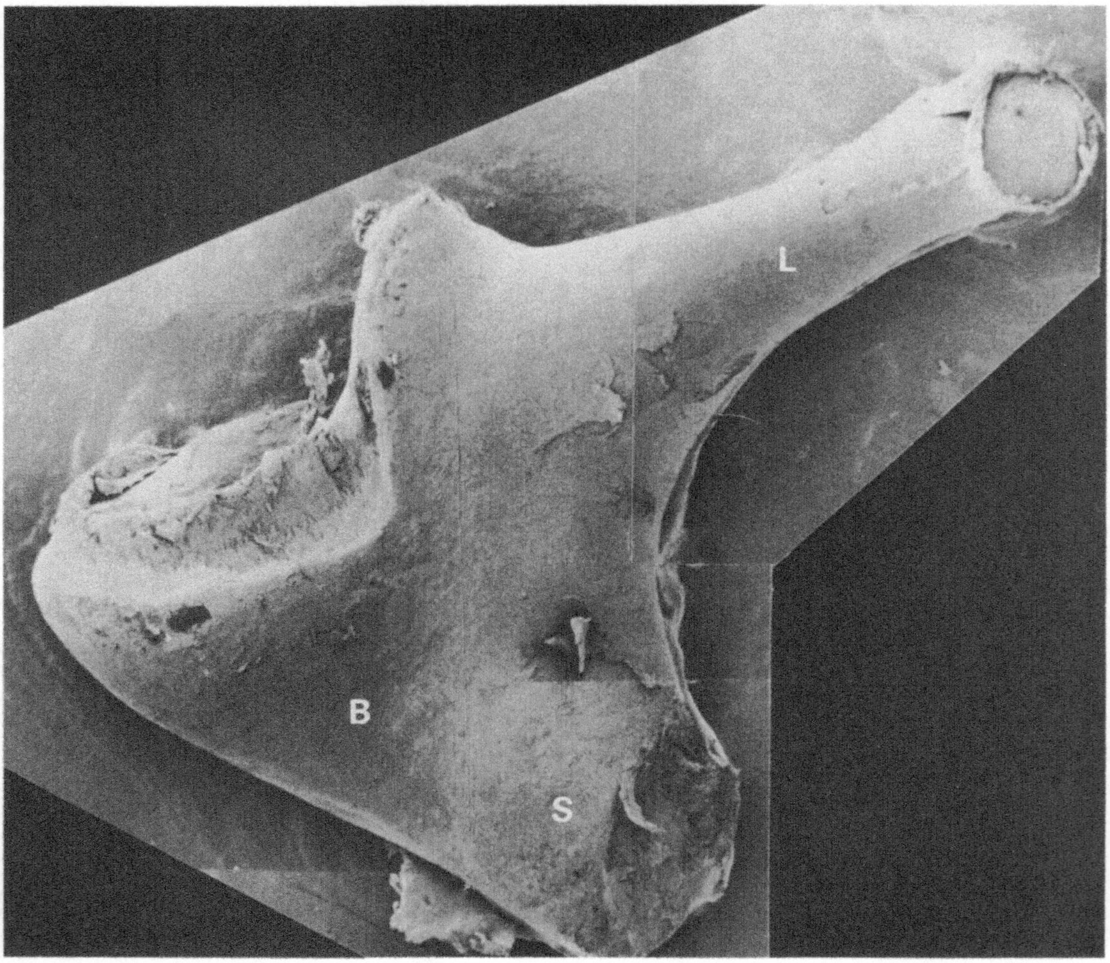

Figure 7 Incus (human). B: body, corpus; S: short leg, crus breve; L: long leg, crus longum

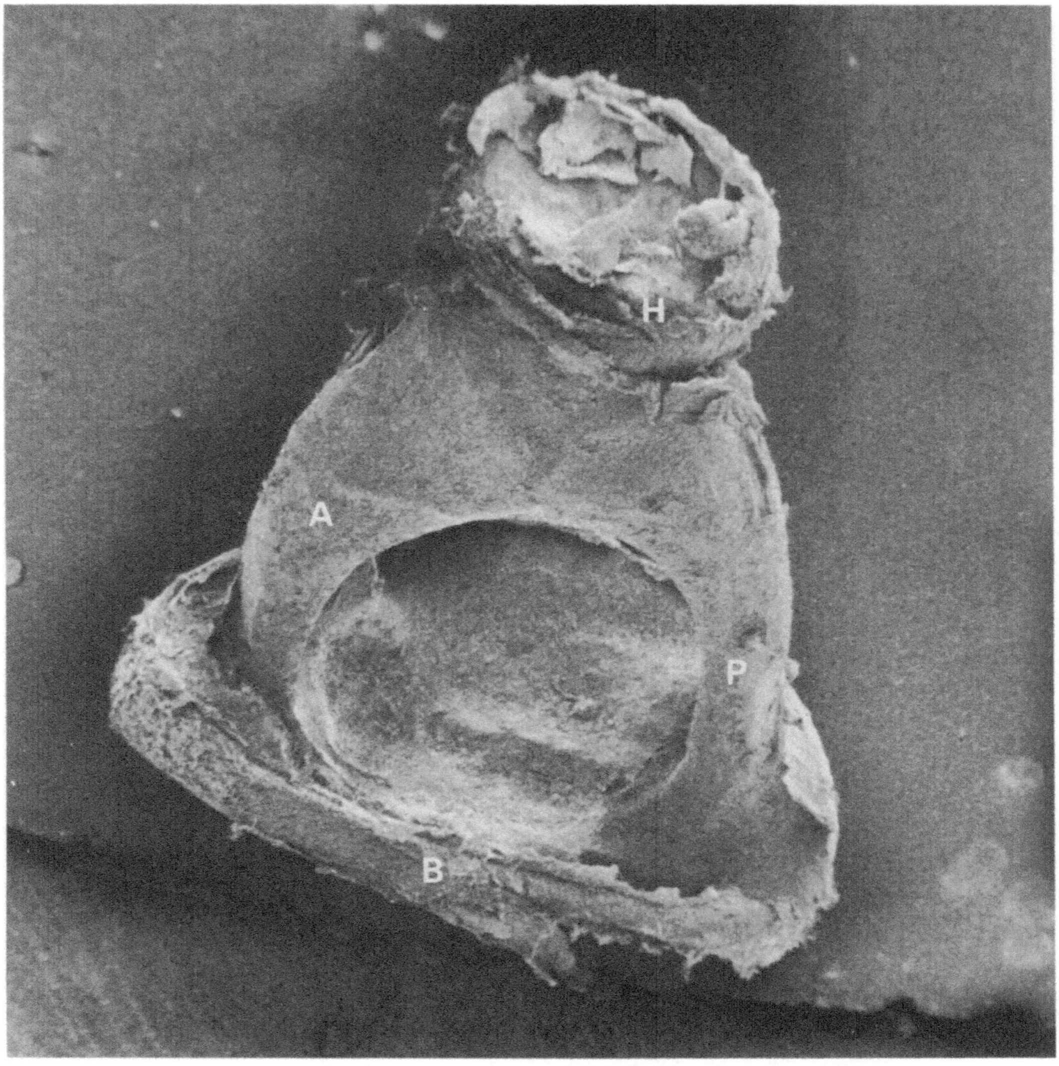

Figure 8 Stapes (human). B: footplate, basis stapedis; H: head, capitulum stapedis; P: posterior crus, crus posterius; A: anterior crus, crus anterius (× 30)

The auditory ossicular chain

The malleus, incus and stapes are the smallest bones in the whole body and the incudomallear and incudostapedial articulations are the smallest joints in the body. Vibrations of the tympanic membrane are transmitted to the ossicles. The malleus and incus perform a pendulum movement, while the stapes has a piston-like movement. The ossicles also amplify the sound intensity slightly by acting as a lever, and considerably because of the great difference in area between the tympanic membrane and the stapes foot plate.

a

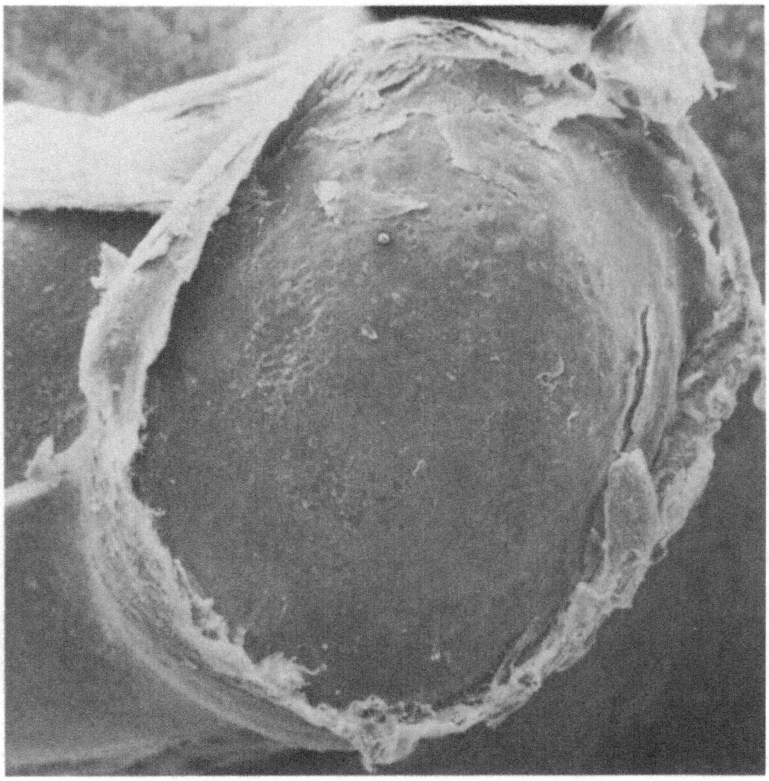

Figure 9 Incudostapedial joint (human). (**a**) The joint surface of the incus. A structure like a ligament is seen in the periphery. The joint surface of the incus is slightly convex as seen in this figure, while the joint surface of the stapes is concave (× 115). (**b**) Secretory activity is observed (× 3400). (**c**) A fibrous structure forms a network underneath the secretion (× 3400)

b

c

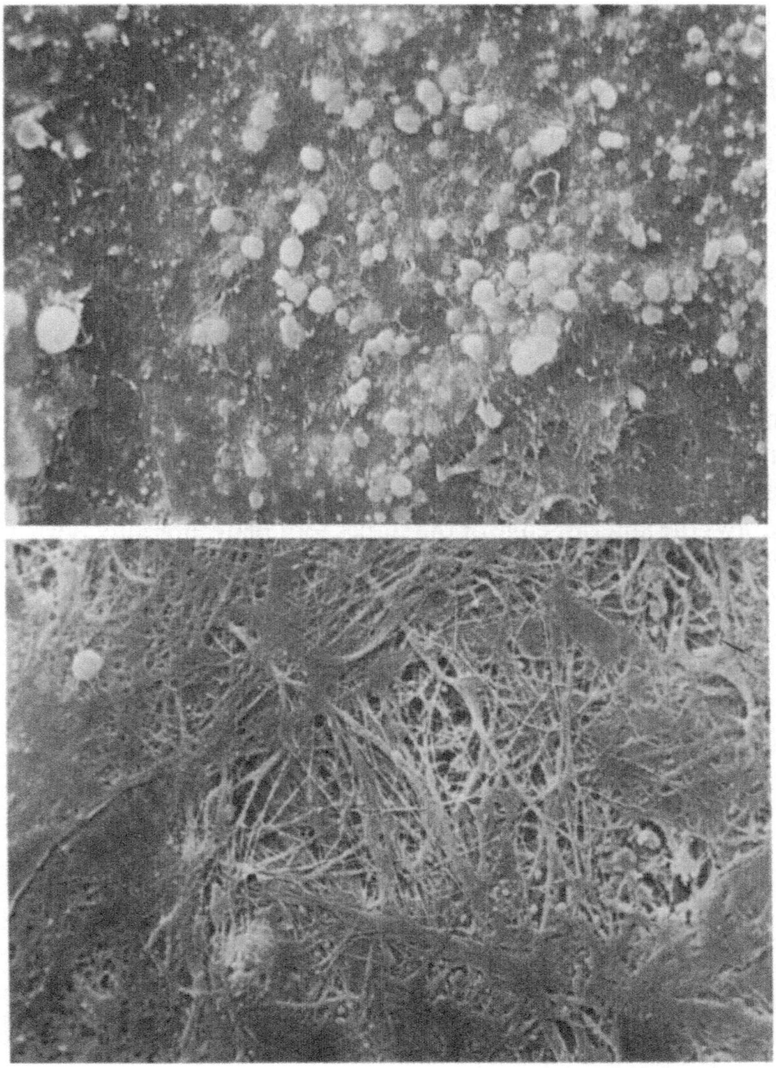

Figure 9

The auditory muscles

(1) *Tensor tympani muscle*

This muscle arises from the superior face of the cartilagenous part of the auditory tube and semicanal of this muscle. It turns laterally 90 degrees at the cochleariform process and attaches to the upper portion of the manubrium of the malleus. Nerve supply is from the third branch of the trigeminal nerve. Muscle function is to tighten the tympanic membrane.

(2) *Stapedius muscle*

This muscle is located in the hollow of the pyramidal eminence. Its tendon ends at the upper portion of the posterior crus of the stapes. This muscle is supplied by the stapedial branch of the facial nerve and it draws the anterior edge of the stapes foot plate laterally. Both muscles prevent transmission of intense vibration to the inner ear.

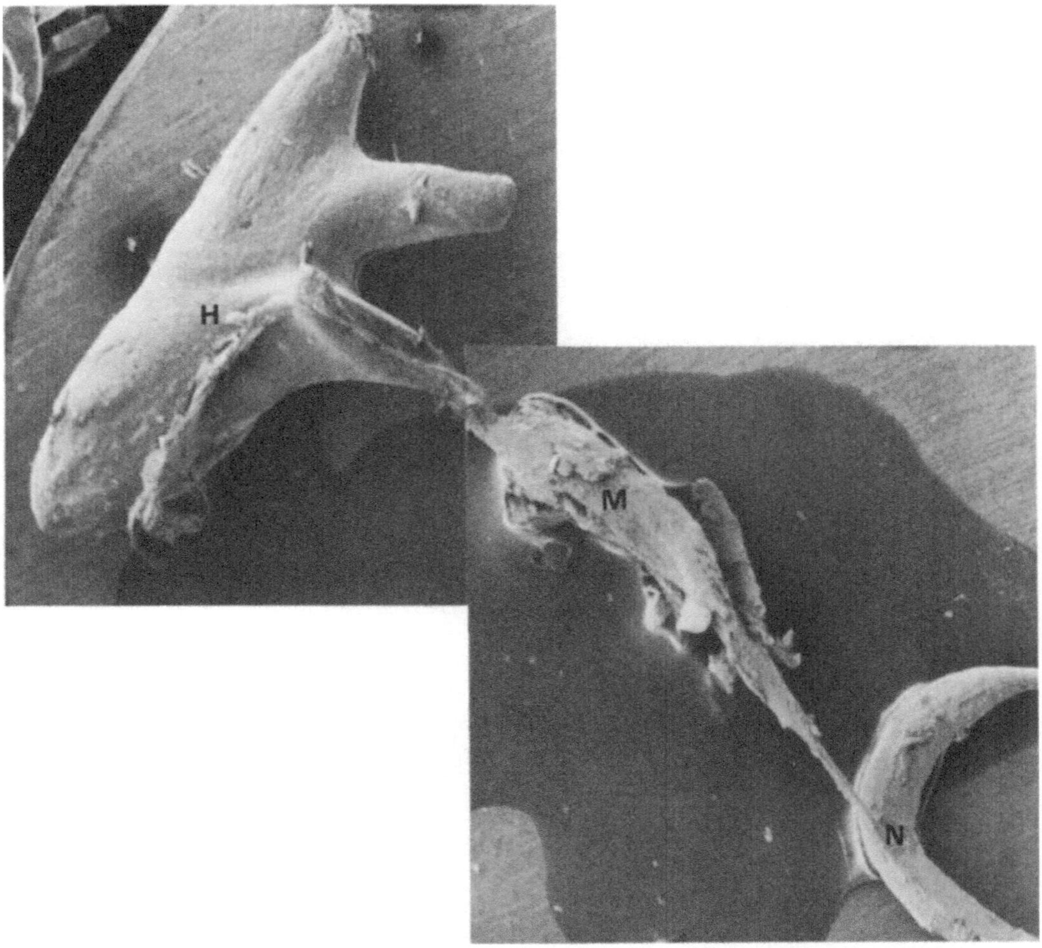

Figure 10 Tensor tympani muscle (guinea pig). In guinea pig, the malleus is fused with the incus (H). Tensor tympani muscle (M) which attaches to the manubrium of the malleus receives nerve supply from the trigeminus nerve (N) (× 20)

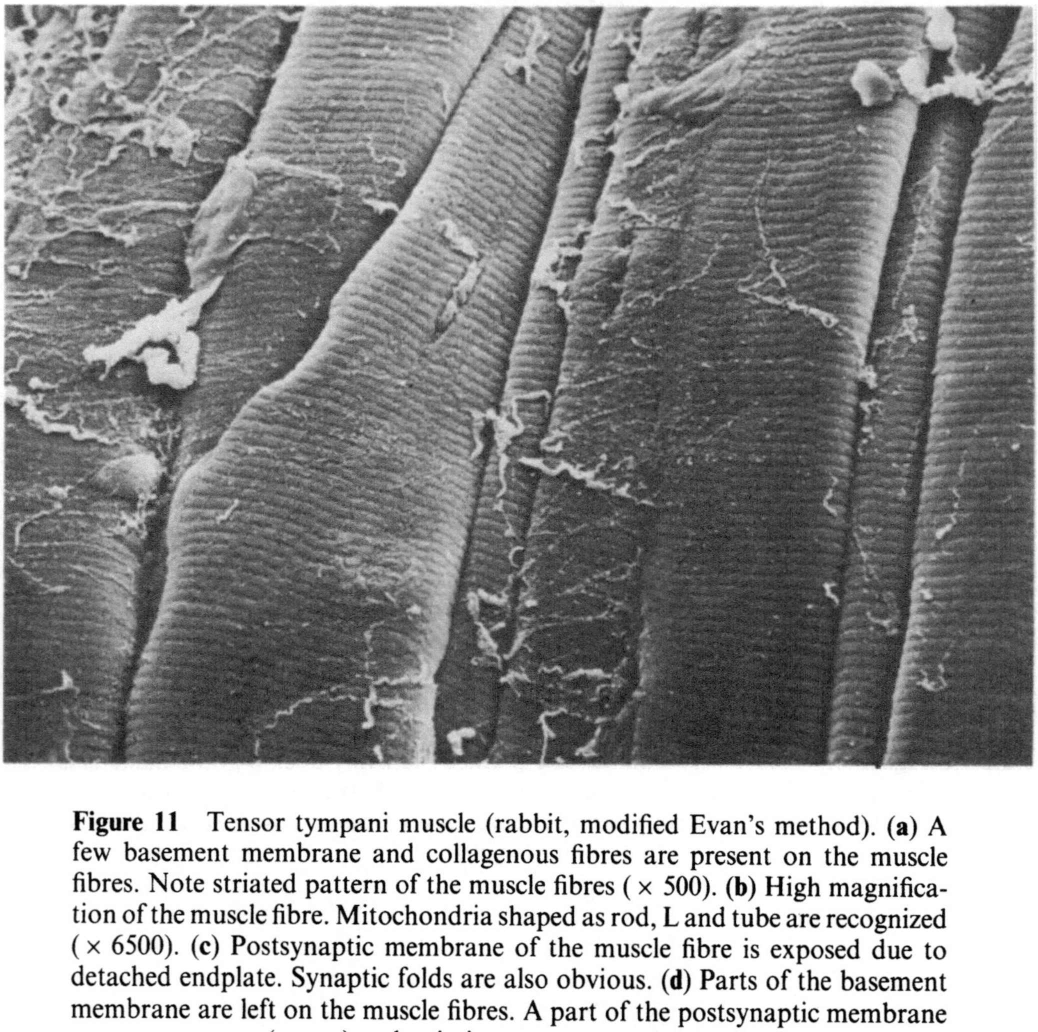

Figure 11 Tensor tympani muscle (rabbit, modified Evan's method). (**a**) A few basement membrane and collagenous fibres are present on the muscle fibres. Note striated pattern of the muscle fibres (× 500). (**b**) High magnification of the muscle fibre. Mitochondria shaped as rod, L and tube are recognized (× 6500). (**c**) Postsynaptic membrane of the muscle fibre is exposed due to detached endplate. Synaptic folds are also obvious. (**d**) Parts of the basement membrane are left on the muscle fibres. A part of the postsynaptic membrane (arrow) and striations are present (× 2000)

b

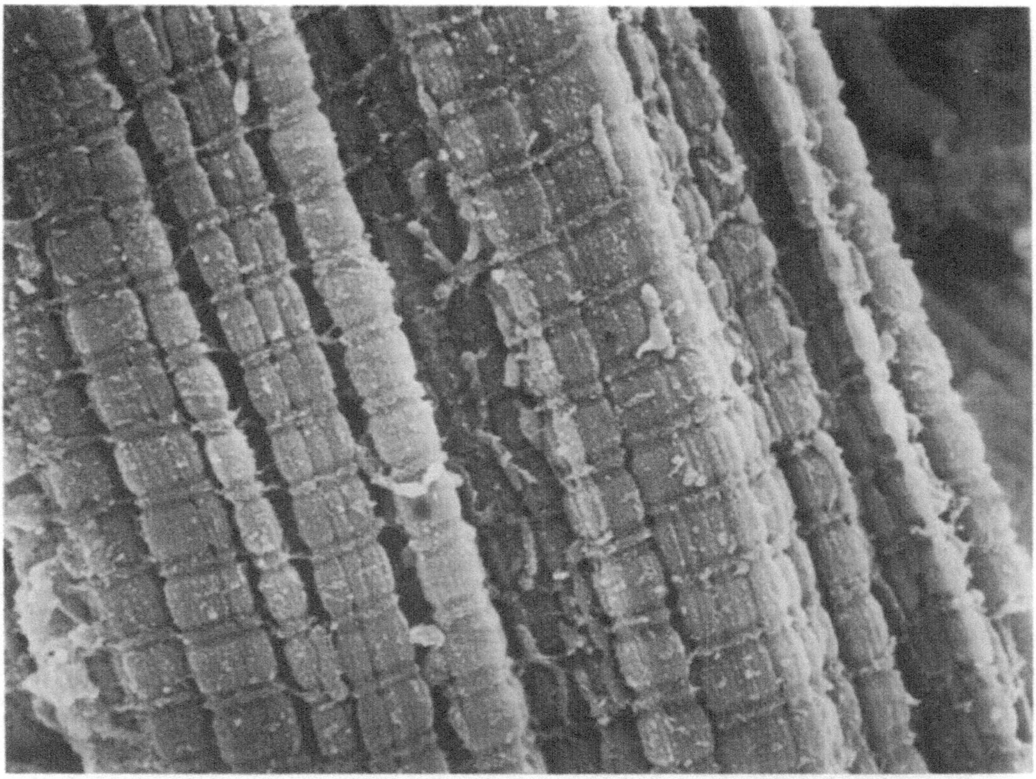

c

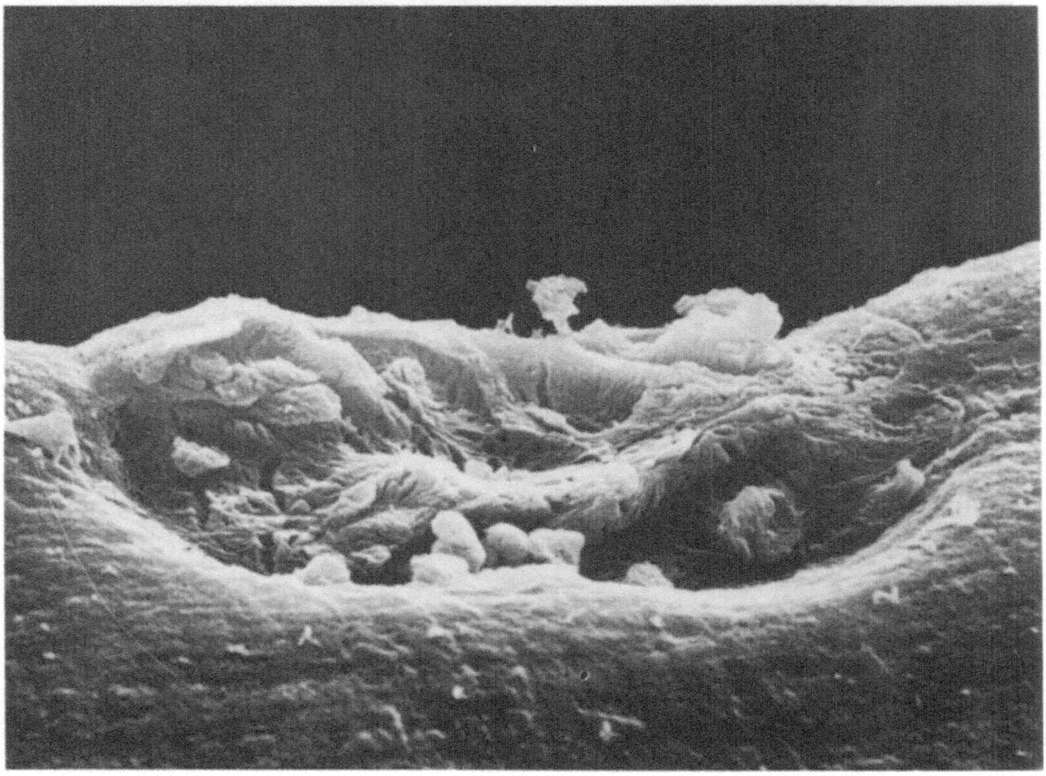

Figure 11

d

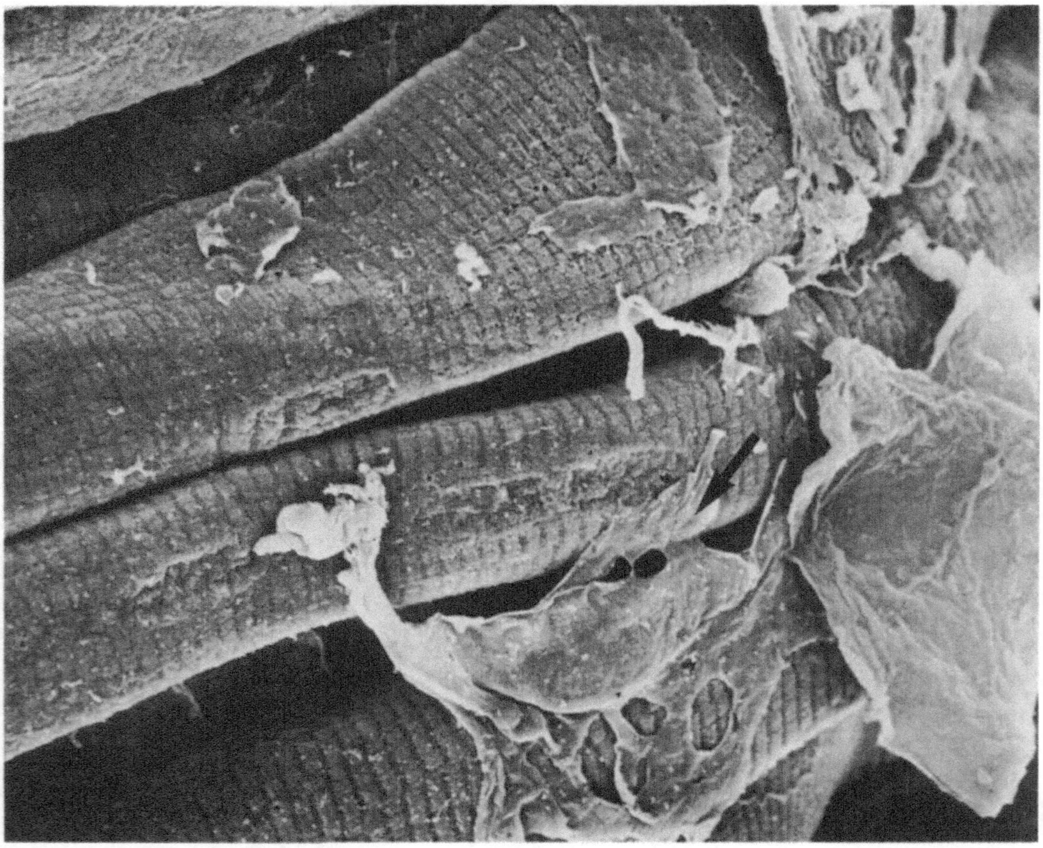

Figure 11

The mucous membrane of the middle ear

This middle ear cavity develops embryologically from the upper respiratory tract, consisting of ciliated cells, non-ciliated cells, goblet cells and others. However, interestingly, distribution of the ciliated cells differs according to the site of the middle ear cavity. SEM study of the human middle ear shows abundant ciliated cells in the hypotympanum with reduction in numbers toward the upper portion of the cavity. Ciliated cells are found also in the mucous membrane of the mastoid cavity. Kawabata schematically showed this distribution of the ciliated cells in humans (Figure 12). Lim and Shimada *et al.* reported similar findings on the distribution of these cells in the mastoid and middle ear cavity. In the mastoid cells, cilia do not show bundle formation and vary considerably in their length.

References

1. Kawabata, I. *et al.* (1969). Ultrastructure of normal human middle ear mucosa. *Ann Otol.*, **78,** 125
2. Lim, D. J. (1974). Functional morphology of the lining membrane of the middle ear and eustachian tube. *Ann. Otol.*, **83** Suppl., 11
3. Shimada, T. *et al.* (1972). Distribution of ciliated cells in the human middle ear. SEM, TEM and light microscope observation. *Ann. Otol.*, **81,** 203

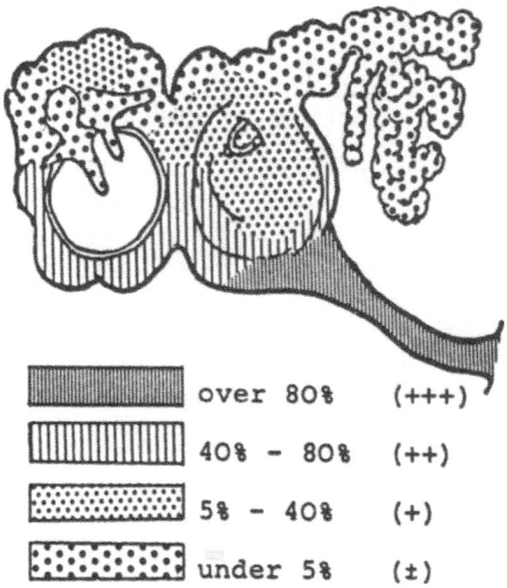

Figure 12 Distribution of the ciliated cell in human middle ear (courtesy of Dr Kawabata)

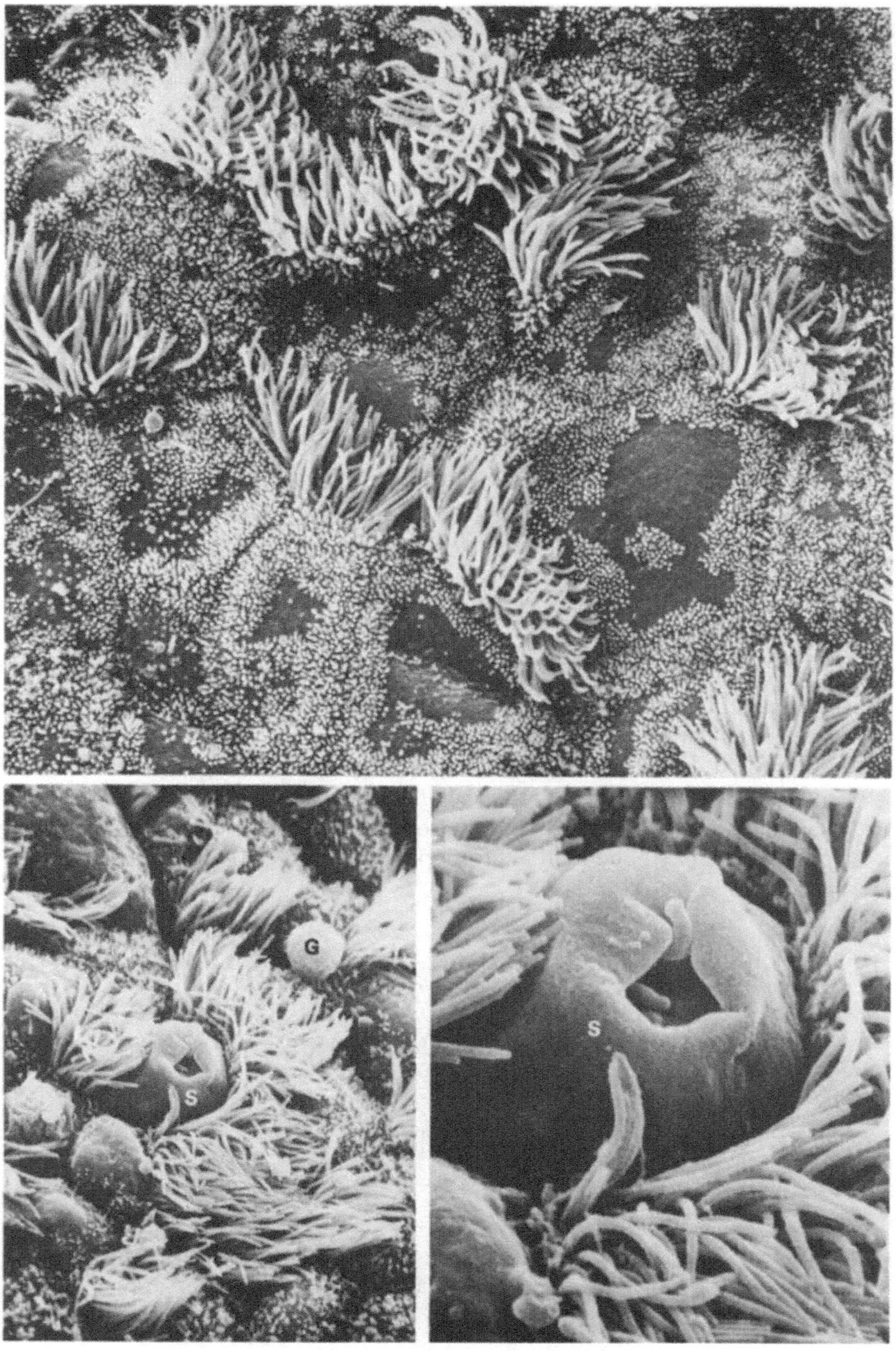

Figure 13 Tympanic membrane (human). (**a**) Ciliated cells on the surface of tympanic membrane. Cilia do not form a bundle, but appear splayed (× 4350). (**b**) and (**c**) Mucosa of the hypotympanum. There are many ciliated cells and non-ciliated cells which look like domes are also observed. S is a secretory cell which completed secretion. The global feature (G) looks like a secreted mucous globule. (**b**) × 2600 (**c**) × 8700

The round window membrane

This membrane, also called the second tympanic membrane by Antonio Scarpa, separates the inner ear from the middle ear and is located in the bottom of the cochlea. The round window membrane is divided into three layers, epithelial, middle and inner layers, from the middle ear to the inner ear side. The epithelial layer continues from the mucous membrane of the promontory, consisting of single layer flat cells which create pentagonal or octagonal patterns on the surface. It differs from the mucous membrane of the promontory in that there are no cilia on the round window membrane. The middle layer is formed by connective tissue, which includes fibrous cells and collagenous and elastic fibres. Fibrous cells have relatively little cytoplasm and in it intracellular organelles are scarce (Kawabata and Ishii, 1972)

Both collagenous and elastic fibres run parallel to the minor axis of the round window membrane. Among these there are coarse and fine fibres which connect the thick parallel ones to each other. Surface structure of median layer is not very clear; however, according to a TEM study by Kawabata (1972), there are a few layers of cells which contact each other with their processes.

References

1. Harty, M. (1963). The secondary tympanic membrane and annular ligament. *Ztsch. Mikr. Anat. Forsch.*, **70,** 484
2. Link, R. (1941). Beitrag zur Histologie der Membran des runden Fensters. *Z. Laryngol. Rhinn. Otol.*, **32,** 295

a b

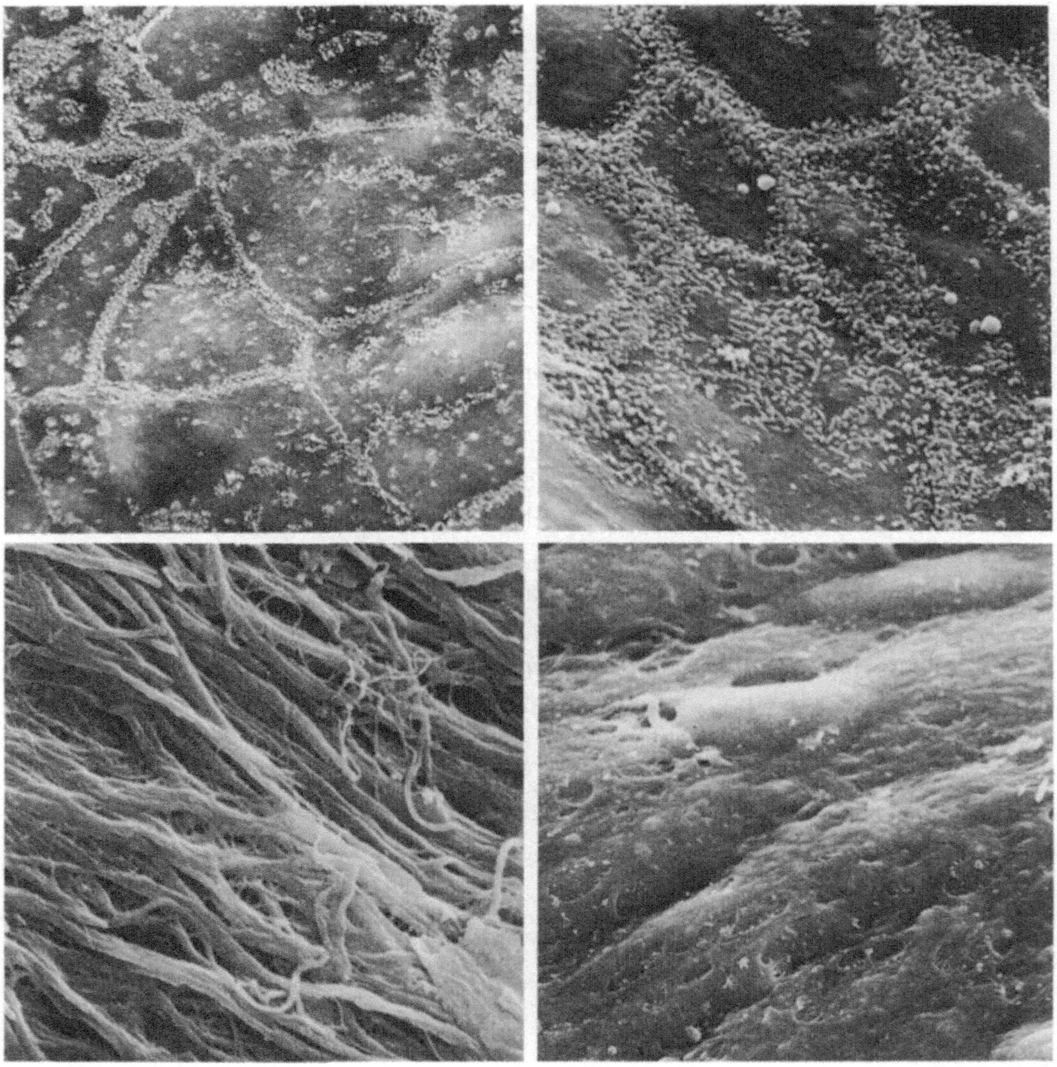

c d

Figure 14 Round window membrane (guinea pig). (**a**) Mucosa of the tympanic side (× 2700), (**b**) same as (a) (× 4200), (**c**) lamina propria (× 4200), (**d**) inner layer (× 7000)

The Eustachian tube

There are several electronmicroscopic studies on the mucous membrane of the Eustachian tube, Shimada and Lim, (1972), Hentzer (1970), Lim *et al.* (1967) and Harada (1977). The mucous membrane is formed by ciliated, non-ciliated, goblet and basal cells. Distribution of the ciliated cells, length of their cilia and surface structure of the non-ciliated cells vary according to the site on the Eustachian tube.

(1) *The bone-cartilage junction* Ciliated cells are densely distributed in this area, showing a carpet-like appearance. Each cilium is long. There are some goblet cells which create bulging surfaces like domes.

(2) *The tympanic portion* Ciliated cells are dense, but less in number than isthmus cells. There are also many goblet cells. Cilia are long and probably serve for the clearance of foreign bodies in the middle ear.

(3) *The pharyngeal portion* Ciliated cells are fewer when approaching the pharyngeal side. Instead, cells with long microvilli increase in number. Goblet cells are still abundant and they secrete mucus. Non-ciliated cells with short microvilli increase in number in this portion.

References

1. Harada, Y. (1977). Scanning electron microscopic study on the distribution of epithelial cells in the Eustachian tube. *Acta Otolaryngol. (Stockholm)*, **83,** 284
2. Hentzer, E. (1970). Ultrastructure of the normal mucosa in the human middle ear, mastoid cavities and Eustachian tube. *Ann. Otol. Rhinol. Laryngol.*, **79,** 1143
3. Lim, D. J., Paparella, M. M. and Kimura, R. S. (1967). Ultrastructure of Eustachian tube and middle ear mucosa in the guinea pig. *Acta Otolaryngol. (Stockholm)*, **63,** 425
4. Shimada, T. and Lim, D. (1972). Distribution of ciliated cells in the human middle ear. *Ann. Otol. Rhinol. Laryngol.* **81,** 203

a

b

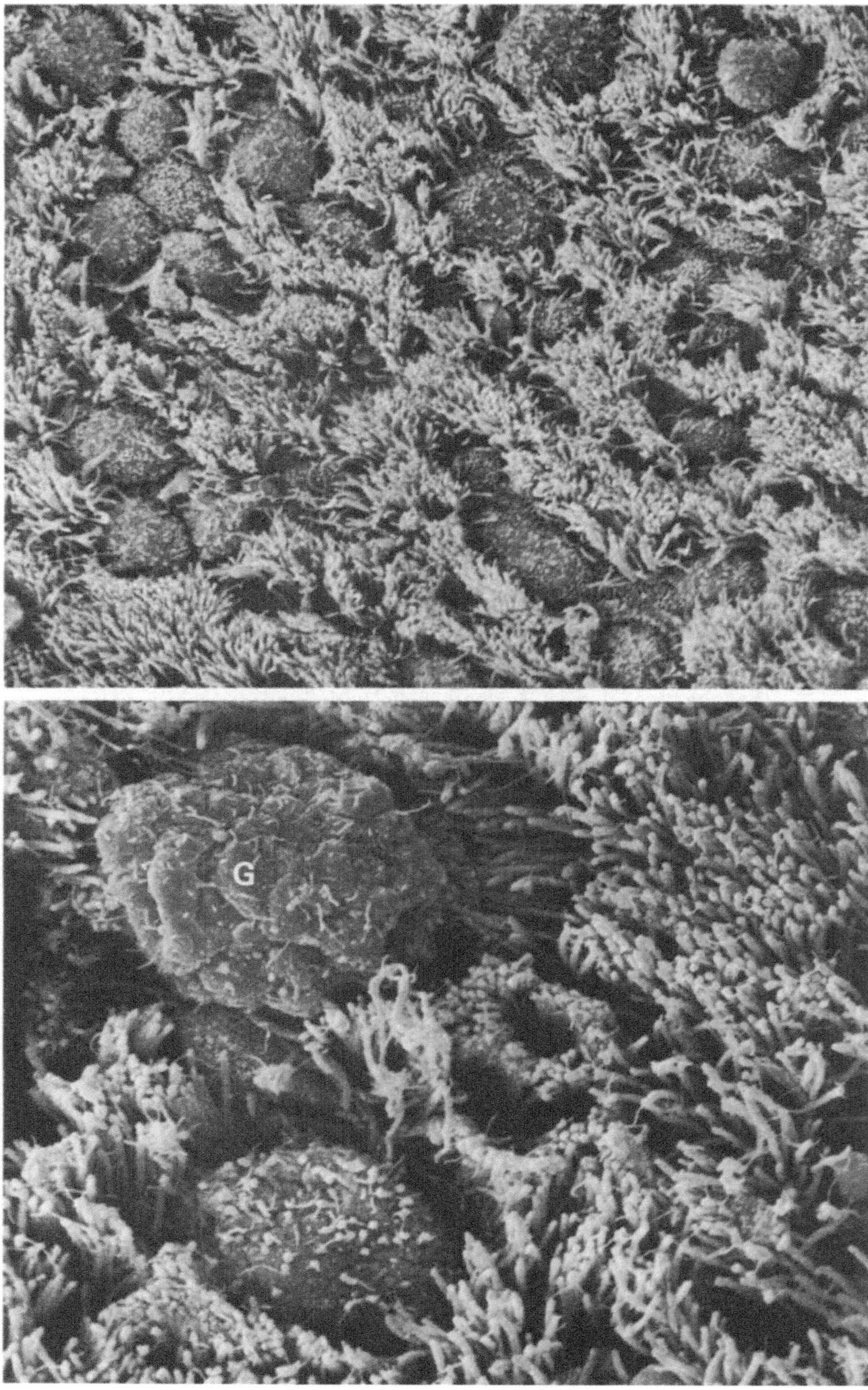

Figure 15 Mucosa of the Eustachian tube (dog). (**a**) Mucosa of the tympanic portion. Numerous goblet cells are seen between the ciliated cells (× 1300). (**b**) Mucous globule (G) is secreted from the goblet cell (× 4000)

a b c

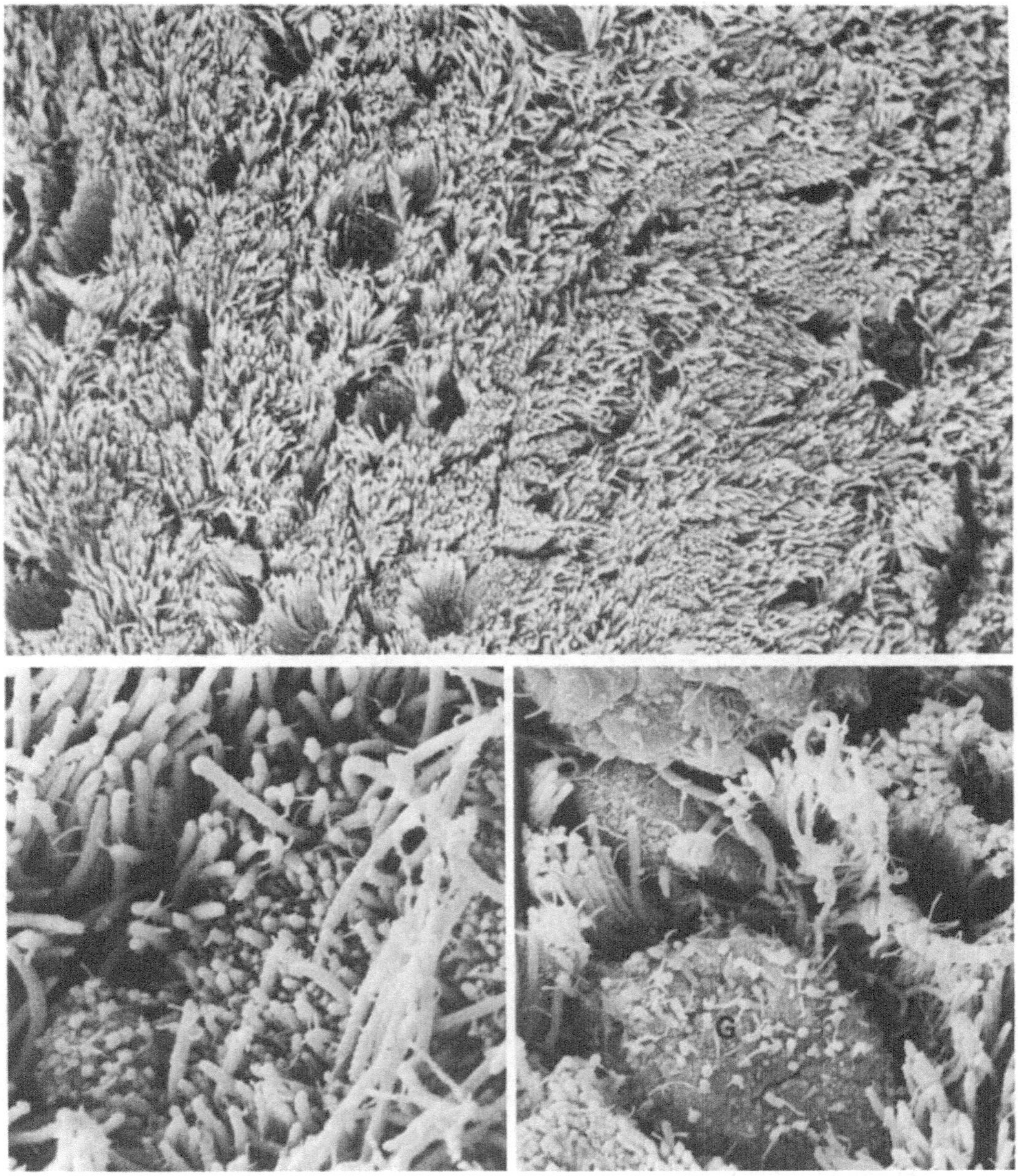

Figure 16 Mucosa of the isthmus (dog). (**a**) Dense distribution of the cilia (× 1600), (**b**) fine filaments are seen on each cilium (× 8000), (**c**) microvilli on the goblet cell (G) (× 4800)

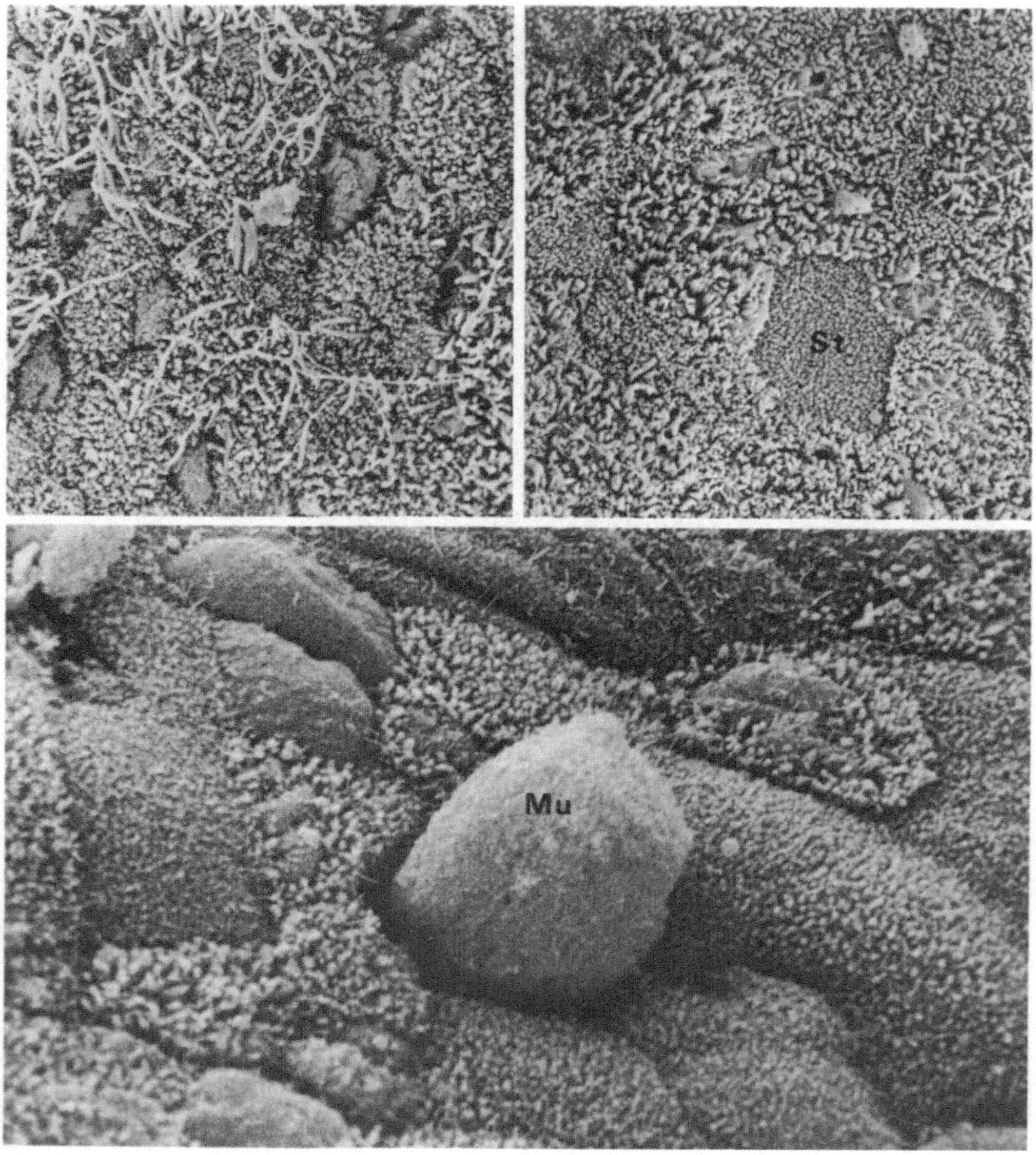

Figure 17 Pharyngeal portion (dog). (**a**) Flat cells covered by microvilli and other cells with a few cilia are observed (× 2400), (**b**) Cells with long microvilli and flat cells (St) are dominant when approaching the pharyngeal orifice. Cells with long cilia are very rarely found (× 2400). (**c**) Mucus (Mu) is secreted from the goblet cell (× 4000)

Figure 18 Cracked surface of the Eustachian tube (dog). (**a**) Cracked surface of the ciliated cell. Cilia are approximately 3 μm long and are covered with mucous blanket. N: nucleus (× 8400). (**b**) Nucleus of the ciliated cell. Mi: mitochondrion (× 8400). (**c**) Cracked goblet cell. Cell body at an active phase is extended and many secretory granules are seen (× 8400). (**d**) Inactive goblet cell (G) is seen between the ciliated cells (C). Basal cells (B) are either triangular or square with large nucleus (N). Usually basal cells form three or four layers on the basement membrane (× 2500). (**e**) Submucosal collagenous fibres. Fibres run along the long axis of the Eustachian tube (× 5000)

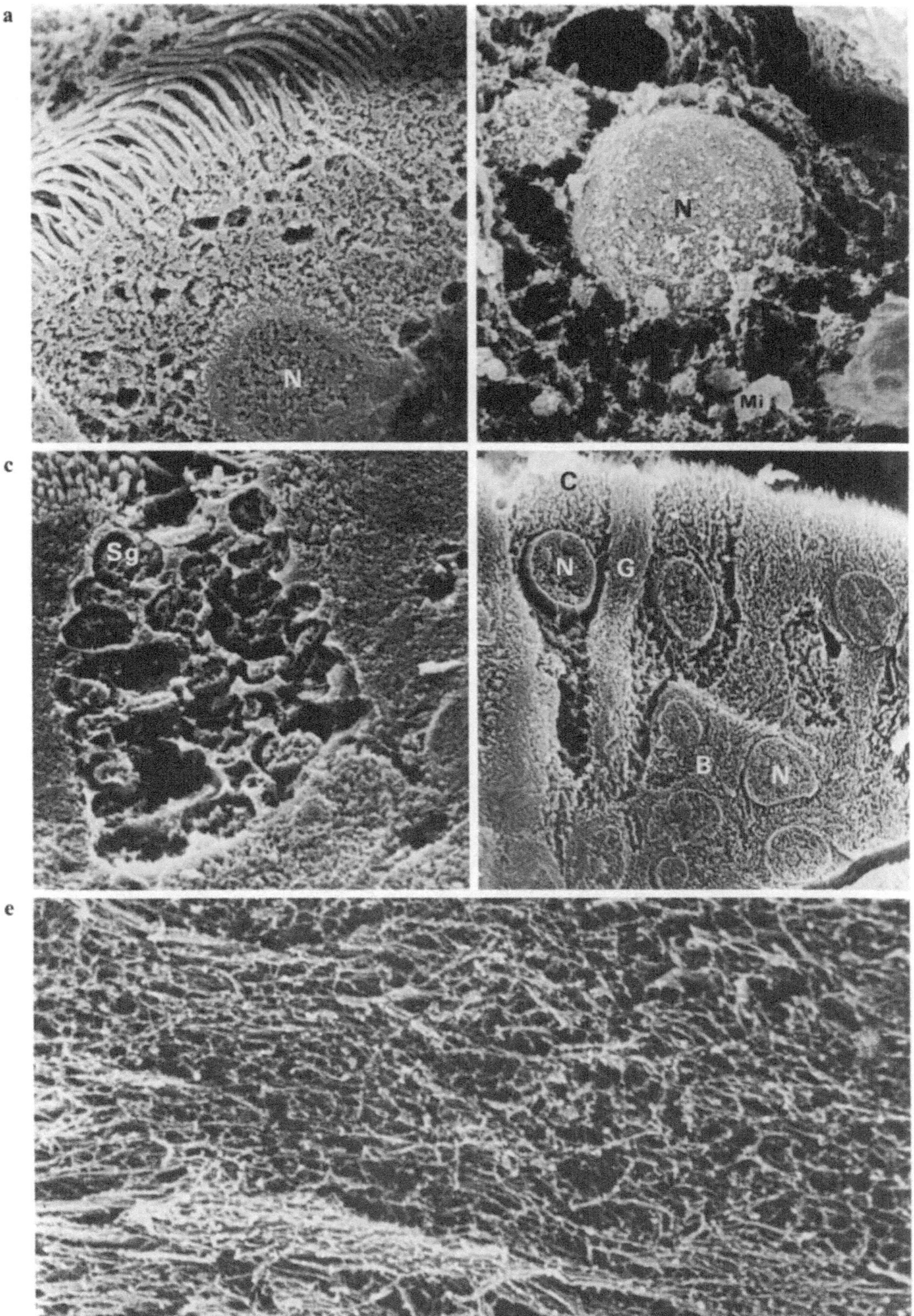

Figure 18

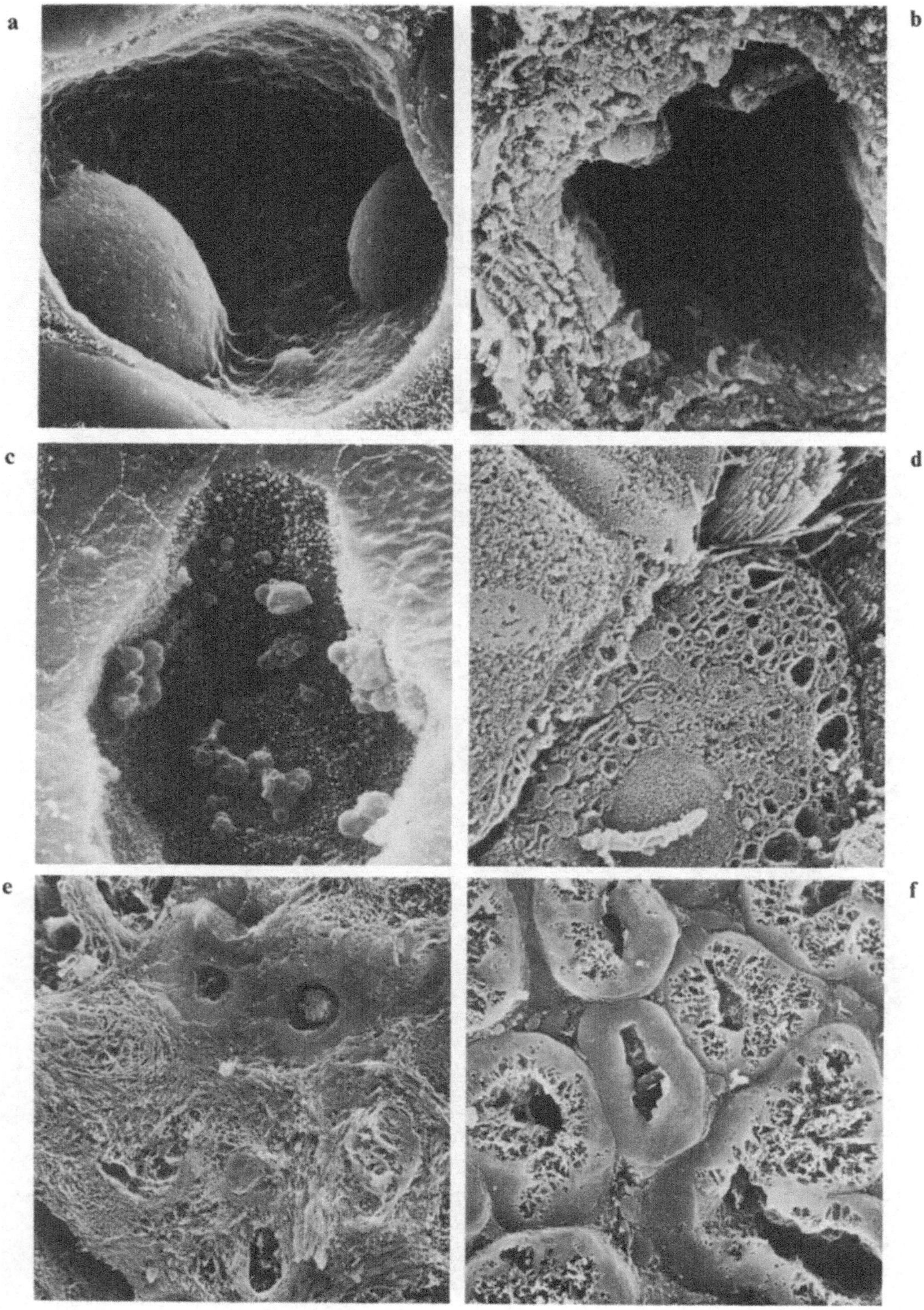

Figure 19 Eustachian tube of the rabbit. (**a**) Cracked surface of Eustachian tube. Secretory granules are found inside the subepitheliar gland. (**b**) Cracked surface of the duct (× 1800). (**c**) Globular substances secreted in the duct (× 2500). (**d**) Cracked ciliated cell; arrow: mitochondria (× 8000). (**e**) Gland cell (arrow) surrounded by the connective tissue (arrow head). (**f**) Cracked secretory glands (× 600)

The Inner Ear and Vestibular Organs

The inner ear

The inner ear is located in the petrous part of the temporal bone. It consists of two parts, the osseous and membranous labyrinths, and functions as two sensory receptors; the cochlea (hearing) and the vestibulum (equilibrium).

Palaeontologically the vestibulum is older than the cochlea. For example, jellyfish has only an otolithic organ as a vestibular apparatus, a lamprey lacks a lateral semicircular canal and a frog lacks a cochlea. A bird has a cochlea not spiral, but straight, of which the sensory epithelia are called the basilar papilla. Only mammals have turns of the cochlea, but the number of turns varies according to species. Humans have $2\frac{3}{4}$ turns, whales, $\frac{1}{2}$; horses, 2; cats, 3 and guinea pigs, 4. Since the surface preparation technique was developed by Engström, many researchers have been involved in the complicated inner ear study. SEM study of the inner ear was initiated by Barber and Boyde who did work on the otolith in 1968.

Reference

1. Barber, V. C. and Boyde, A. (1968). Scanning electron microscopic studies on cilia. *Z. Zelforsche*, **84**, 269

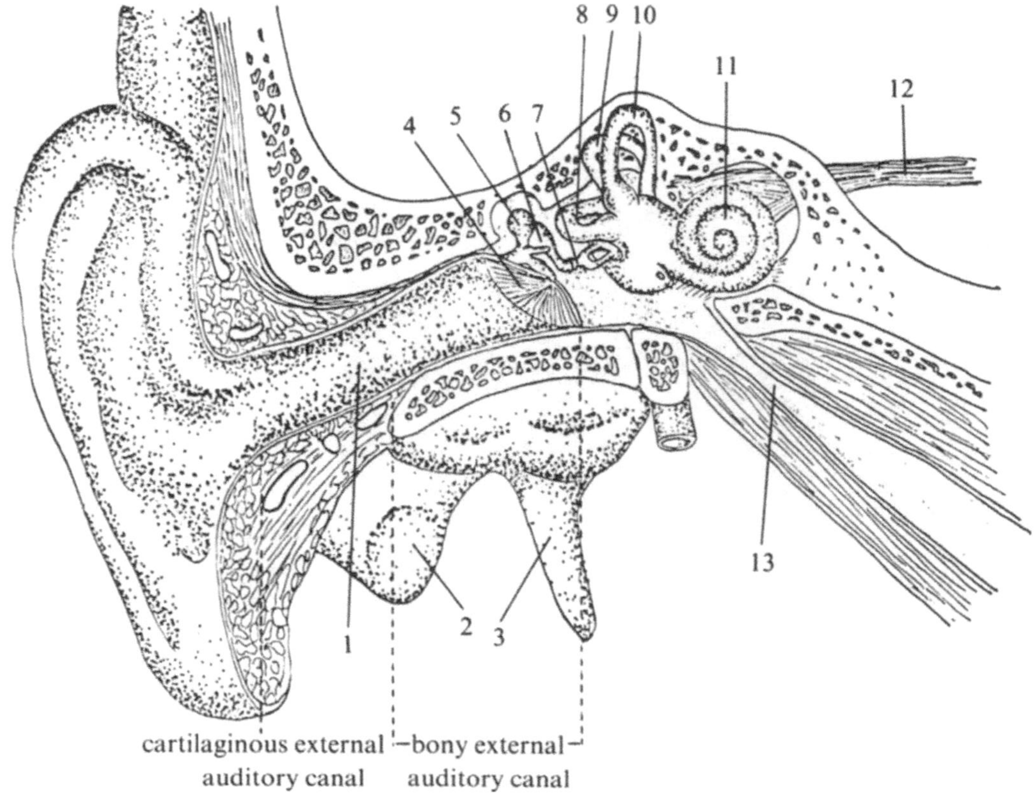

Figure 20 Schema of the middle and inner ear. (1) external auditory canal, (2) mastoid process, (3) styloid process, (4) tympanic membrane, (5) malleus, (6) incus, (7) stapes, (8) horizontal semicircular canal, (9) posterior semicircular canal, (10) anterior semicircular canal, (11) cochlea, (12) cochlear and vestibular nerve, (13) Eustachian tube

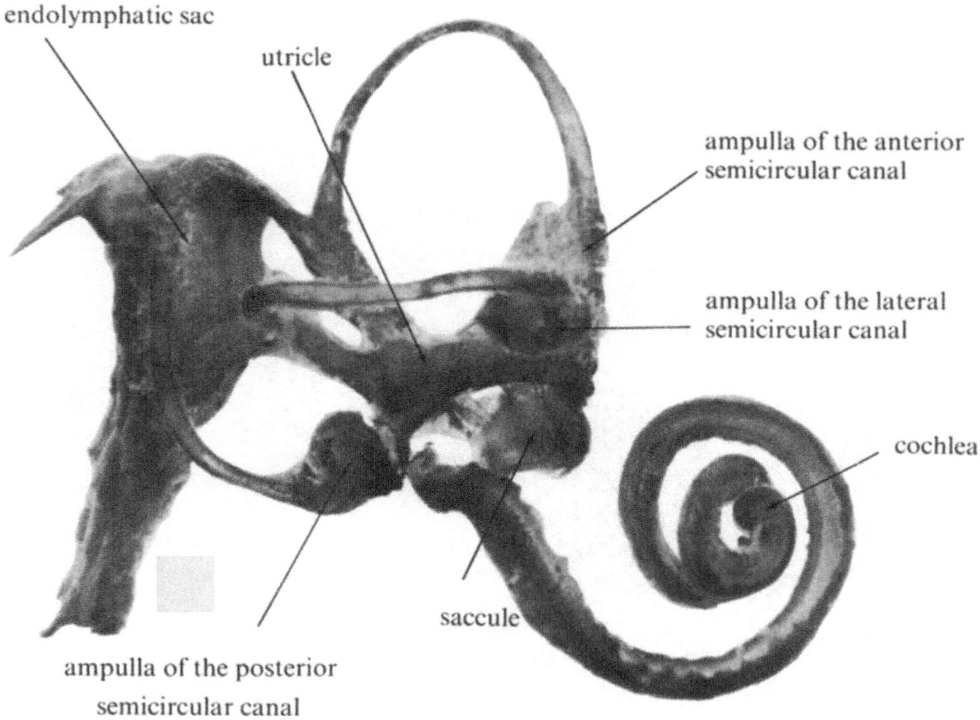

Figure 21 Membranous labyrinth (human). Bony wall of the osseous labyrinth is removed to expose the membranous labyrinth (courtesy of Dr Watanuki)

Figure 22 (**a**) Osseous labyrinth (bat). R: round window, O: oval window, C: cochlea, Cr: crus commune, S: anterior semicircular canal, L: horizontal semicircular canal, P: posterior semicircular canal (× 30). (**b**) Cochlea and vestibulum (cat). Three and half turns of the cochlea, utricle (U), saccule (Sc) and round window membrane (Rm) are exposed (× 12)

a

b

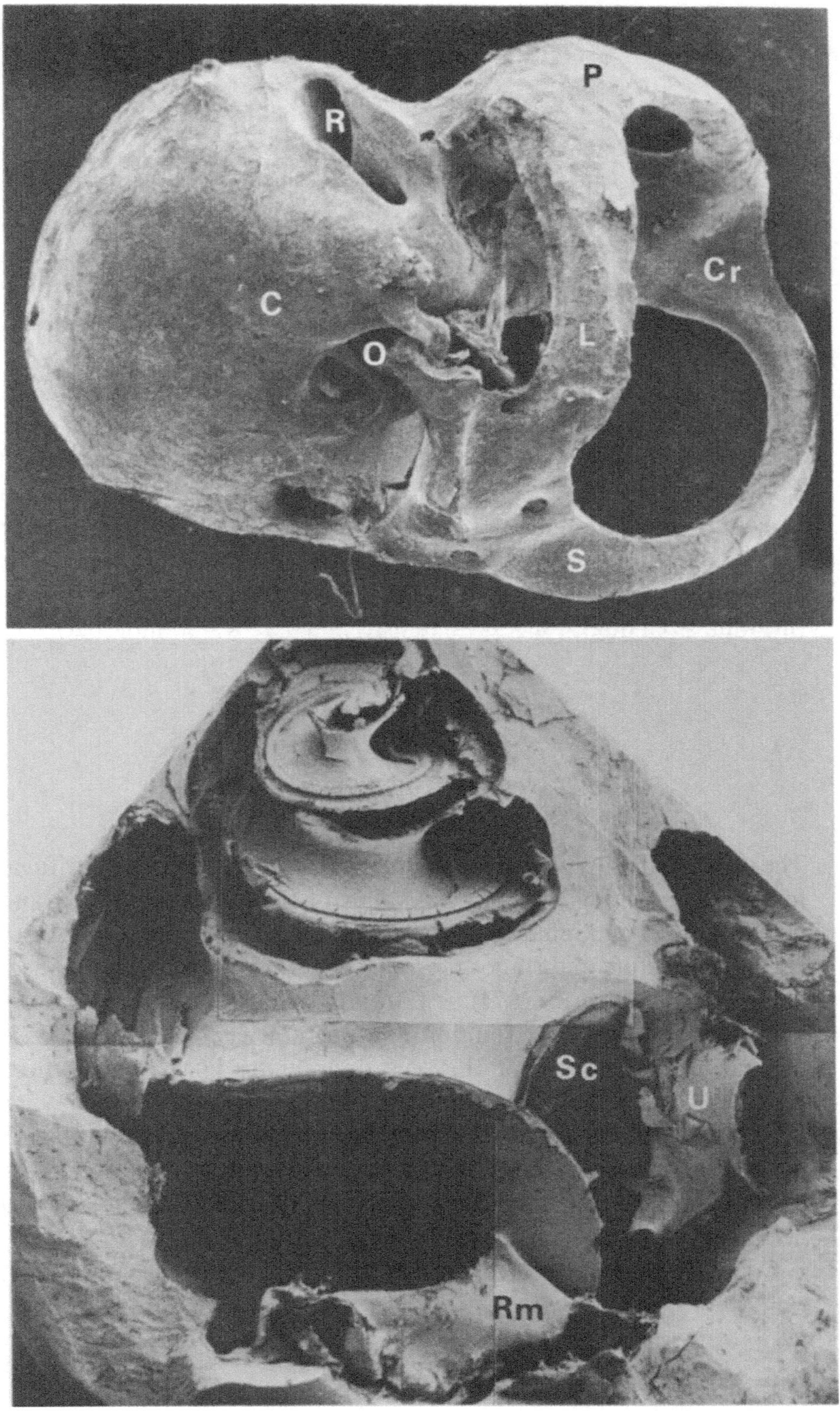

Figure 22

The otolithic organs

The otolithic organs are divided into the utricle and saccule. Birds have a lagena which is also called the third otolithic organ.

The utricle belongs to pars superior of the inner ear, while the saccule belongs to pars inferior. The two develop during different periods, but the basic structures, which are otolith, otolithic membrane, sensory hair, sensory cell and nerve, are identical.

The macula sacculi is located in the recessus sphericus, and the macula utriculi in the recessus utriculi, creating a 90 degree angle to each other. In a human, in upright head position, the macula sacculi is in the vertical plane and the macula utriculi in the horizontal plane. The macula utriculi is shell- (human, monkey, guinea pig, mouse, bat and frog) or kidney-shaped (cat, dog and bird). Its size varies among species. The axis of the macula utriculi is 2.2 × 2.2 mm (human), 1.25 × 0.7 mm (medium sized dog), 1.0 × 0.7 mm (cat) and 0.23 × 0.22 mm (bat).

The function of the otolithic organs

The otolithic organs perceive gravity, linear acceleration and centrifugal force, thus affecting the muscular tonus of the body, extremities and ocular muscles and influencing positional sensation of the body. As an effect, the posture and smooth movement of the body are maintained.

Historically, Breuer (1874) first reported that otolithic organs were stimulated by linear acceleration and postural change. Mach (1875) reported some changes of the sensations under linear acceleration. Kreidl (1893) succeeded in creating equilibrium disturbance in crayfish by magnetic stimulation after the otoconia were replaced by iron sand. Magnus and de Kleyn (1923) demonstrated that the otolithic organs are involved in the vestibular tension reflex of the body, extremities and neck, compensatory ocular movement and standing reflex.

Counterrolling of the eyes was first found by Hunter (1786). In 1934,

Maxwell and Ulrich provoked counterrolling in fish by direct stimulation of the otoconia and Miller and Graybiel (1972) stated that counterrolling did not occur under agravic conditions.

There are three main hypotheses on the excitatory mechanism of this organ, which depend on shearing, traction and pressure. This is still under discussion even today. However, it is generally agreed that the otoconia shear sensory hairs, thus producing depolarization, hyperpolarization and finally excitement of the nerve. Considering the anatomical relationship of the plane in which the utricle and the saccule are located, it is easy to understand that the utricle responds to horizontal acceleration and the saccule to vertical acceleration (Hasegawa).

The striola of the utricle and the saccule are arranged in U-and L-shapes respectively. This creates overlap of the sensory perception among the two and there exist differences in perception between type I and type II sensory cells, all of which make the physiological mechanisms of the otolithic organs complicated and leave many questions unsolved.

a

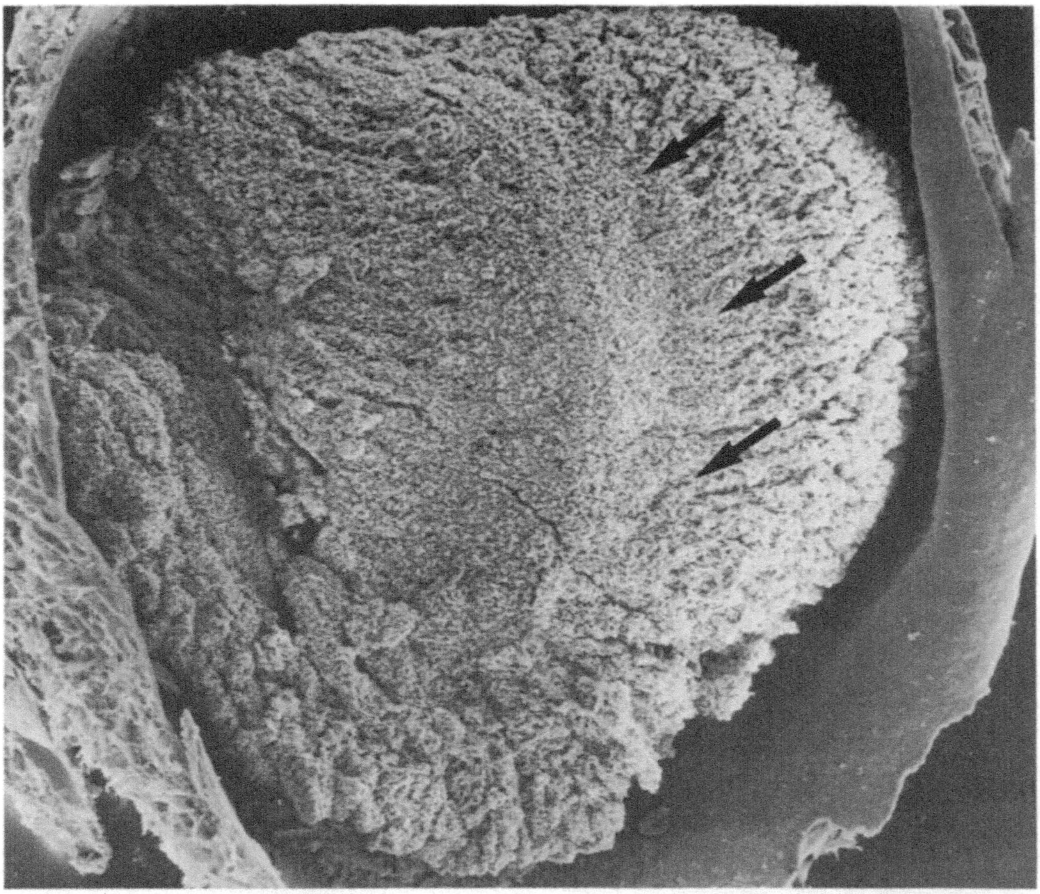

b

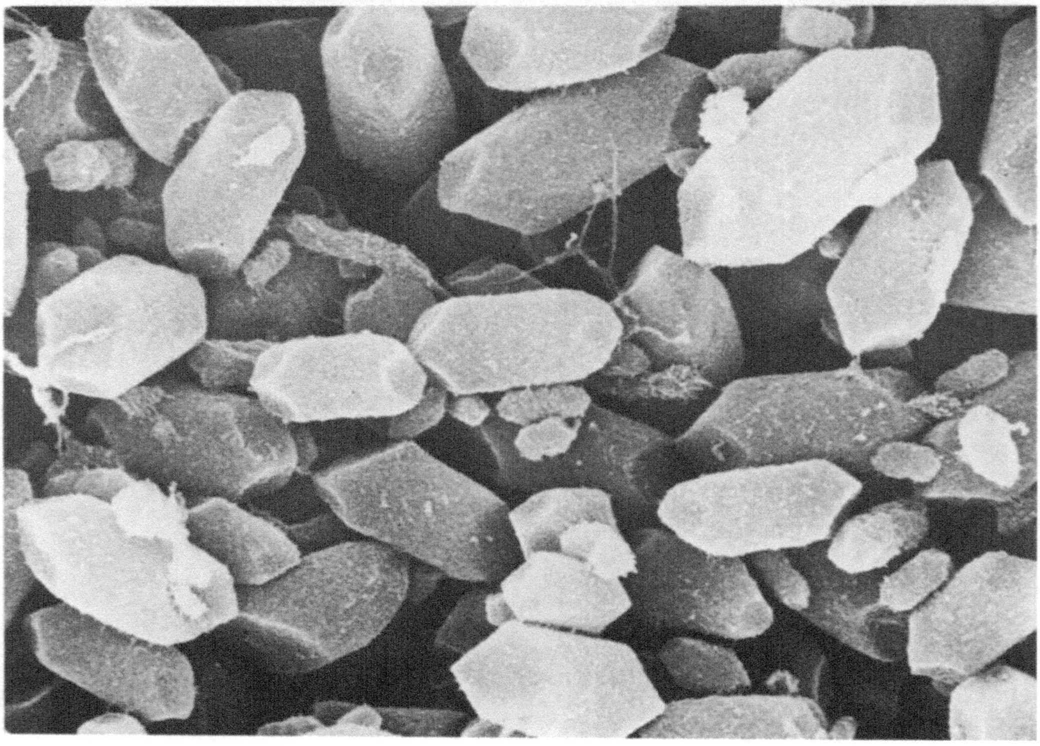

Figure 23

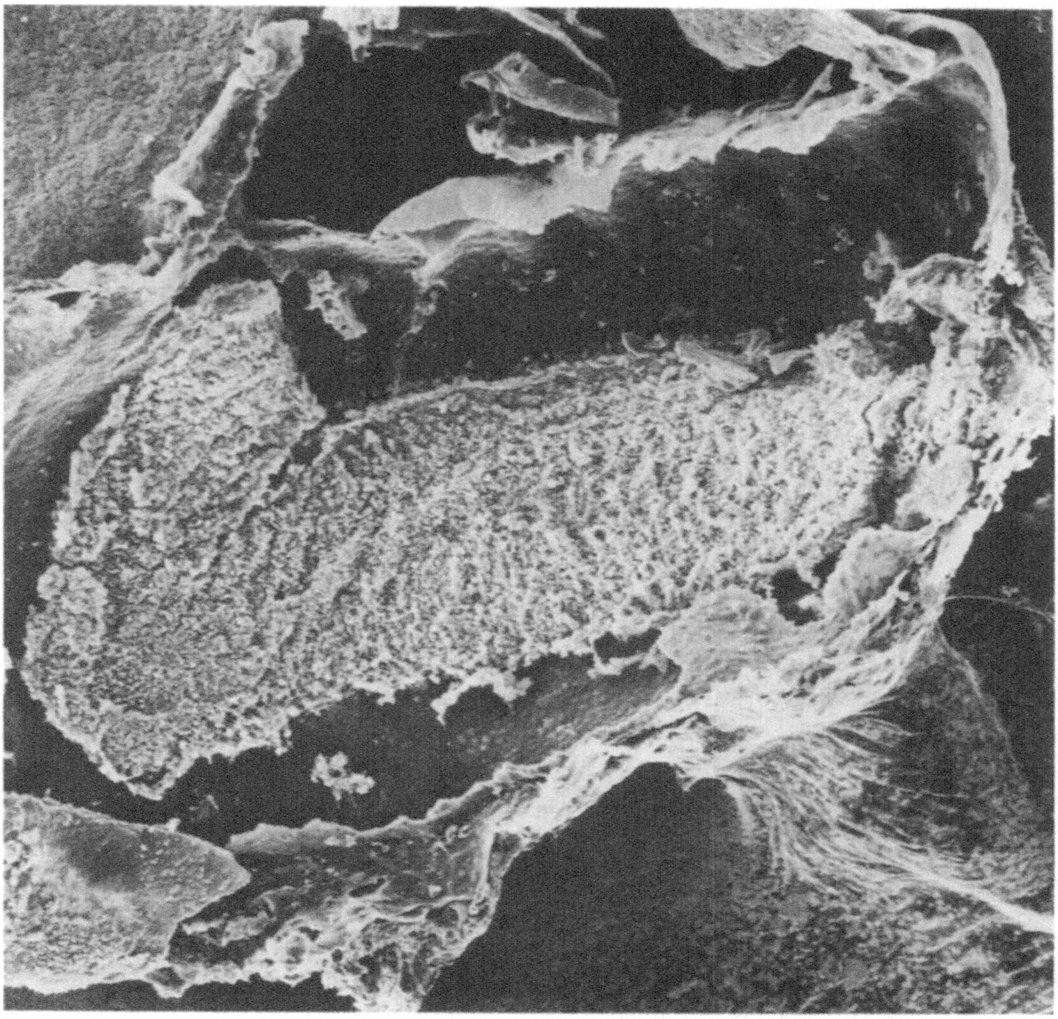

Figure 24 Saccular macula (guinea pig). The saccular macula of the guinea pig is L-shaped and is especially thick at the striola portion (× 170)

Figure 23 Otolithic layer of the utricular macula (guinea pig). (**a**) The thickness of the otolithic layer of the guinea pig is not even. It is especially thin at the striola portion (arrow). Small otoconia are predominant on the surface of the otolithic layer (× 150). (**b**) Otoconia of various size. The length of otoconia is 3-5 μm in general. The bodies of otoconia are rounded and three terminal faces at each end are rhombohedral. The angle formed between the faces is approximately 110°. (× 8000)

The shape and composition of otoconia

Otoconia are composed of calcium carbonate. The shape and the size of the otoconia vary among the species and even among individuals of the same species. The general shape is cylindrical with pyramidal ends. The angle of the peak of the pyramid varies among species, such as 90° in a frog, 110° in a guinea pig and 120° in a human. Also the shape of the otoconia is sometimes different according to diet.

Kolmer (1927) reported that the otoconia have their nuclei in the centre and this finding was supported by Lindeman (1969). However, it is open to discussion whether this is a true nucleus, because it is observed that the small global substance with calcium concentration, which is considered to be a future nucleus, is secreted from the supporting cells of the macula. The crystal forms of the otoconia are calcite and aragonite. According to Carlström and Engström (1955) and Sasaki (1970), calcite belongs to warm-blooded animals and aragonite to cold-blooded animals.

References

1. Carlström, D. and Engström, H. (1955). The ultrastructure of statoconia. *Acta Otolaryngol. (Stockholm)*, **45**, 14
2. Kolmer, W. (1927). Gehörorgan. In Möllendorff, W. (ed.). *Handbuch der Mikroskopischen Anatomie des Menschen*, p. 250
3. Lindeman, H. (1969). Regional differences in structure of the vestibular sensory regions. *J. Laryngol.*, **83**, 1

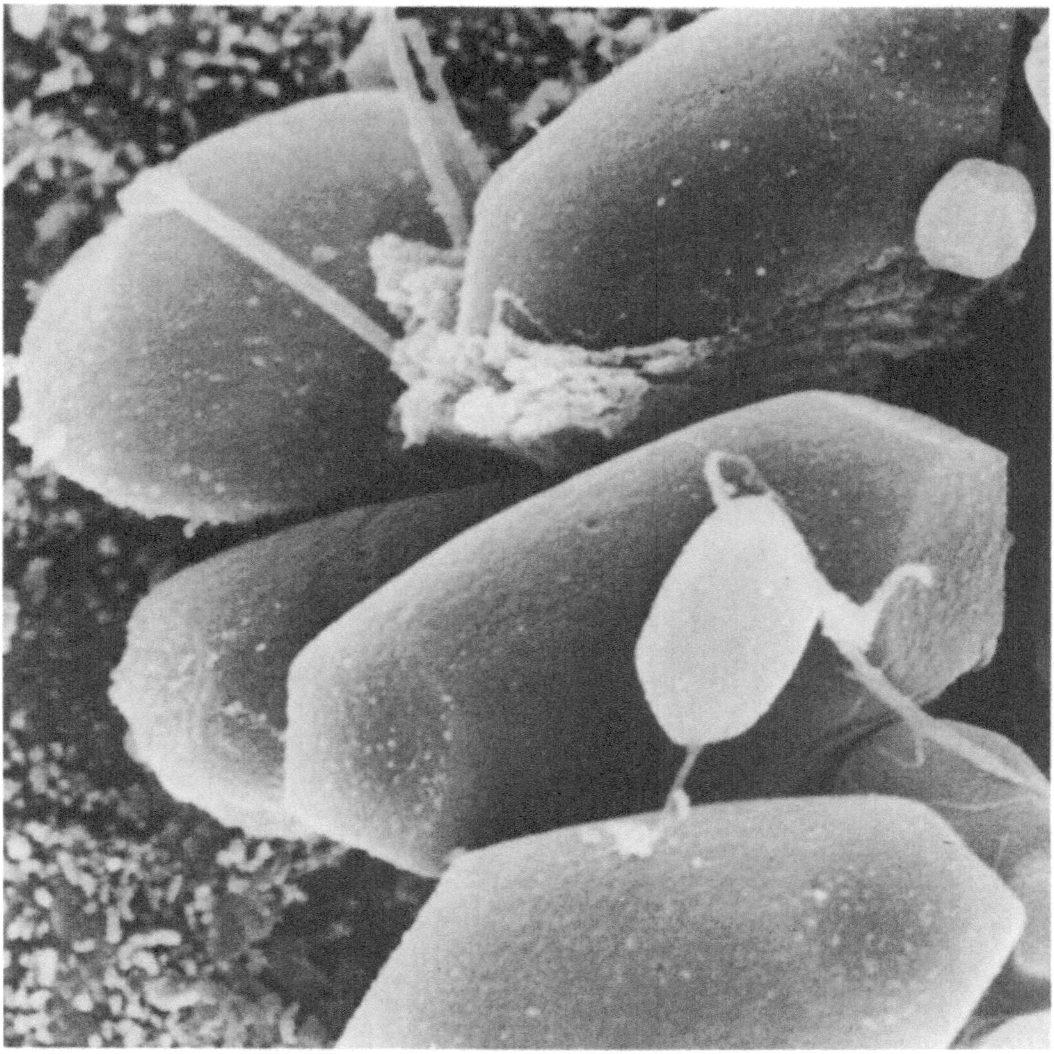

Figure 25 Otoconia (human). Otoconia from the Ménière's disease patient who underwent labyrinthectomy. Each otoconium is shaped like a crystal which has pyramidal ends, with angles of 110–120° at the apices (× 6000)

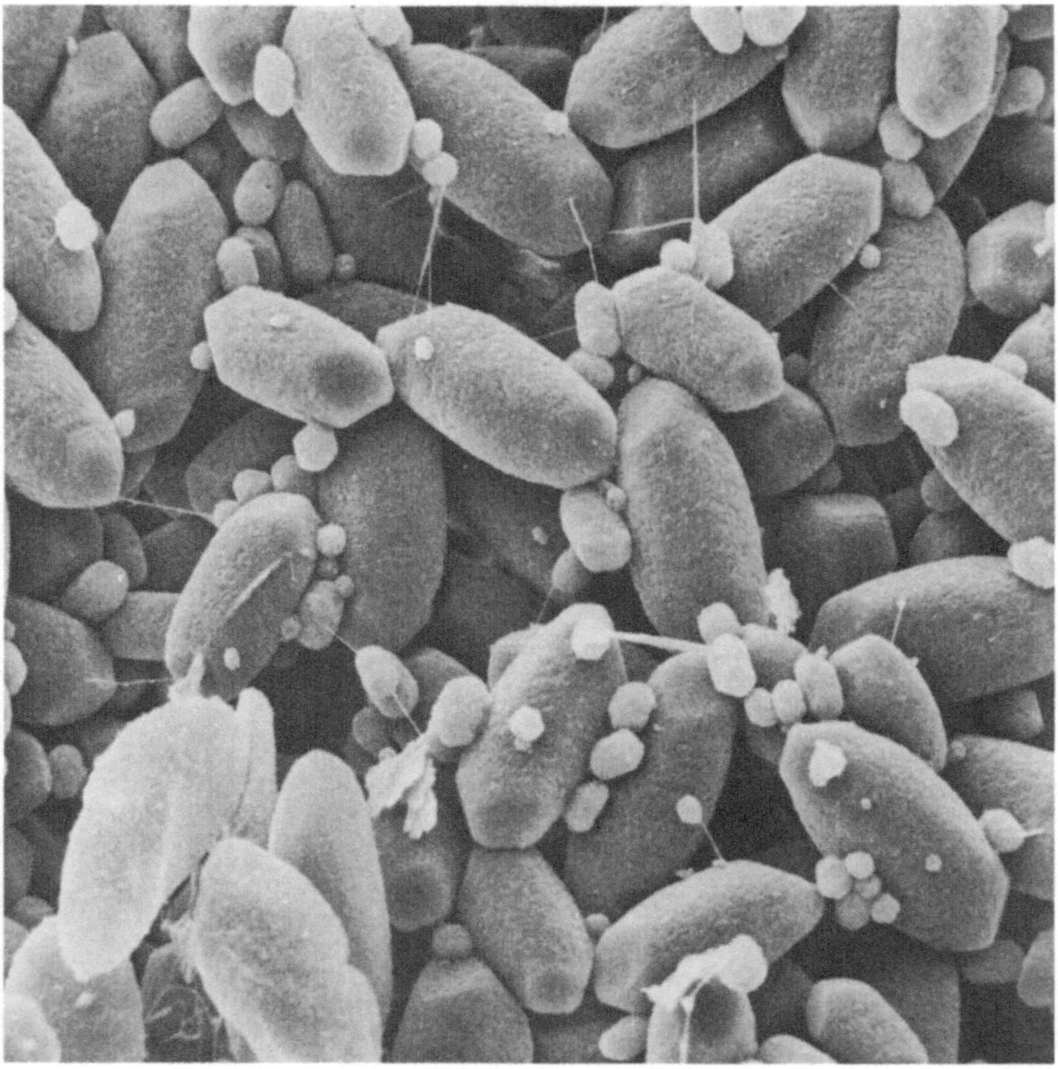

Figure 26 Otoconia (pigeon). The otoconia of the pigeon are grain-shaped and relatively large. Small otoconia are attached to these large ones with gelatinous substance (× 7200)

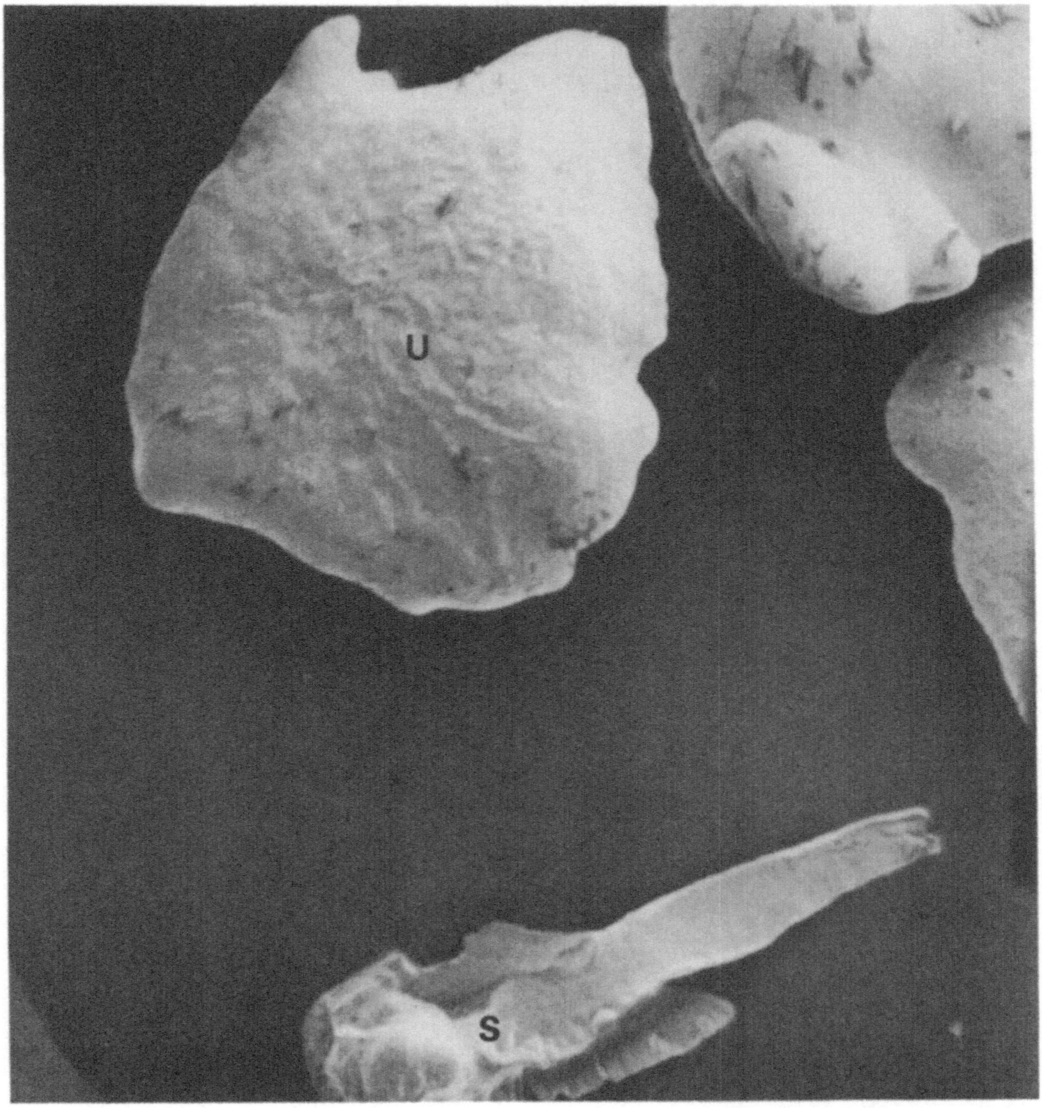

Figure 27 Otoconia of the goldfish. These are three otoconia: utricular, saccular and lagena otoconia. Each otoconium is composed of a large mass of $CaCO_3$. U: utricular otoconium, S: Saccular otoconium (× 30)

a

b

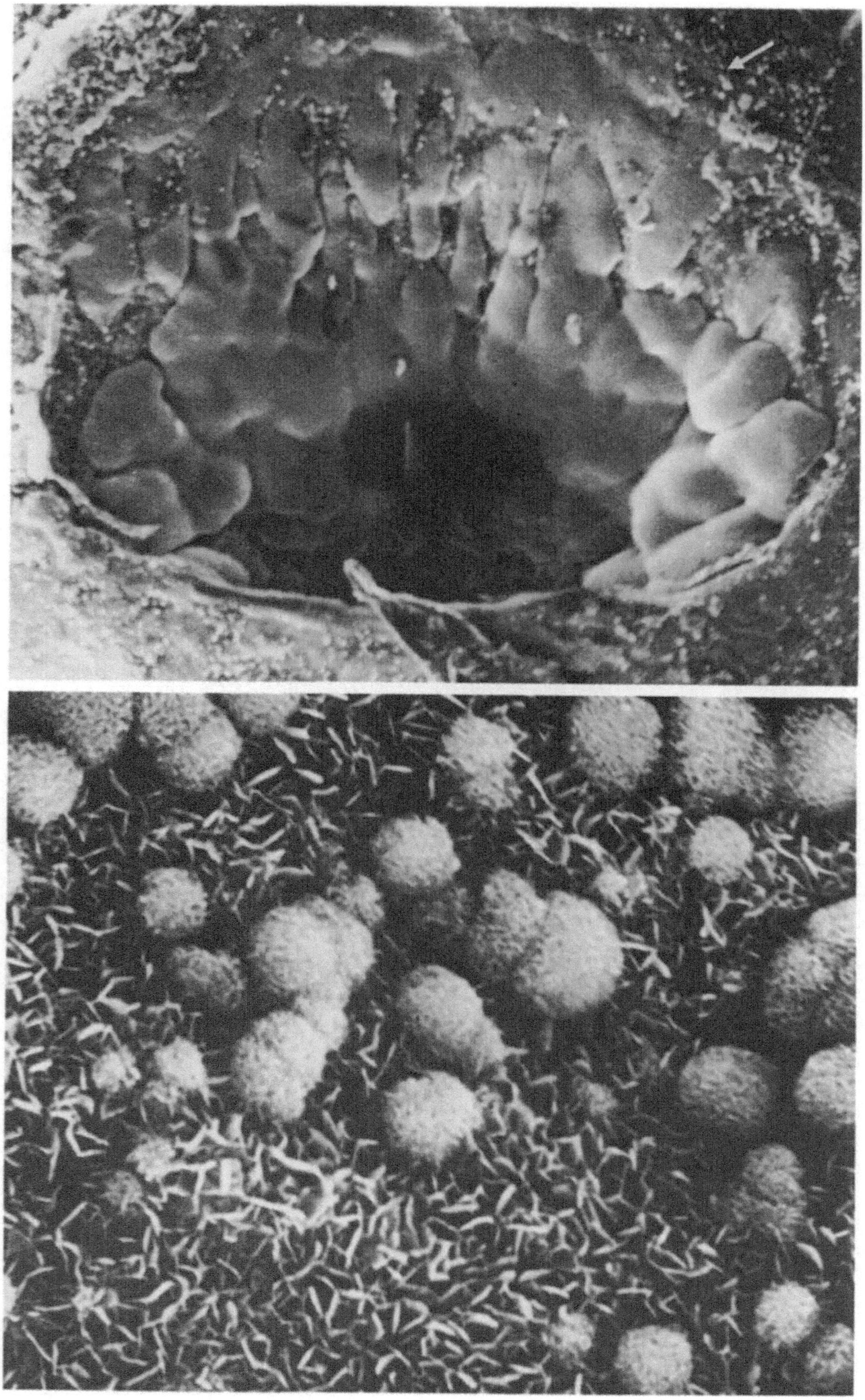

Figure 28 Otoconia of the goldfish. (**a**) Utricular otoconia (sensory epithelia side) (× 30), (**b**) High magnification of a part of Figure 28 (a) (arrow) (× 3900)

a

b

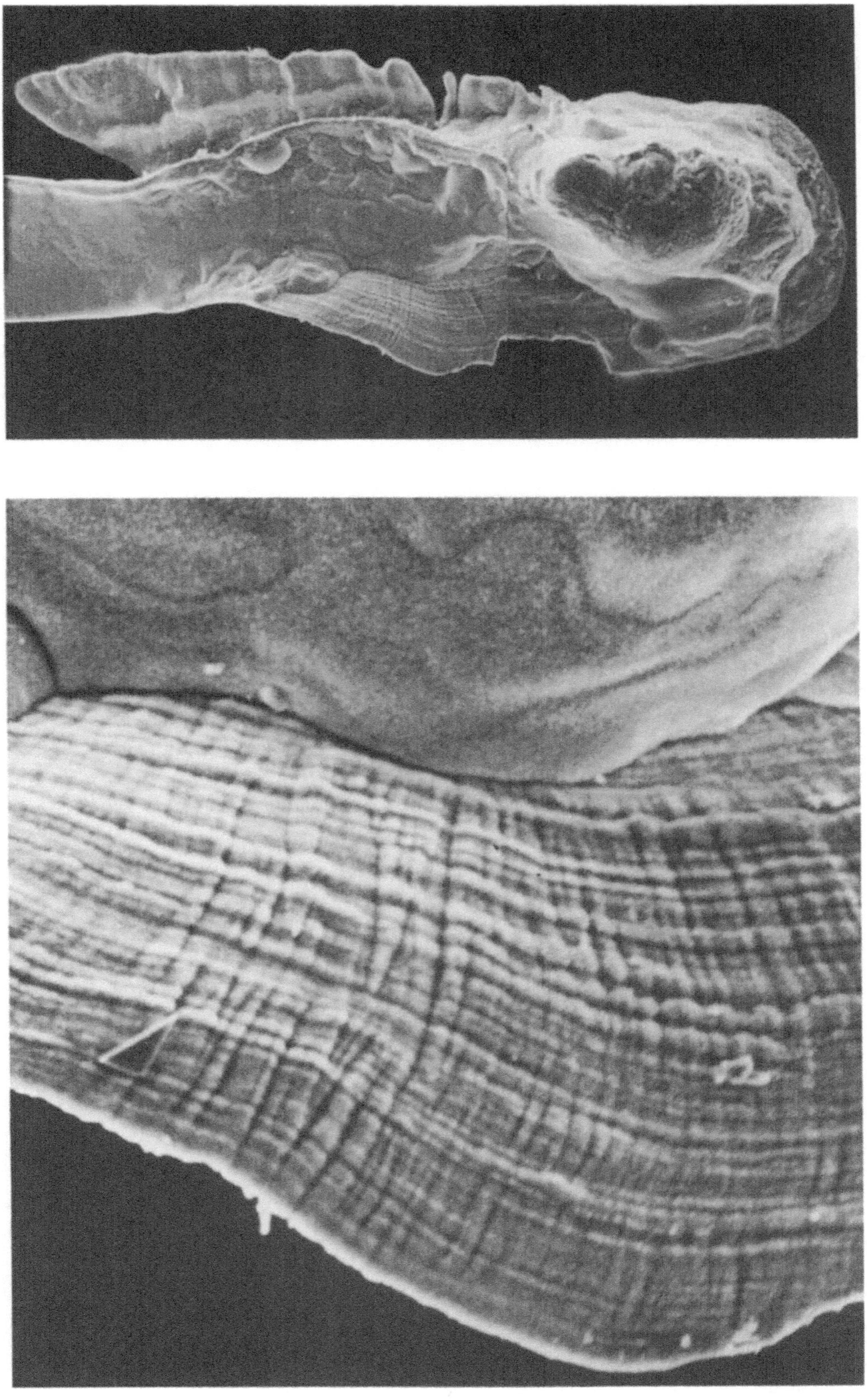

Figure 29 Otoconia of the goldfish. (**a**) Saccular otoconia (× 80), (**b**) high magnification of the marginal portion (× 450)

Microanalysis of the otoconia and standard calcite

Both otoconia and standard calcite are crystals of $CaCO_3$. X-ray m: croanalysis shows 40% concentration of Ca in both materials. Th remaining 60% is CO_3. 40% concentration of Ca in the otoconia is als calculated by the following equation.

	atomic weight
$CaCO_3$	100.08
Ca	40.08

$$\frac{40.08}{100.08} = 40\%$$

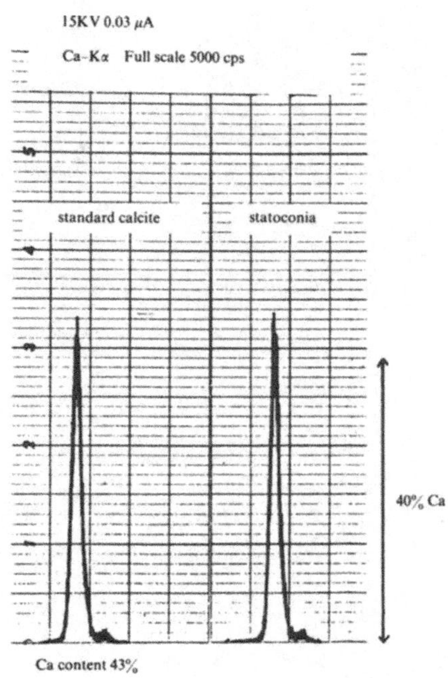

Figure 30 Microanalysis of the calcite and the otoconium

a

b

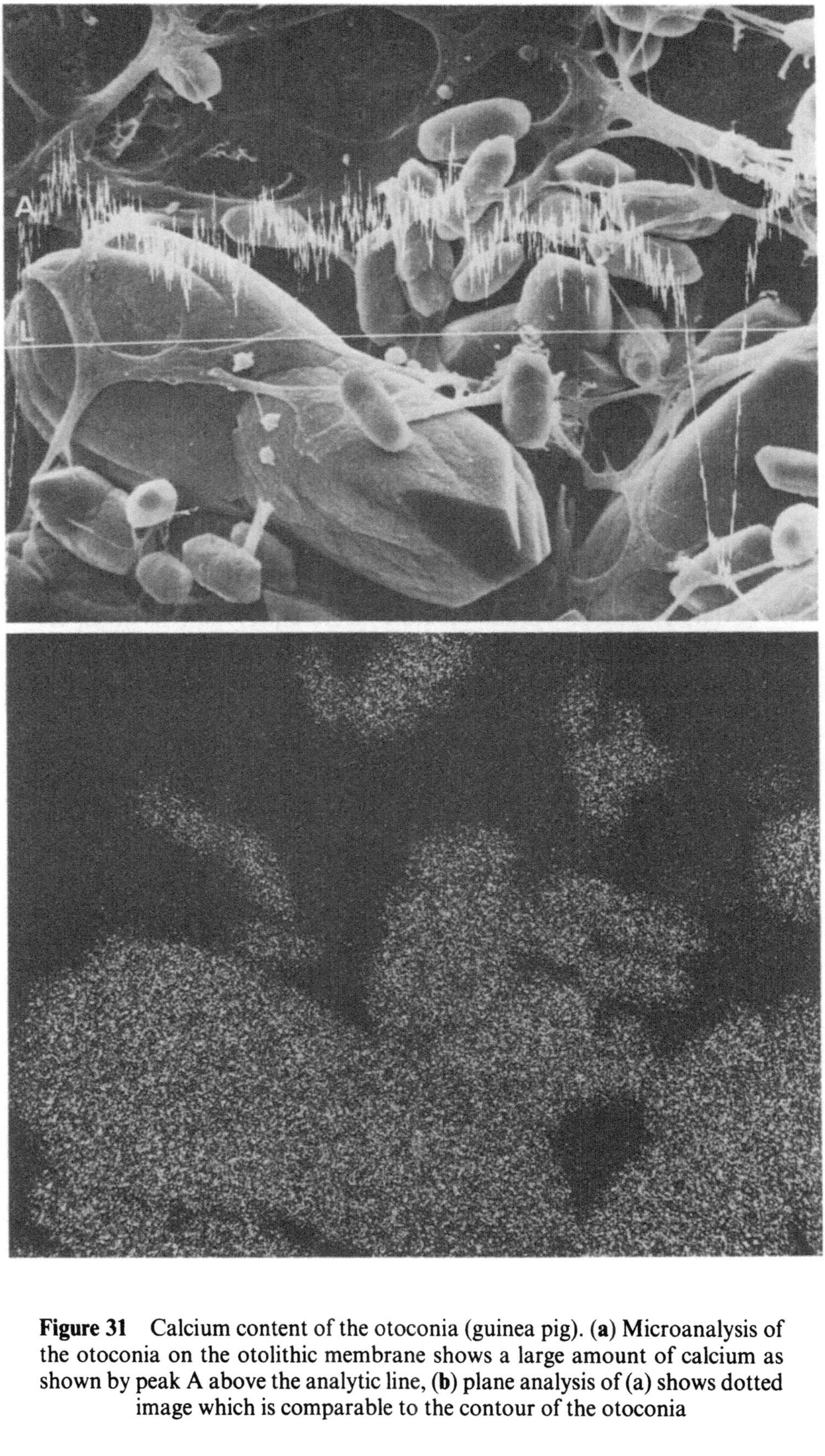

Figure 31 Calcium content of the otoconia (guinea pig). (**a**) Microanalysis of the otoconia on the otolithic membrane shows a large amount of calcium as shown by peak A above the analytic line, (**b**) plane analysis of (a) shows dotted image which is comparable to the contour of the otoconia

The otolithic membrane

The first reports on the otolithic membrane were done by Tenglia (1925) and Brock (1926). Wittmaak (1956) studied it in the guinea pig, rabbit and dog; Johnsson and Hawkins (1967) in the human and Lindeman (1969 a,b) in the guinea pig. Igarashi and Kanda (1969) recognized cupular zone 1 and cupular zone 2, which are called marginal and medial zones respectively by Marco, Fernandez *et al.* (1971). These findings are from TEM speciemens. SEM specimens show that cupular zone 1 corresponds to the part in which otoconia are embedded in the gelatin-like substance and that cupular zone 2 is a membrane of mesh-like structure which was observed by Lim (1971, 1973), Harada (1971) and Hoshino (1973). The numerous small holes of the membrane are especially predominant in the striola. Sensory hairs are impressed in this membrane, but the tops of the hairs do not reach the otoconia through the membrane (Harada, 1971).

Another structure of the otolithic membrane is the veil, which connects the membrane with the sensory epithelium (Lim, 1973). The veil is a fibrous filament which comes out of the supporting cells of the sensory epithelia, and probably serves like the trabeculum of the tectorial membrane. The part where the veil is generally found is called the subcupular space by Vilstrup (1951), Dohlman (1971) and Igarashi and Kanda (1969).

References

1. Dohlman, G. F. (1971). The attachment of the cupulae, otolith and tectorial membranes to the sensory cell areas. *Acta Otolaryngol.* (*Stockholm*), **71,** 89
2. Harada, Y. (1975). Scanning electron microscopic studies on the morphological relation of vestibular sensory hair bundles to cupula and otolithic membrane. *Minerva Otorhinolaryngologica,* **25,** 86
3. Igarashi, M. and Kanda. T. (1969). Fine structure of the otolithic membrane in squirrel monkey. *Acta Otolaryngol.* (*Stockholm*), **68,** 43
4. Johnsson, L. G. and Hawkins, J. E. (1967). Otolithic membrane of the saccule and utricle in man. *Science,* **157,** 1454
5. Lim, D. J. (1971). Vestibular sensory organs. *Arch. Otolaryngol.*, **94,** 69

6. Lim, D. J. (1973). Formation and fate of the otoconia. *Ann. Otol. St. Louis*, **82,** 23
7. Lindeman, H. (1969a). Studies on the morphology of the sensory regions of the vestibular apparatus. *Adv. Anat. Embryol. Cell. Biol.*, **42,** 1
8. Lindeman, H. (1969b). Regional differences in structure of the vestibular sensory regions. *J. Laryngol.*, **83,** 1
9. Marco, J. Fernandez, S. and Romar, R. (1971). Ultrastructure of the otoliths and otolithic membrane of the macula utriculi in the guinea pig. *Acta Otolaryngol. (Stockholm)*, **71,** 1
10. Vilstrup, T. (1951). On the formation of the otolith. *Ann. Otol.*, **60,** 974
11. Wittmaak, K. (1956). *Die Ortho und Pathoviologie des Labyrinthes.* (Stuttgart: Georg Thieme)

a

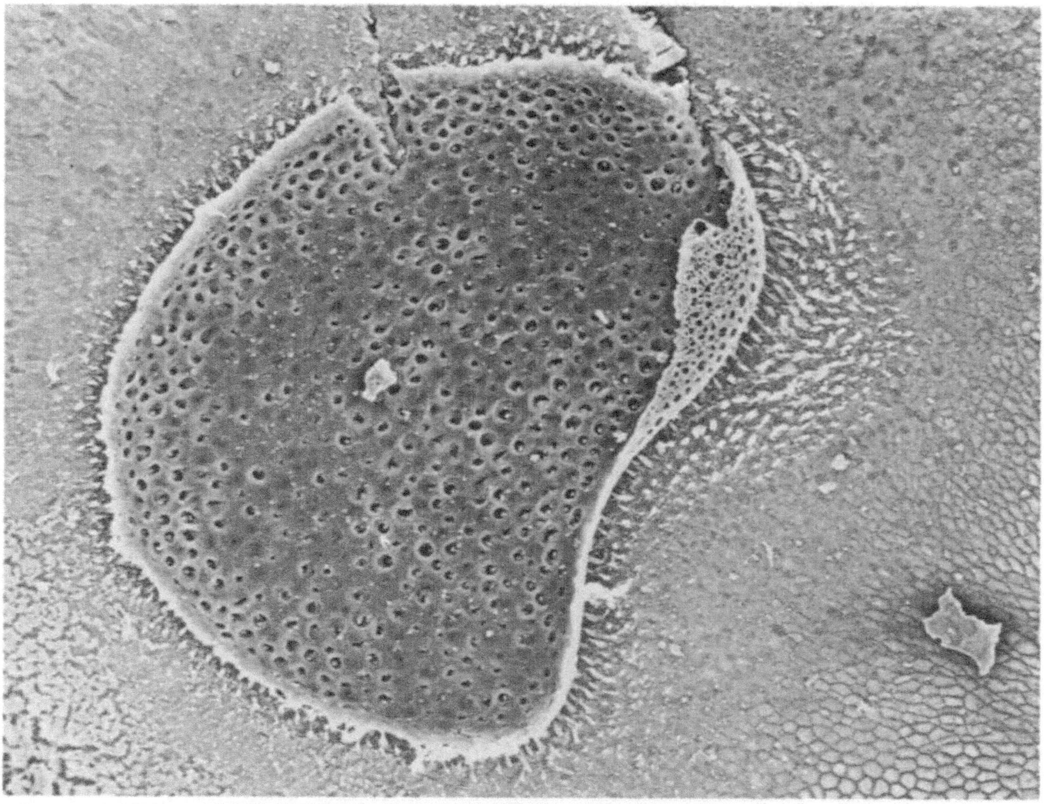

b

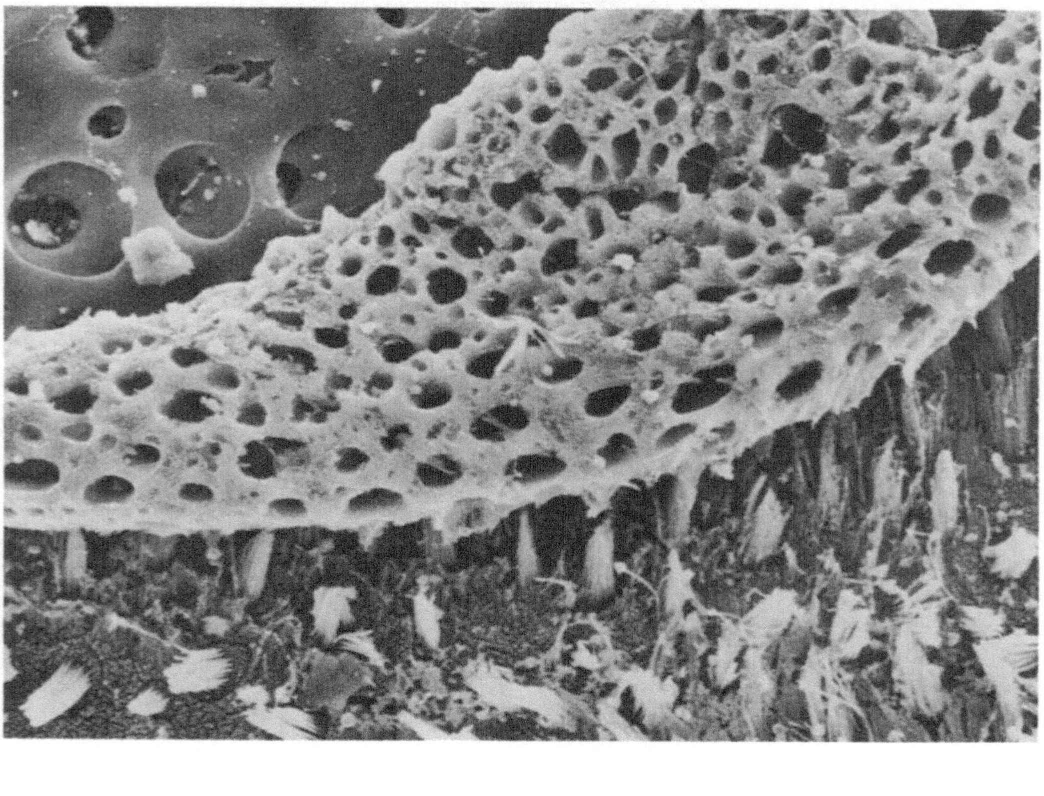

Figure 32

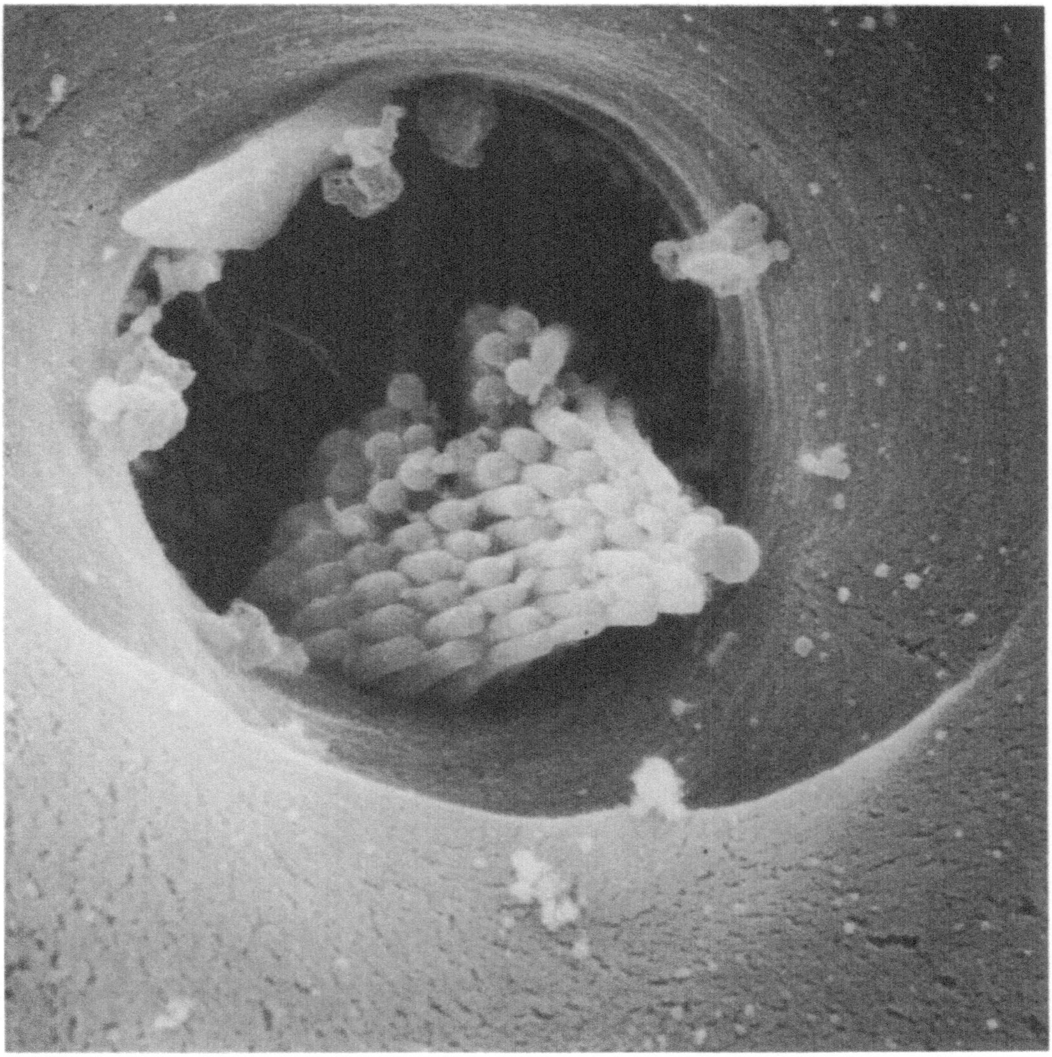

Figure 33 High magnification of Figure 32A (× 30 000)

Figure 32 Saccular otolithic membrane (frog). (**a**) Surface of the otolithic membrane. Numerous small holes are found. (× 300), (**b**) Sensory cilia are embedded in the hole of otolithic membrane (× 1500)

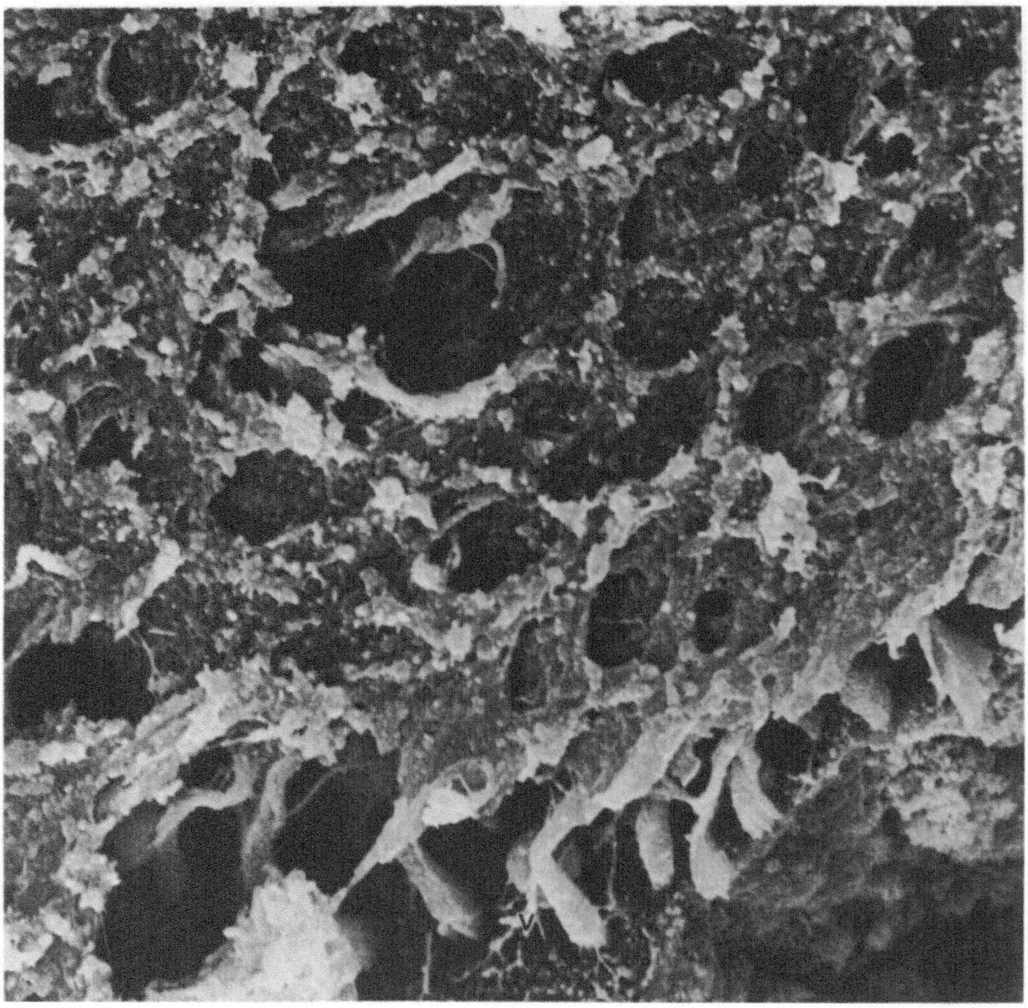

Figure 34 Otolithic membrane and the sensory cilia (pigeon). Some sensory cilia are embedded in the small holes of the otolithic membrane. The top of another cilia touches the gelatinous substance of the membrane. Mesh like substance, which is termed 'veil' (V) by Dohlman, extends from the microvilli on the sensory cell border to the otolithic membrane (× 4500)

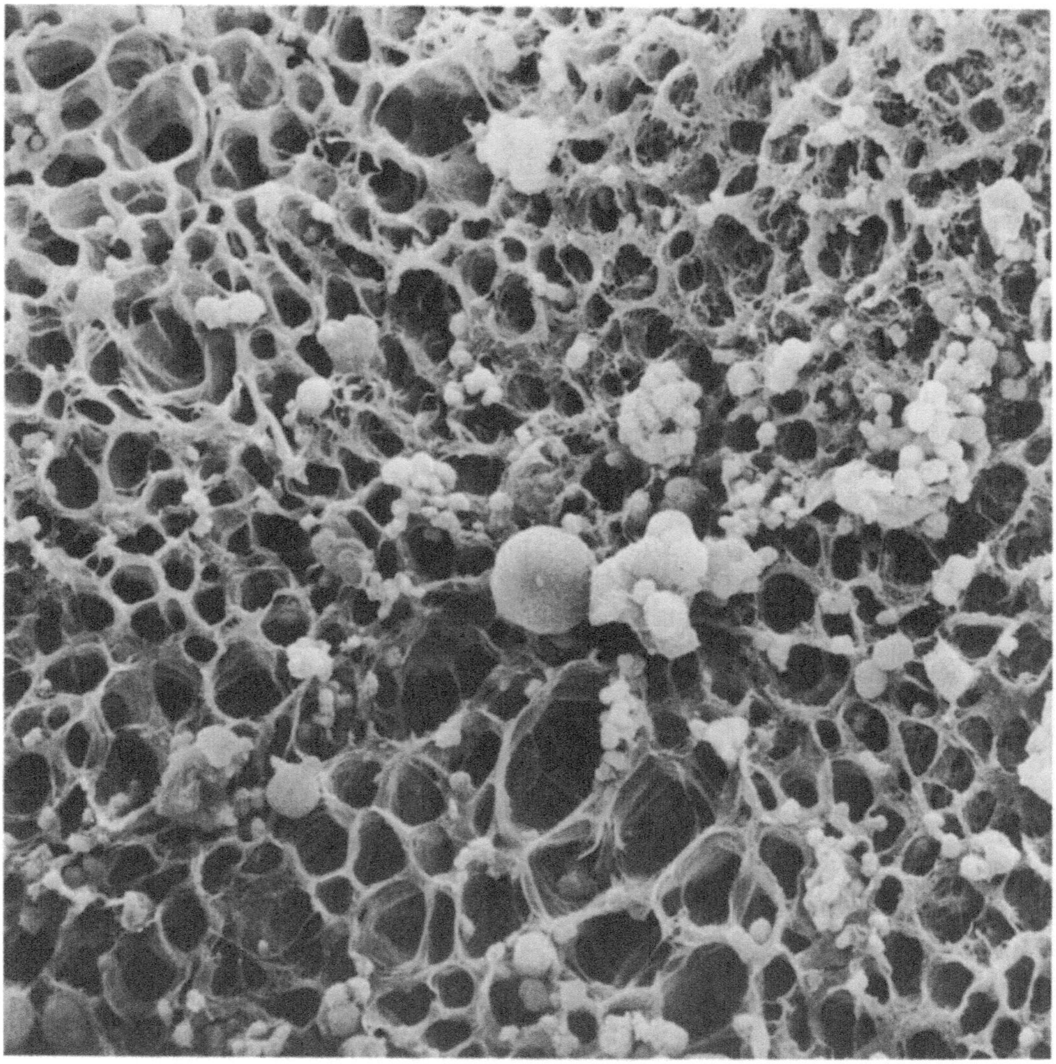

Figure 35 The undersurface of the otolithic membrane facing the sensory epithelia (cat). The undersurface of the otolithic membrane appears like honeycomb, because of the numerous holes. A part of the sensory cilia enters the holes. The average diameter of the hole is 5–6 μm. Also global substances with diameter 1–9 μm are found to be attached to these small holes ($\times$ 1600)

The formation area of the otoconia

Previously it was considered that otoconia are produced in the endolymphatic sac (Vilstrup, 1951). However, according to the recent studies by Harada (1978, a, b), it is found that otoconia are produced not in the endolymphatic sac but in the supporting cells of the macula. When he observed the otolithic membrane from the sensory cell side, a global substance was found to attach to the mesh-like structure with diameters of about 5–6 μm. X-ray microanalysis revealed abundant calcium in this global substance. The same substance was found in the epithelia of the macula. This substance presumably become the nuclei of the otoconia. Calcium analysis of the endolymphatic sac only showed the same amount of calcium as found in the vestibular wall cells, and no specific finding indicating secretion of calcium was observed (Harada, 1978c).

References

1. Harada, Y. (1978a). The formation and absorption area of the statoconia. *L. Clin. Electron Microscopy*, **II,** 827
2. Harada, Y (1978b). Formation area of the statoconia. *Equilibrium Res.*, **37,** 217
3. Harada, Y. (1978c). Metabolic disorder of otoconia and the vestibular dark cells. *Equilibrium Res.*, **37,** 1
4. Vilstrup, T. (1951). On the formation of the otoliths. *Otol. Rhinol. Laryngol. St. Louis*, **60,** 974

Figure 36 X-ray microanalysis of the undersurface of the otolithic membrane (cat). (**a**) A peak, which derives from the large global substance, is recognized. It is also revealed that these structures contain approximately 20% calcium which is half of the normal content of otoconia (× 4000), (**b**) The global substance and the granular products in (**a**) turned into white dotted image by plane analysis, indicating high calcium concentration (× 4000)

a

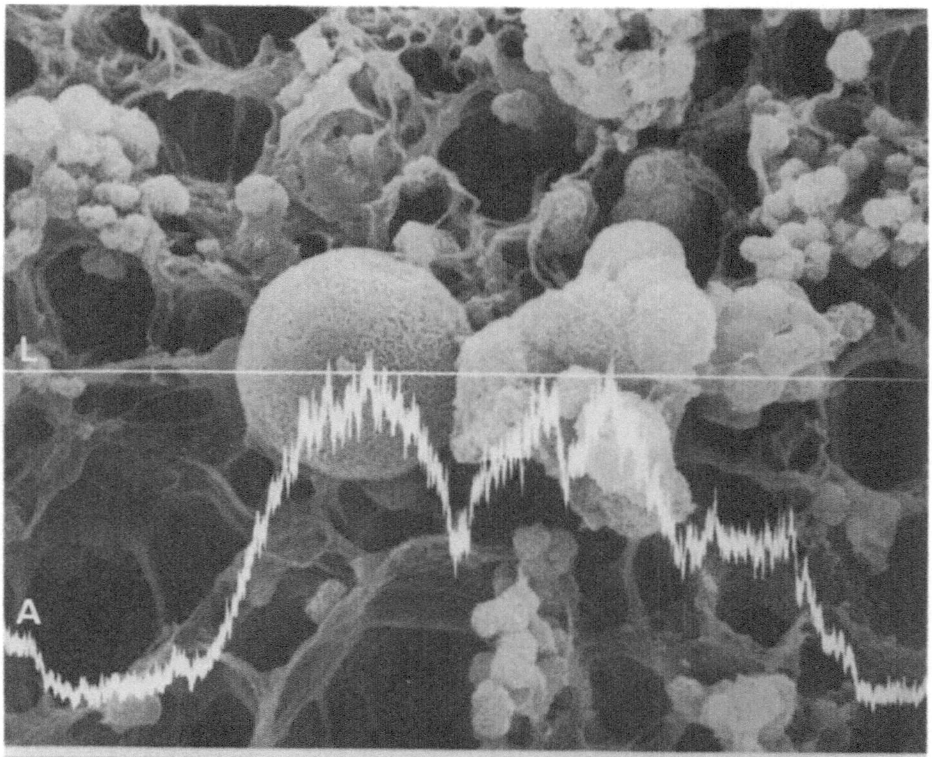

b

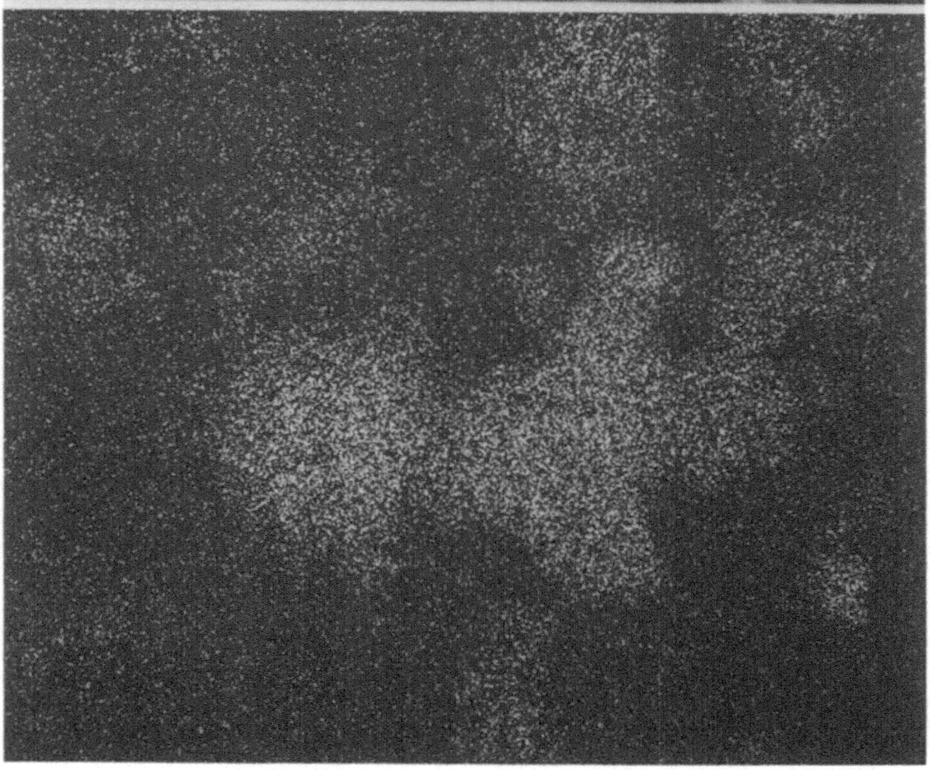

Figure 36

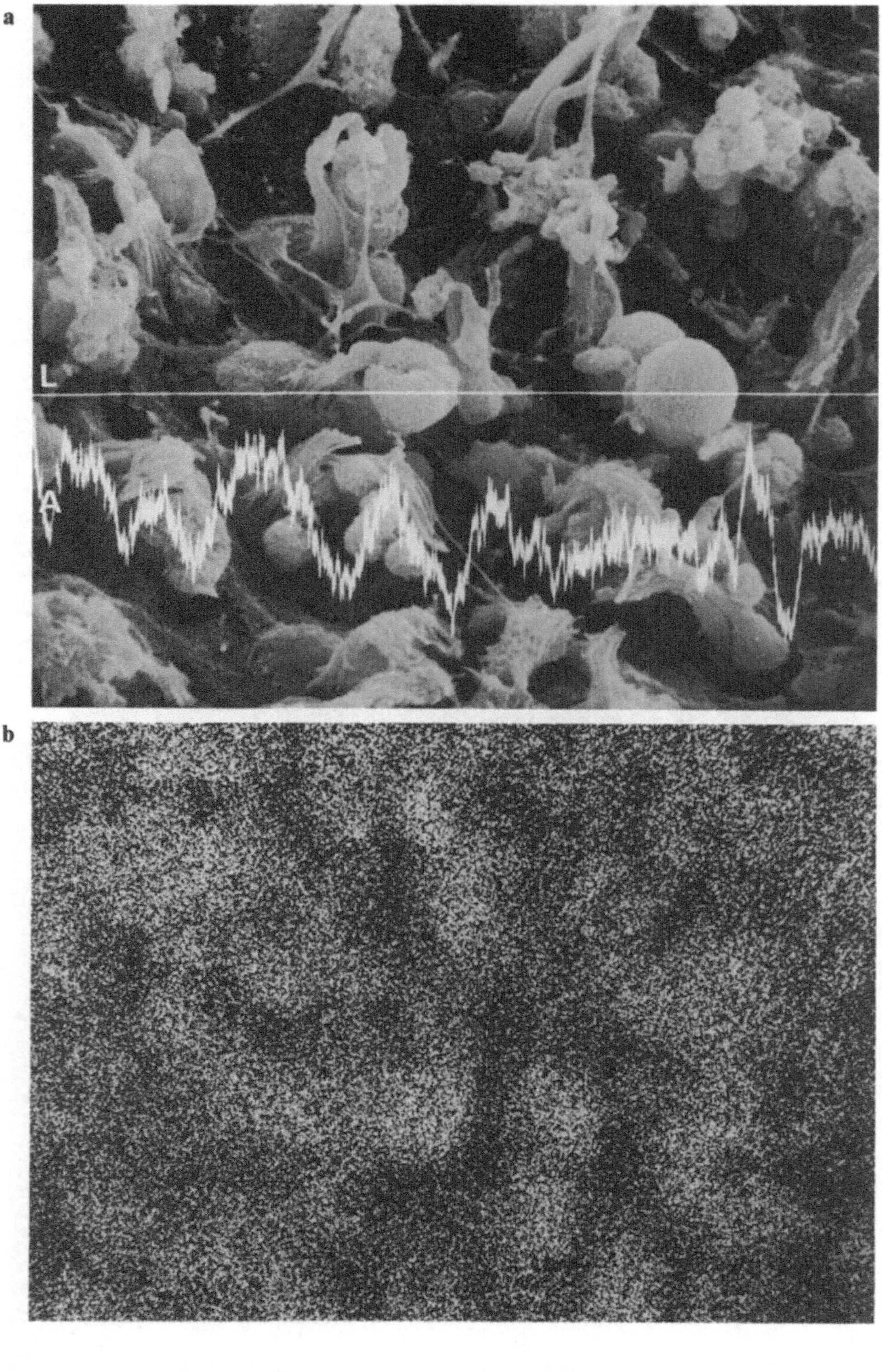

Figure 37 Calcium analysis of the utricular sensory epithelium (cat). Calcium is identified both in line and plane analysis. L: analysis line; A: trace showing calcium content (× 4000)

a

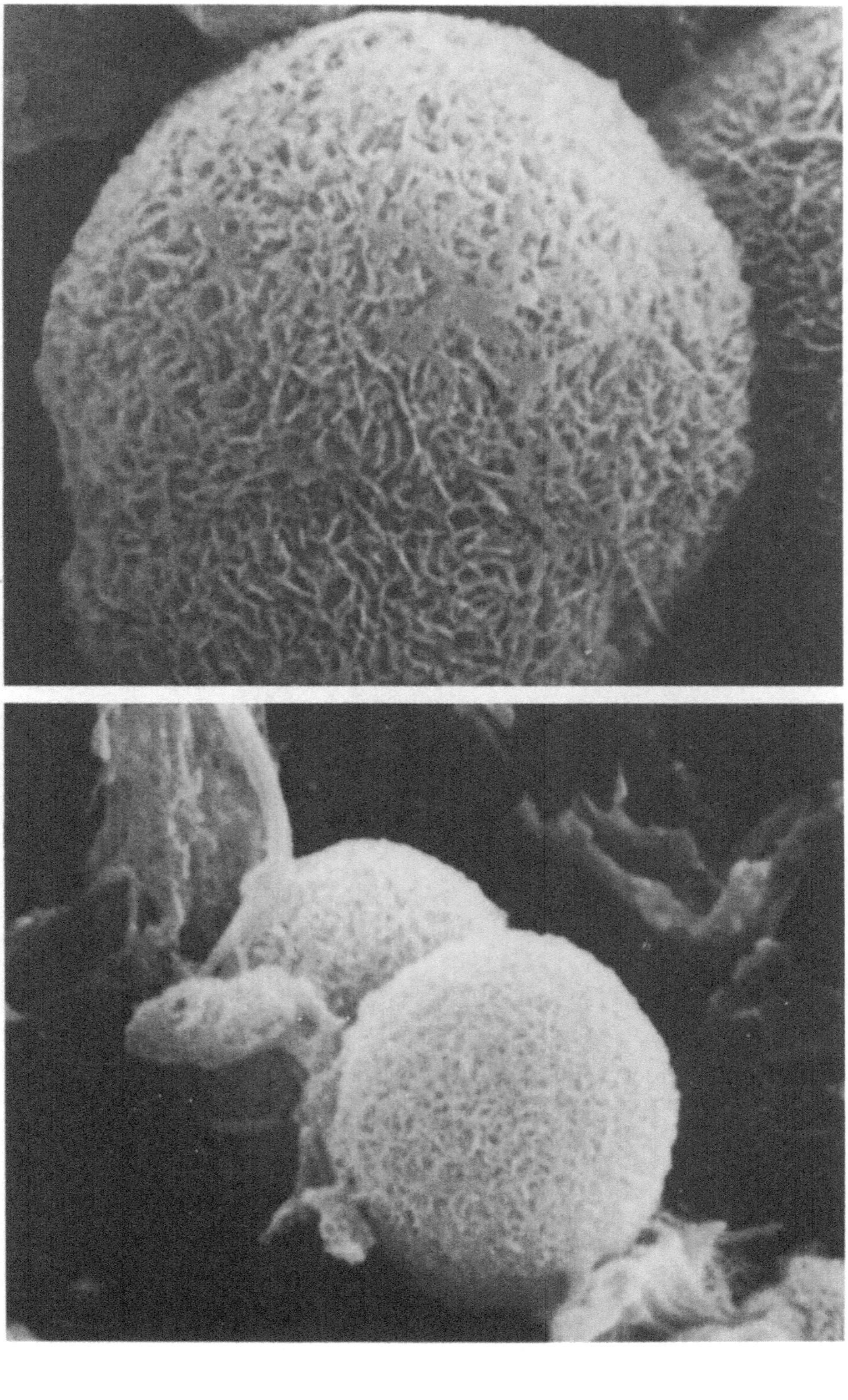

b

Figure 38 (**a**) Global substance in the undersurface of the otolithic membrane (× 26 000), (**b**) global substance on the supporting cells of the sensory epithelia (× 20 000)

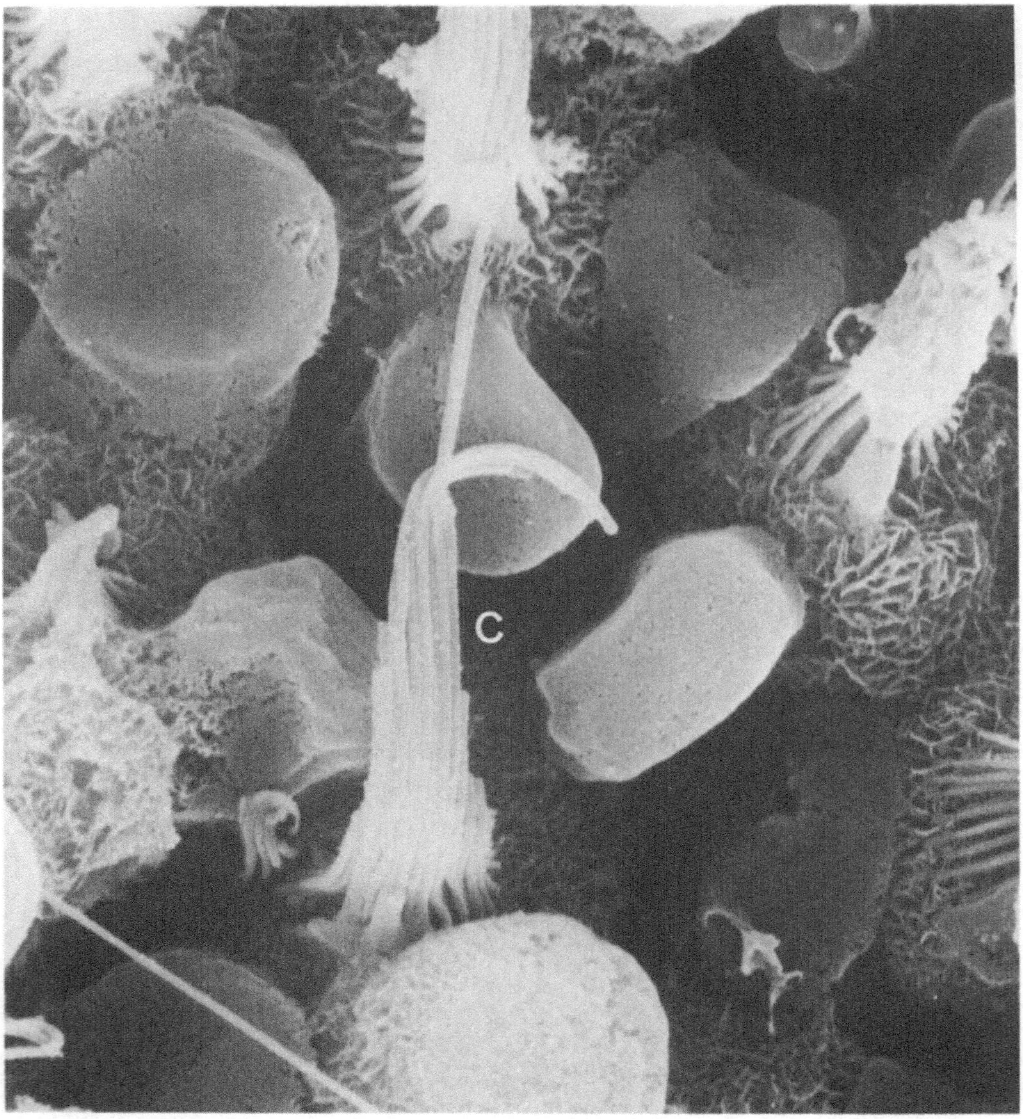

Figure 39 Sensory epithelia of the utricular macula (guinea pig). A number of protrusions are seen around the sensory cilia (C) (× 8000)

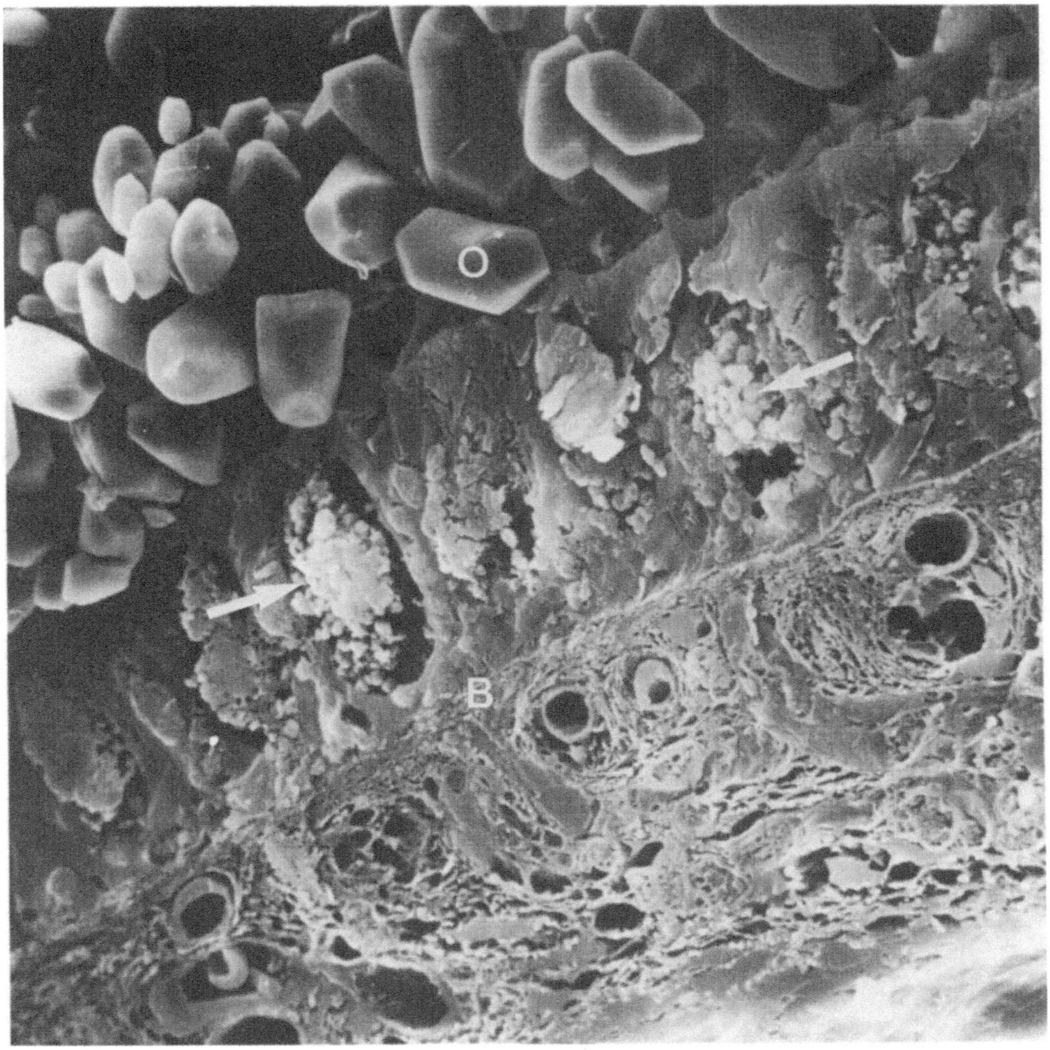

Figure 40 Cracked surface of the utricular macula (guinea pig). Small granules are present in the cell body of the sensory epithelia (arrow). O: otoconia; B: basilar membrane (× 1600)

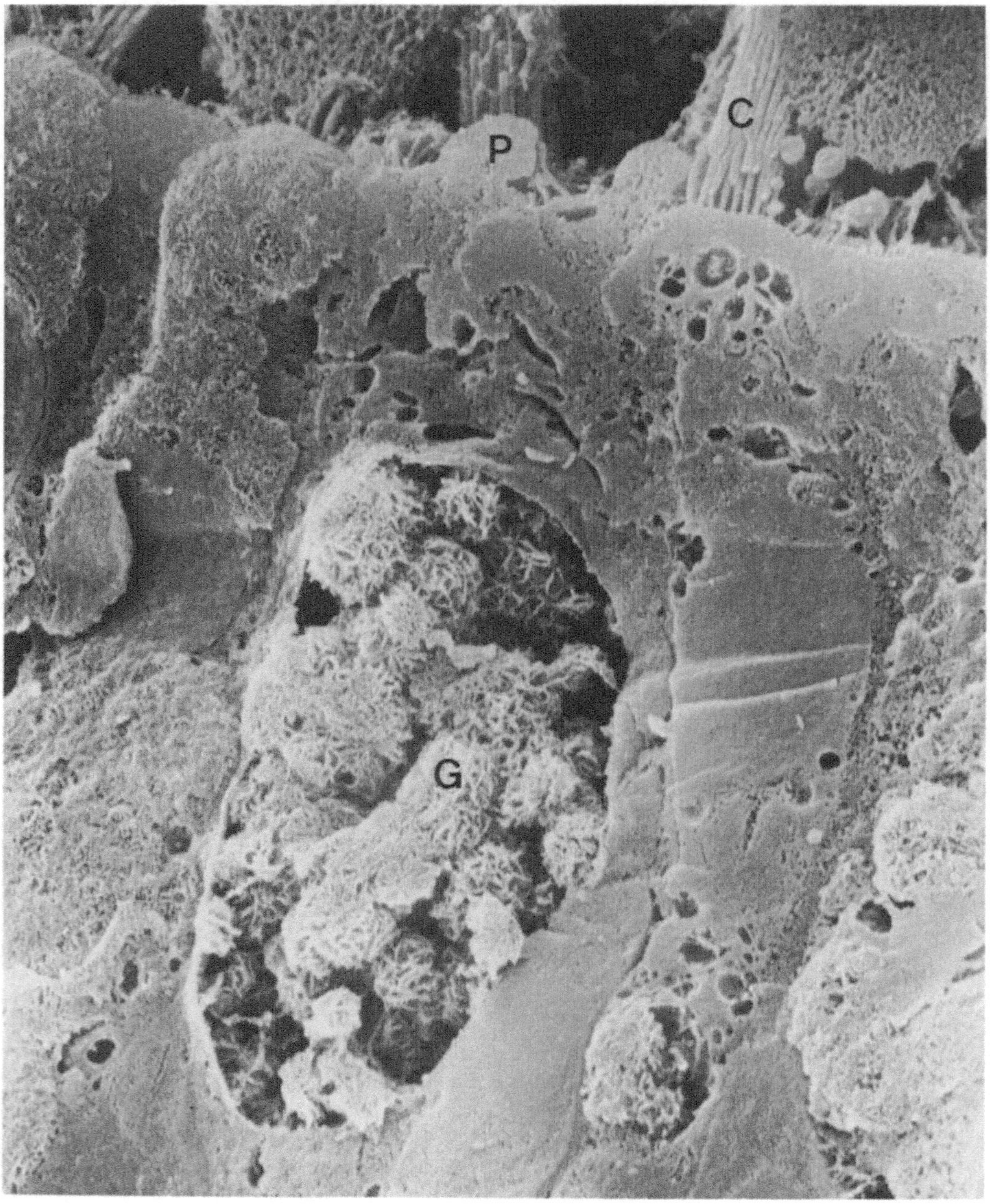

Figure 41 Cracked sensory epithelium of the utricular macula (guinea pig). High magnification of Figure 40. G: granules; C: sensory cilia; P: protrusion (× 9000)

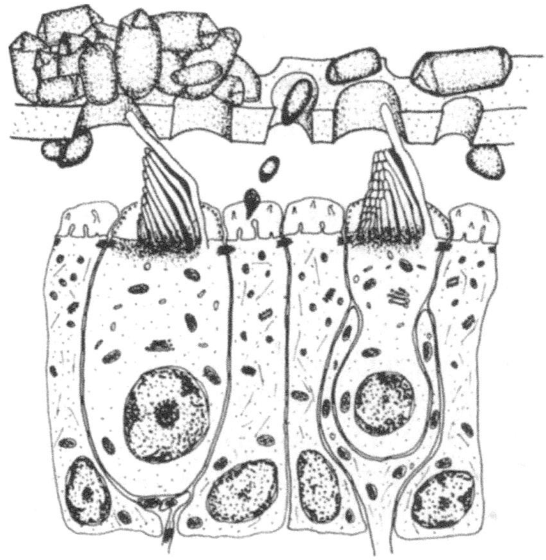

Figure 42 A schema showing the process of the otoconia formation. A global substance containing $CaCO_3$ is first produced from the macular supporting cell. Then this substance becomes an otoconial crystal after passing through the hole in the otolithic membrane. In this process, contribution of carbonic anhydrase is possible, but still remains unclear

The absorption area of the otoconia

There are very few studies on absorption area and metabolism of the otoconia. Lim (1973) found fragmented otoconia attached to the dark cells of the perimacular epithelium of the utricle. Harada (1977, 1978) analysed this fragmented otoconia with the X-ray microanalyser and confirmed that otoconia were decalcified and absorbed in the dark cell area. Further, he reconfirmed this finding by the study of otoconia affected by dihydrostreptomycin (1978).

In conclusion, the otoconia metabolizes by itself and is produced by the macular supporting cells, while it is absorbed by the dark cells. These findings provide important clues when one considers the mechanisms of the cures of benign paroxysmal positional vertigo and labyrinthine concussion, and also cupulolithiasis which was described by Schuknecht. Organic material, which is the remnant of decalcification, is finally absorbed by pinocytotic activity of the dark cells (Harada, 1978).

References

1. Harada, Y. (1978a). Metabolic disorder of otoconia and the vestibular dark cells. *Equilibrium Res.*, **37,** 1
2. Harada, Y., Sugimoto, Y. (1977). Metabolic disorder of otoconia after streptomycin intoxication. *Acta Otolaryngol.* (*Stockholm*), **84,** 65
3. Harada, Y. (1978b). Morphological changes in the vestibular sensory organs after streptomycin intoxication. *Scanning Electron Microscopy*, **II,** 1077
4. Lim, D. J. (1973). Formation and fate of the otoconia. *Ann. Otol. Rhinol. Laryngol. St. Louis.*, **82,** 23
5. Schuknecht, H. F. C. (1968). Cupulolithiasis. *Arch. Otolaryngol.* (*Chicago*), **90,** 765

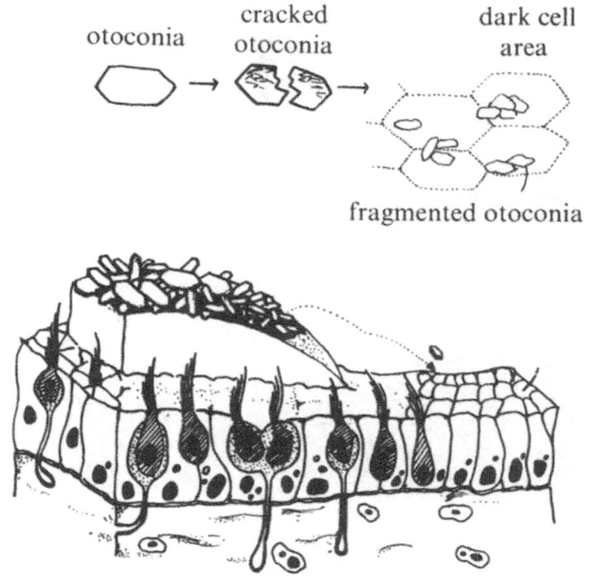

Figure 43 A schema showing the absorption of the otoconia

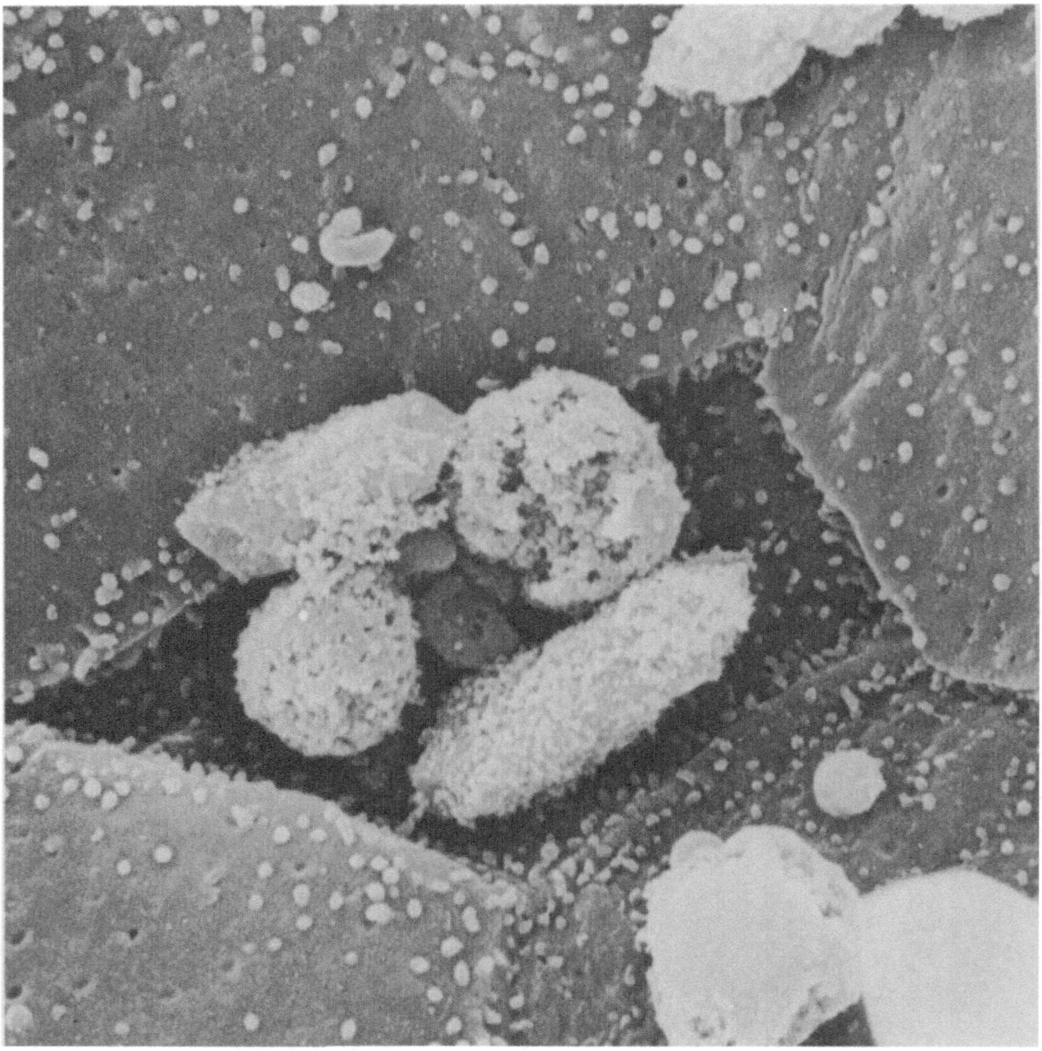

Figure 44 The dark cell portion of the utricle (guinea pig). It is observed that deformed otoconia are attached to the cells. The dark cell surface is generally square or octagonal with a clear cell border (× 14000)

Figure 45 X-ray microanalysis of the otoconia on the utricular dark cells (guinea pig). (**a**) Fragmented otoconia generally have a small amount of calcium, although a large otoconium still contains some calcium as shown by the peak. L: analysis line; A: trace showing calcium content (× 5500). (**b**) The plane analysis shows a dotted image which corresponds to the large otoconia.

a

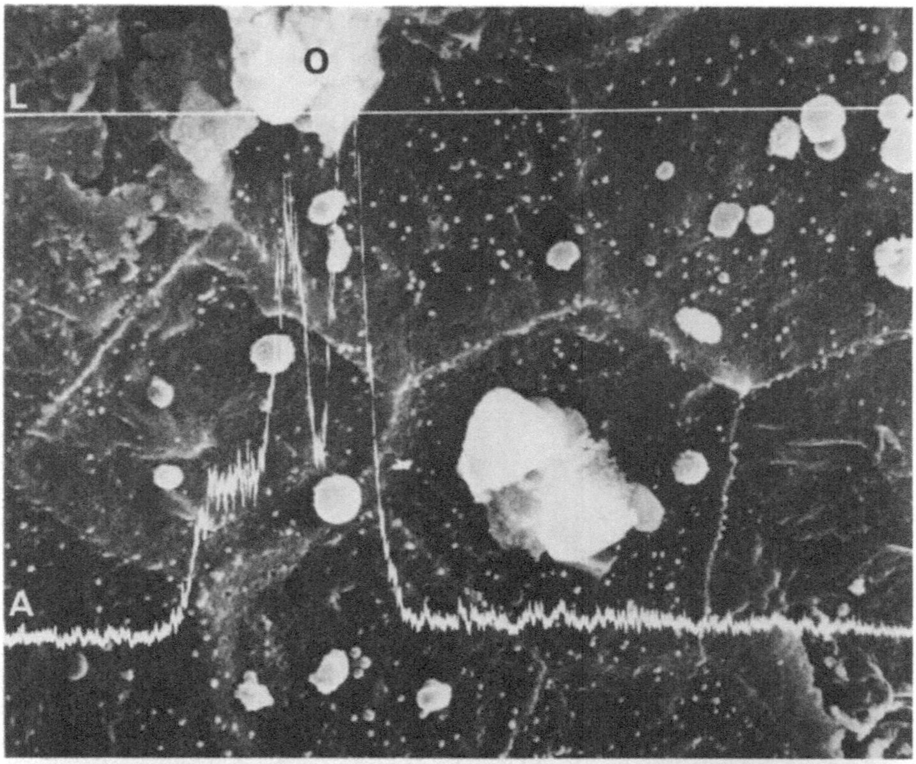

b

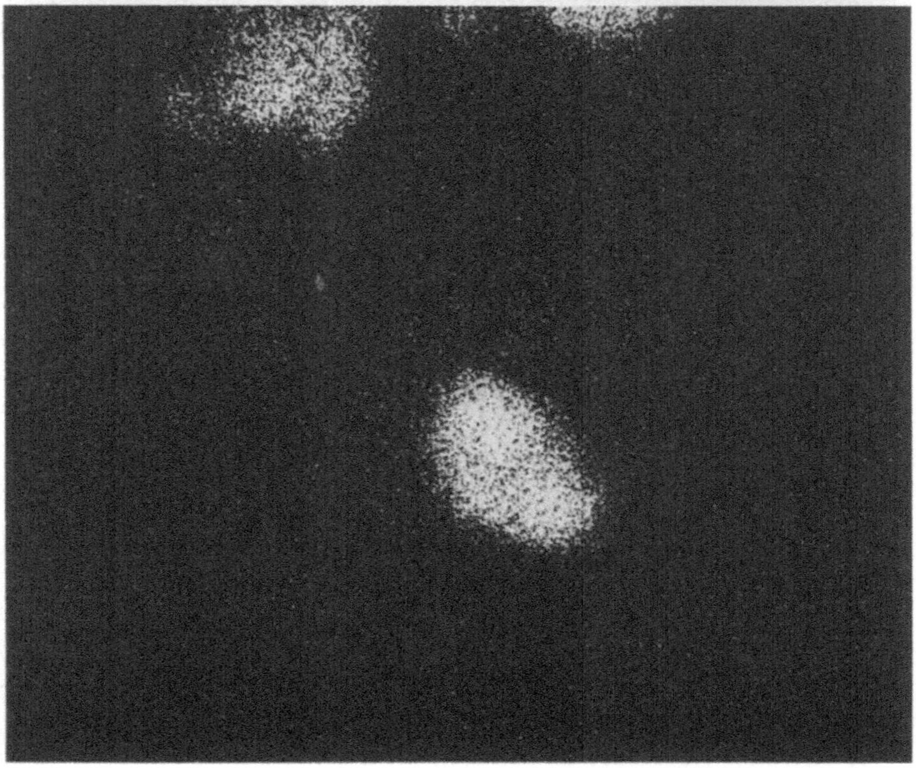

Figure 45

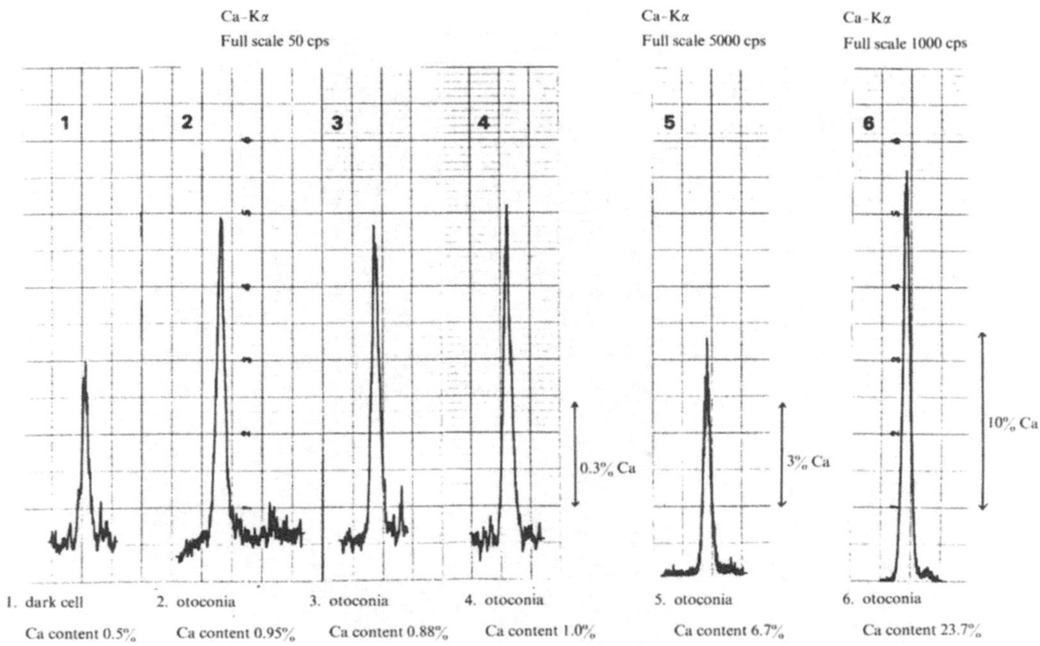

Figure 46 Calcium analysis of the utricular otoconia (guinea pig) and the dark cell in Figure 44. Otoconia detached from the otolithic membrane were scattered on the dark cells after dihydrostreptomycin injection. Different portions as indicated by numbers from 1 to 6 (Figure 47) show different amounts of calcium. For instance, portion 1 (dark cell) contained 0.5% Ca. Otoconium (6) which has fairly good shape contained 23.7% Ca, while the deformed otoconium (2) only 0.95% Ca

---

Figure 47 (**a**) Line analysis reveals a peak on line A which corresponds to an otoconium (5), (**b**) Plane analysis of (a). White dots accumulate in the otoconia with high amounts of calcium (× 6500)

a

b

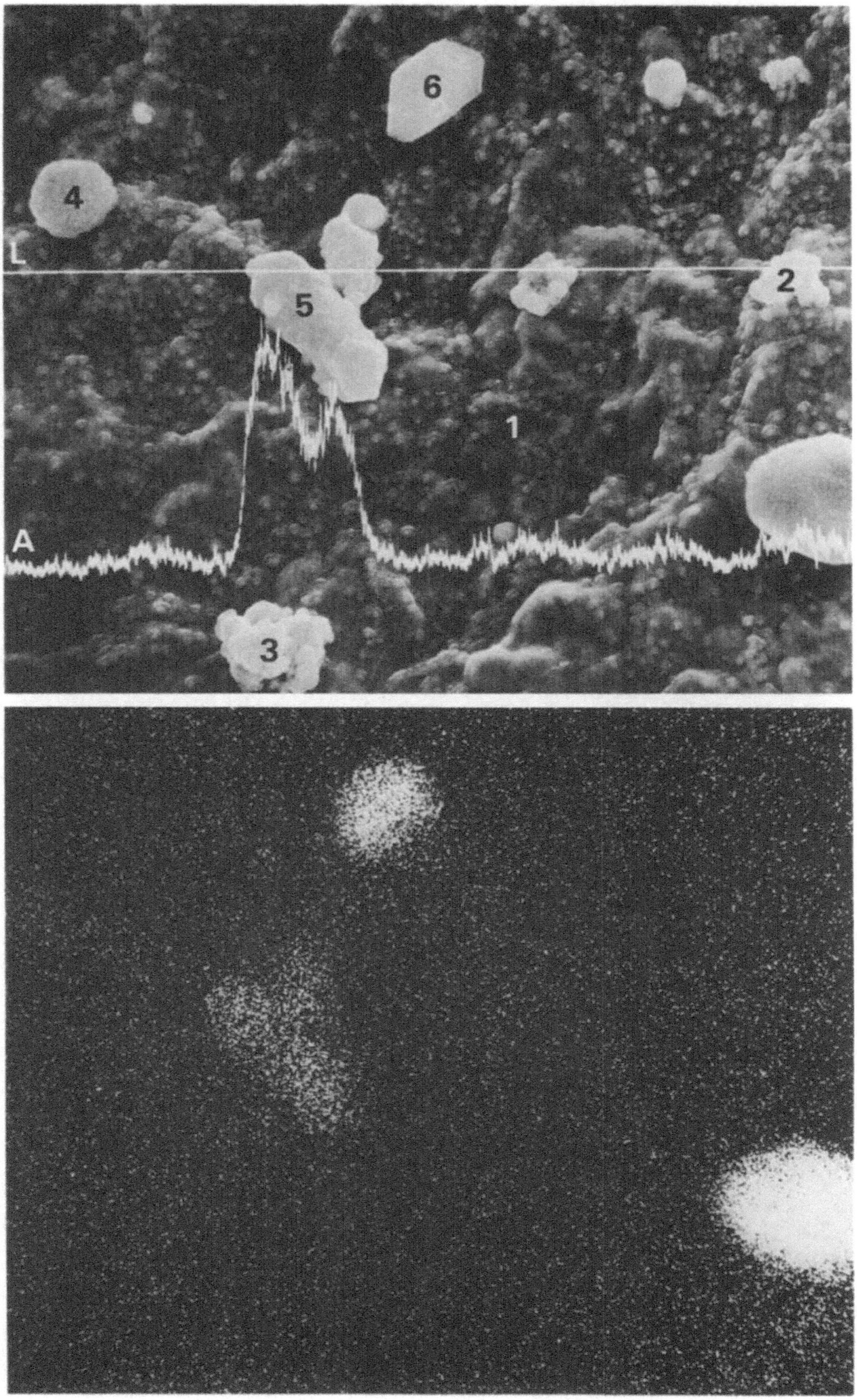

Figure 47

a

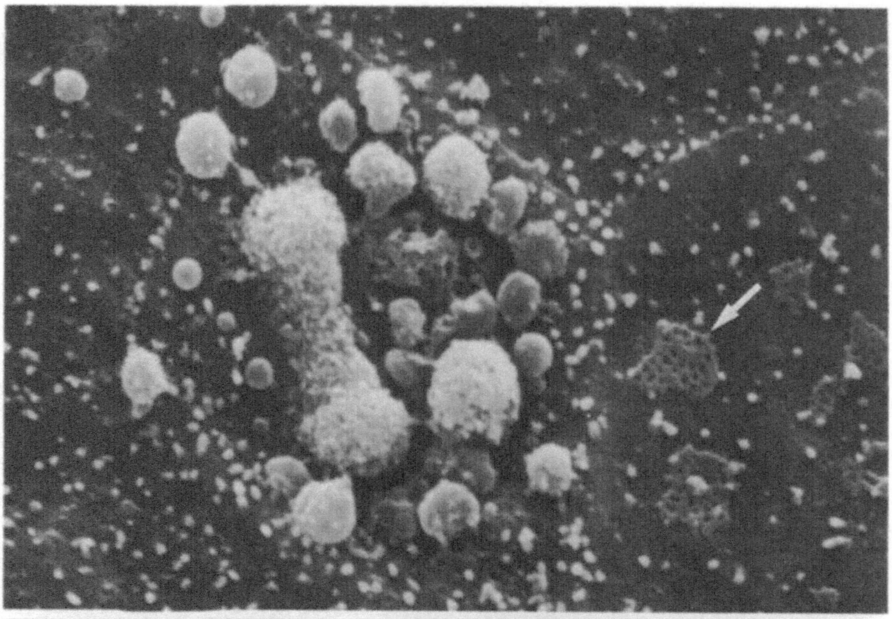

b

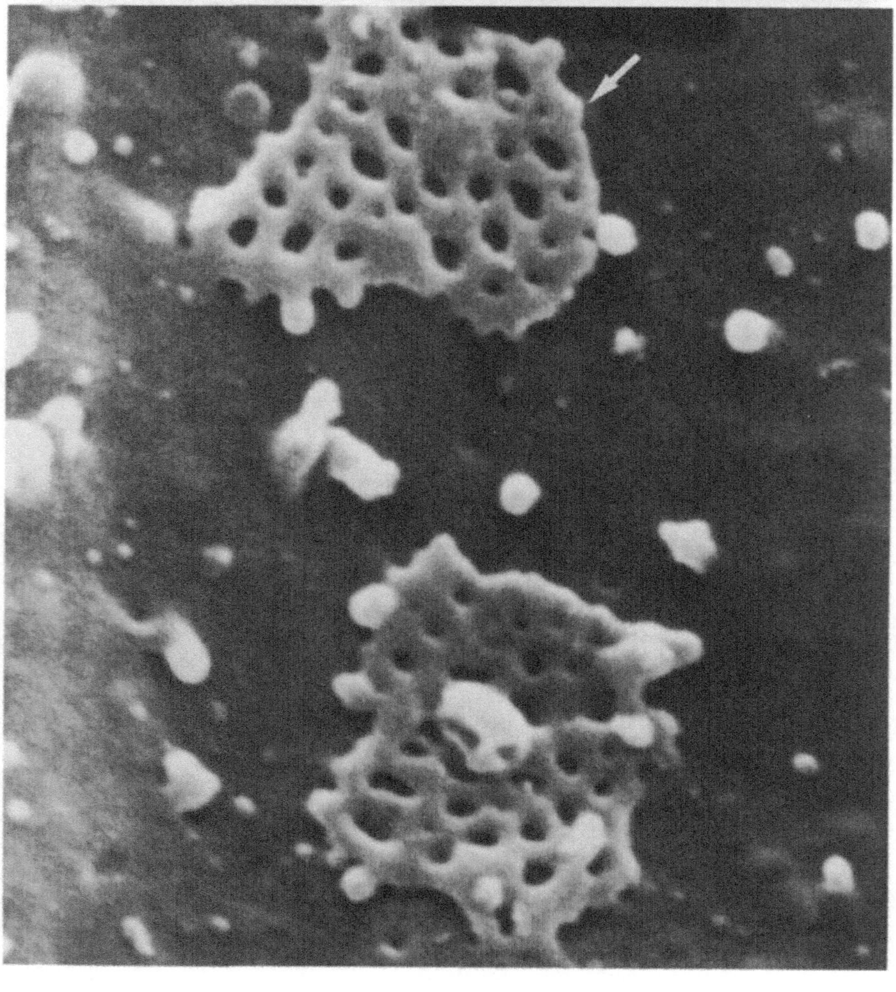

Figure 48 (**a**) Deformed otoconia which appear granular, like pumice stone attached to the surface of the dark cell. Mesh work substances are also found on this area (arrow) (× 6000), (**b**) high magnification of mesh work substances with micropores (× 40 000)

The sensory cells

(1) *Hair cell type I*

This cell is flask-shaped with a long neck and a round bottom which contains the nucleus. The bottom extends two thirds of the depth of the sensory epithelial layer. The cell body, except for the uppermost portion, is surrounded by the afferent nerve chalice. The surface of the type I cell is larger than that of the type II cell. On top of the cell, there are 60-100 stereocilia with their base in the cuticular plate. There is only one kinocilium, and this lacks the cuticular plate. The stereocilia are a group of cilia which increase their length stepwise, resulting in a stair or pipe organ shape (Lim, 1969).

The kinocilium is the longest and is located next to the longest stereocilia. The kinocilia of the macula and semicircular canals show a regular arrangement. Namely, they are located closer to the canal side in the anterior and posterior canals (Flock, 1965). In the utricular macula, each kinocilium is situated closer to the striola and in the saccular macula closer to the side farthest from the striola. This location of the kinocilium is closely related to electrophysiological excitability and polarization (Trincker, 1957; Lowenstein and Wersäll, 1959; Flock and Wersäll, 1962).

The kinocilium is slightly thicker than the stereocilia and its inner structure is of one pair of central fibrils and nine pairs of surrounding fibrils. In the type I cell, underneath the cuticular plate are mitochondria vesicles, Golgi apparati, lysosomes and nuclei. Under the nucleus, there are mitochondria, ribosomes and small number of vesicles.

(2) *Hair cell type II*

This cell is cylindrical and the surface is smaller than that of the type I cell. The arrangement of the cilia is the same as on the type I cell. Intracellular organs are distributed more homogeneously than in the type I cell. They are mitochondria, vesicles, Golgi apparati and ribosomes. Type I cells have a nerve chalice which surrounds almost the whole cell, while type II cells have a button-like attachment of both afferent and efferent nerve endings. There is a synaptic bar in the subnuclear space, which was found by Smith and Sjöstrand (1969). Mammals and birds have both type I and II cells, but fish and frogs have only type II cells. Generally type II cells are older than type I cells.

References

1. Flock, Å. (1965). Electron microscopic and electrophysiological studies on the lateral line canal organ. *Acta Otolaryngol.* (*Stockholm*), *Suppl.*, **199,** 1
2. Flock, Å. and Wersäll, J. (1962). A study of the orientation of the sensory hairs of the receptor cells in the lateral line organ of fish, with special reference to the function of the receptors. *J. Cell Biol.*, **15,** 19
3. Lim, D. J. and Lance, W. C. (1969). Vestibular sensory epithelia. *Acta Otolaryngol.* (*Stockholm*), **90,** 283
4. Lowenstein, O. and Wersäll. J. (1959). A functional interpretation of the electron microscopic structure of the sensory hairs in the crista of the elasmobranch (*Raha clavata*) in terms of directional sensitivity. *Nature* (*London*), **184,** 1807
5. Smith, C. and Sjöstrand. F. (1969). Structure of the nerve endings on the external hair cells of the guinea pig cochlea as studied by serial sections. *J. Ultrastruct. Res.*, **5,** 523
6. Trincker, D. (1957). Permanent potentials in the semicircular canal system of the guinea pig and their changes in experimental cupula leads. *Pflügers Arch. Ges. Physiol.*, **264,** 351

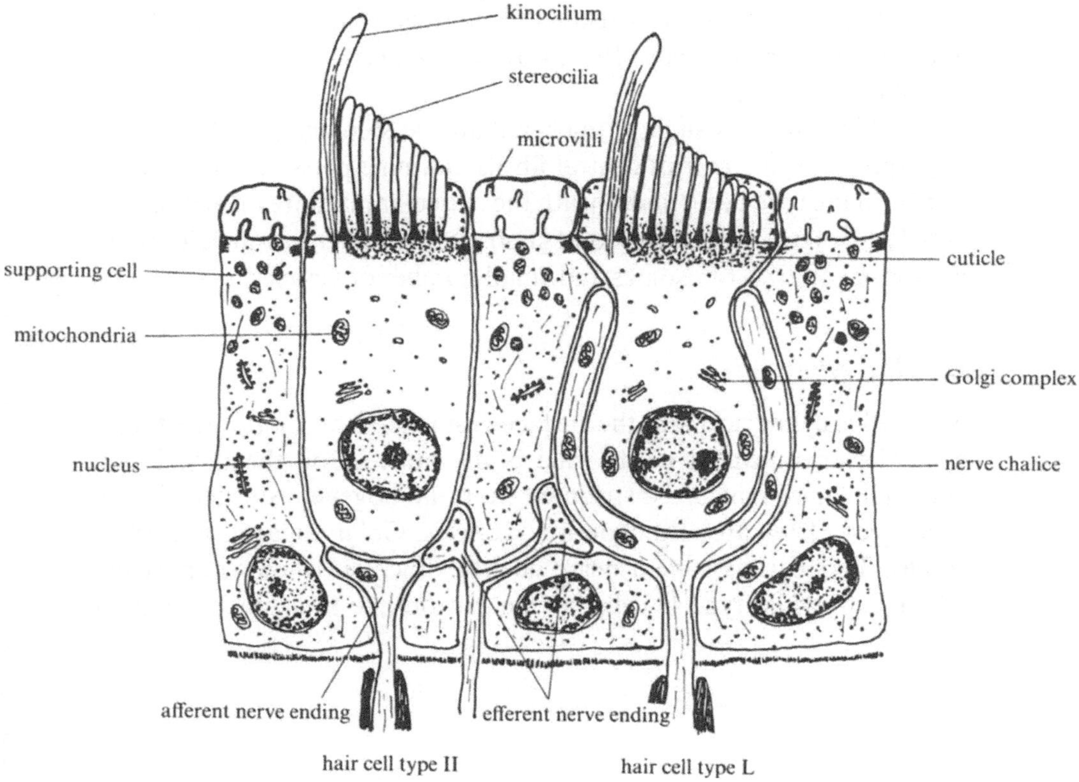

Figure 49 Schema of vestibular sensory cells

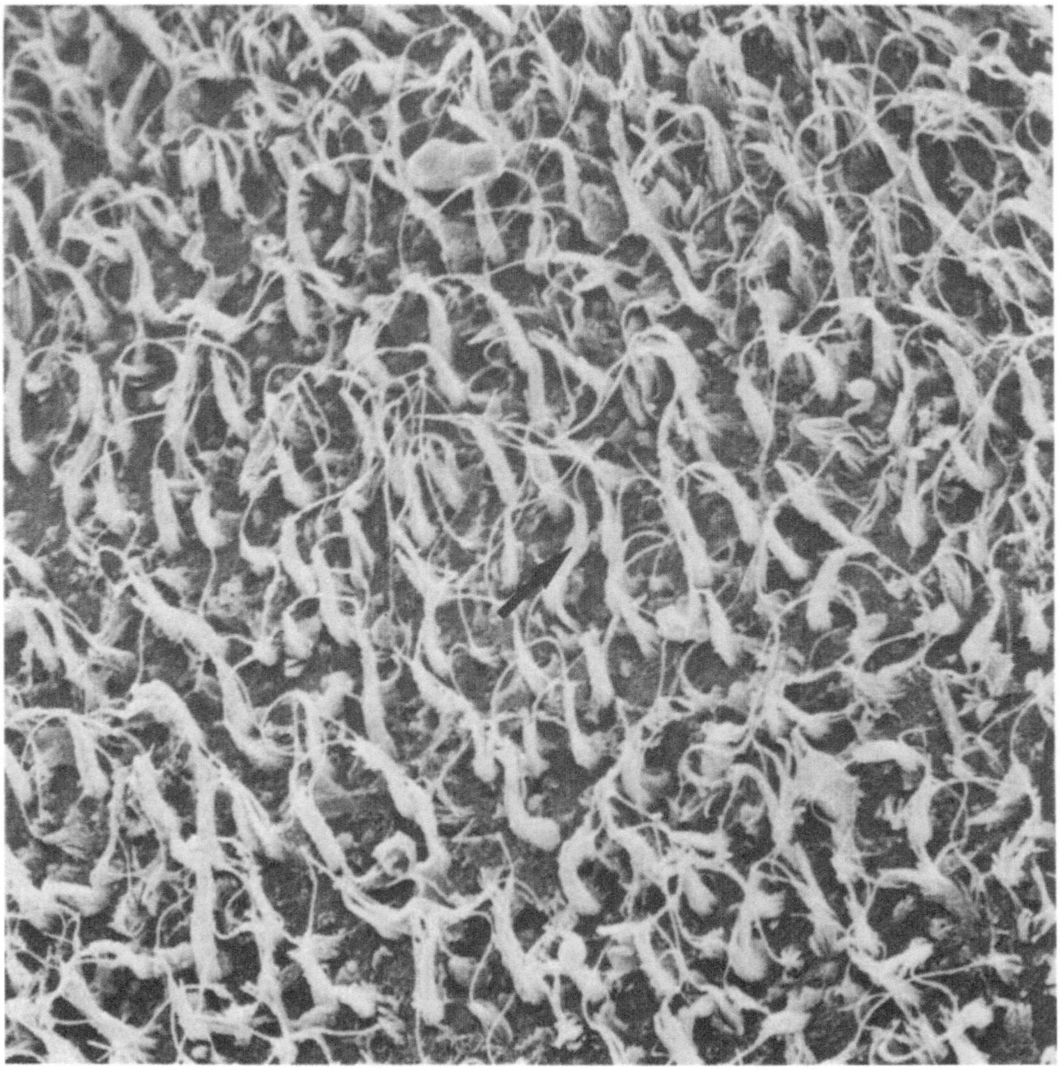

Figure 50 Sensory cilia of the utricular macula (rabbit). Groups of sensory cilia consisting of a long kinocilium and several stereocilia are observed. Polarity of the cilia is indicated by arrow (× 1500)

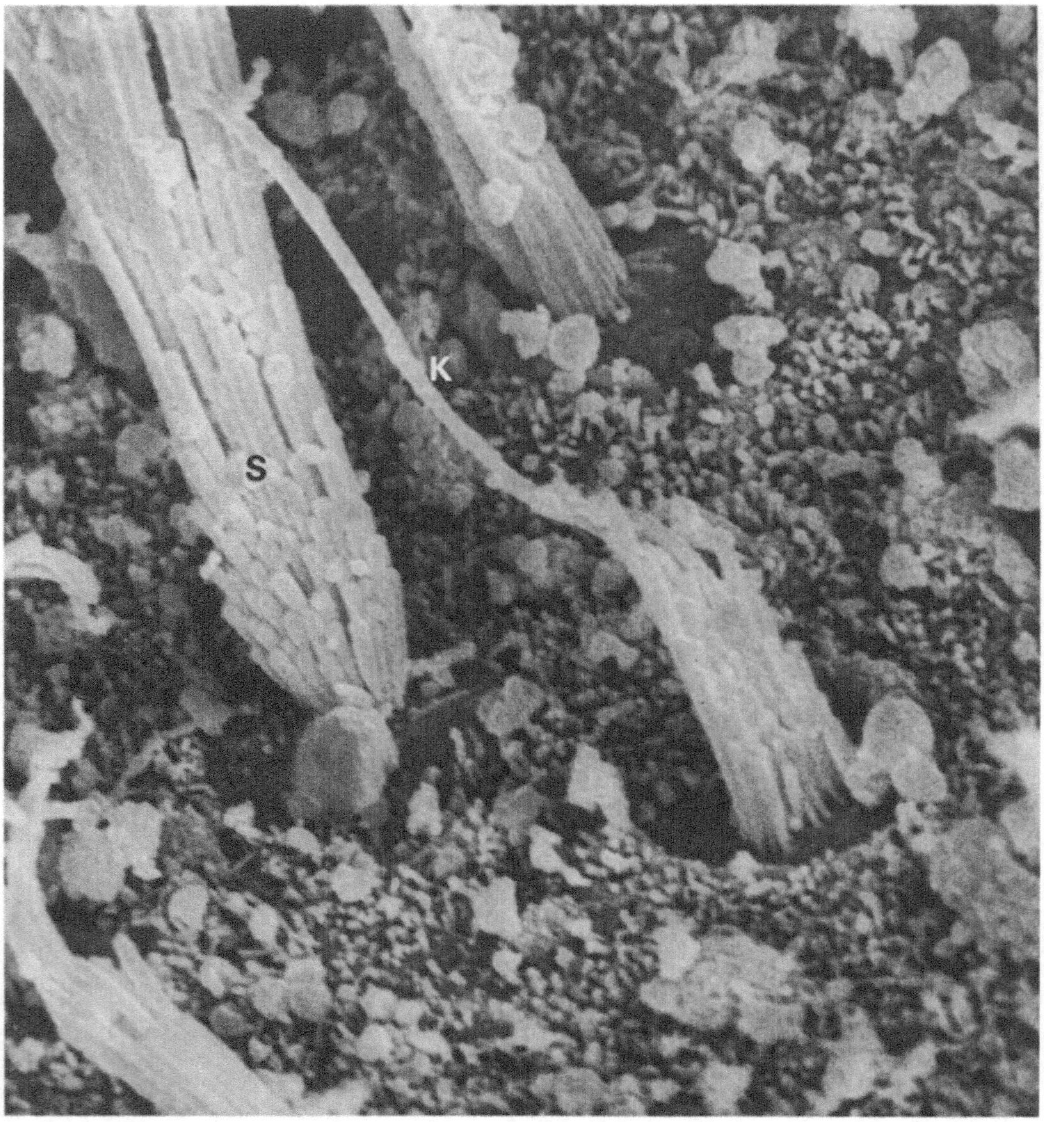

Figure 51 The surface of the sensory epithelium (human). The surface of the utricular sensory epithelium obtained from the acoustic neurinoma patient. Two kinds of the cells, type I cells with long step-like stereocilia (S) and type II cells with a long kinocilium (K) and short stereocilia are seen (× 7500)

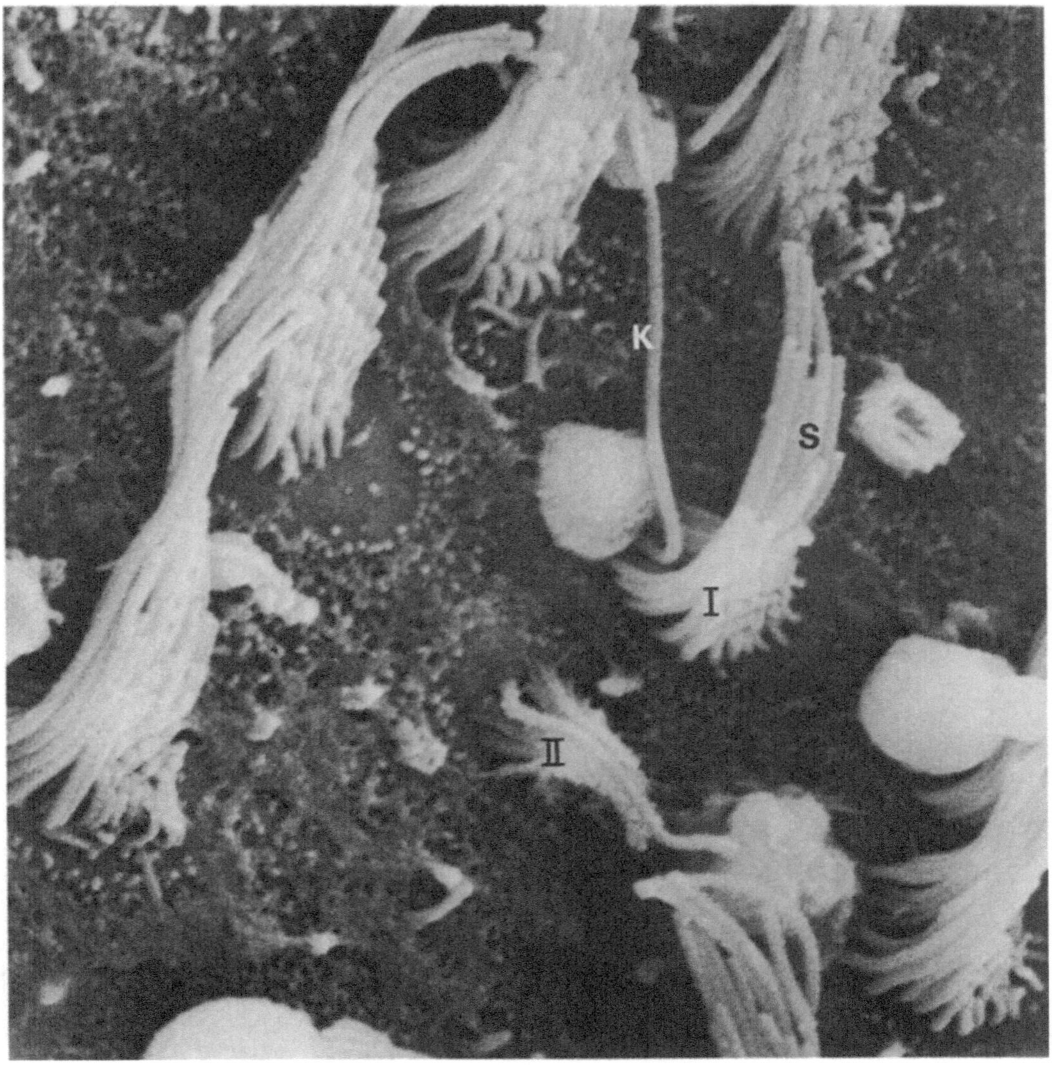

Figure 52 The surface of the sensory epithelia (kite). Sensory cilia are formed by a long kinocilium (K) and step-like stereocilia (S). Type I cell has wider surface than type II cell (× 8400)

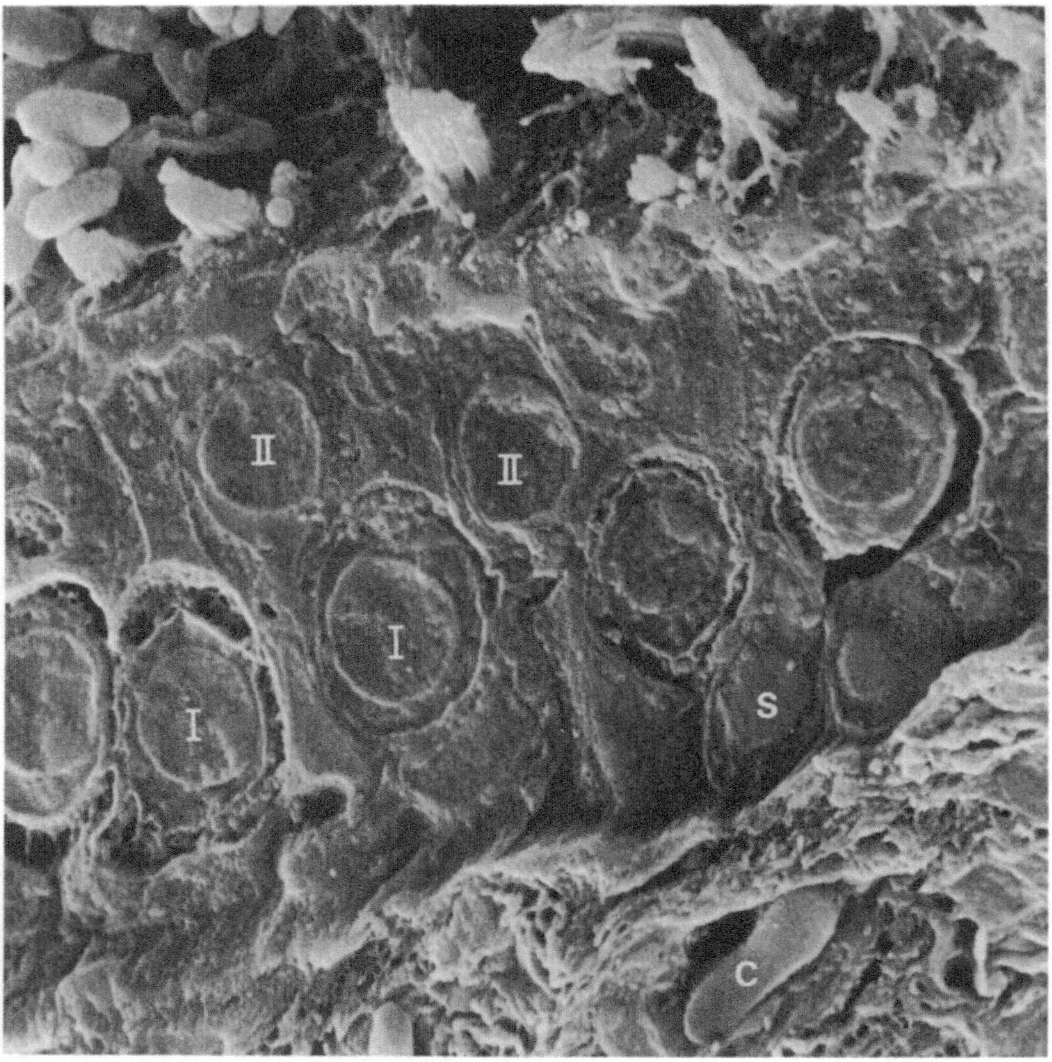

Figure 53 Fractured utricular macula (dog). Flask-shaped type I cell (I) and cylindrical type II cell (II) are shown. Type I cell is surrounded by the nerve chalice. S: supporting cell; C: red blood cell in the vessel (× 4200)

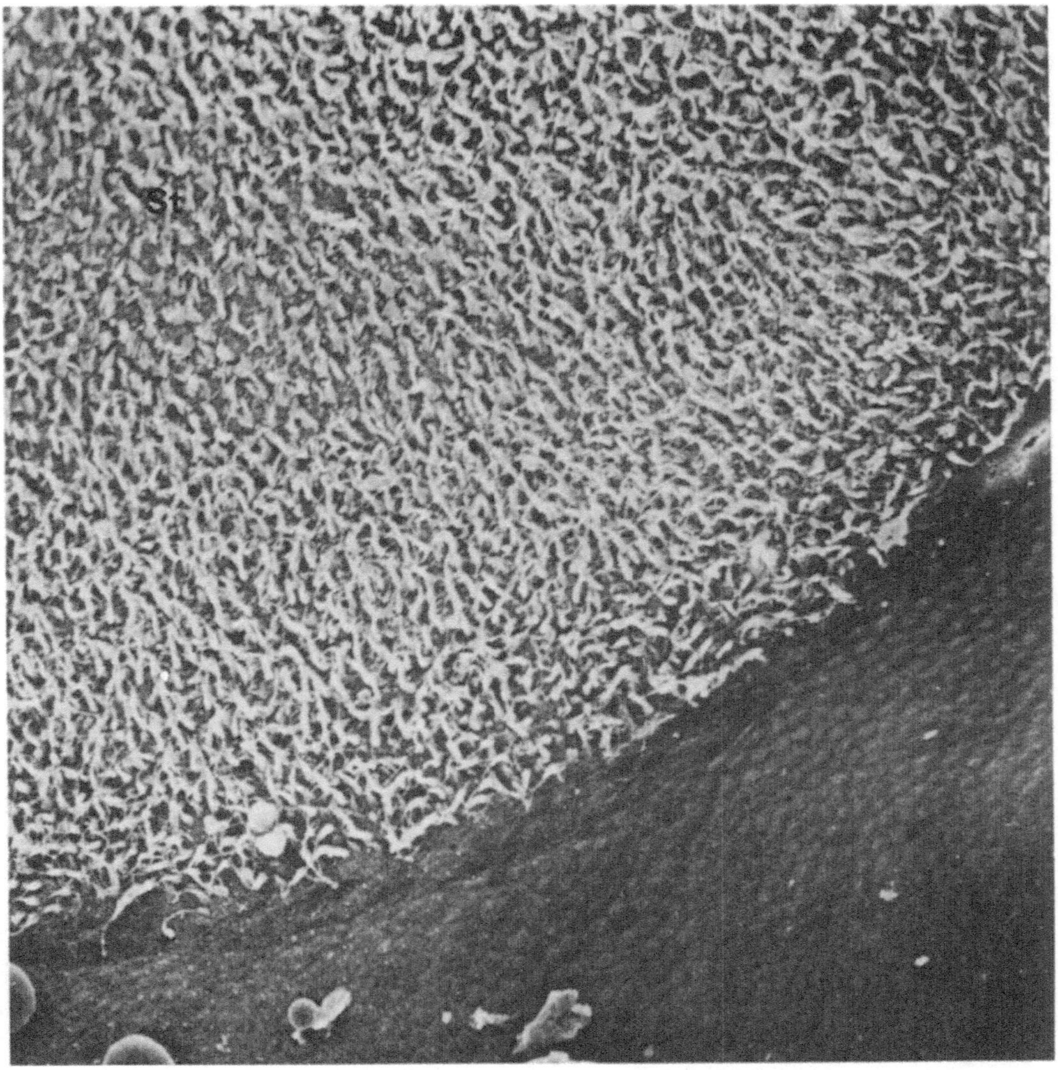

Figure 54 Sensory epithelium of utricular macula (rabbit). Sensory cilia are arranged as pointing towards the striola (St). In the striola, the sensory cells are less densely distributed than in other parts. (× 4200)

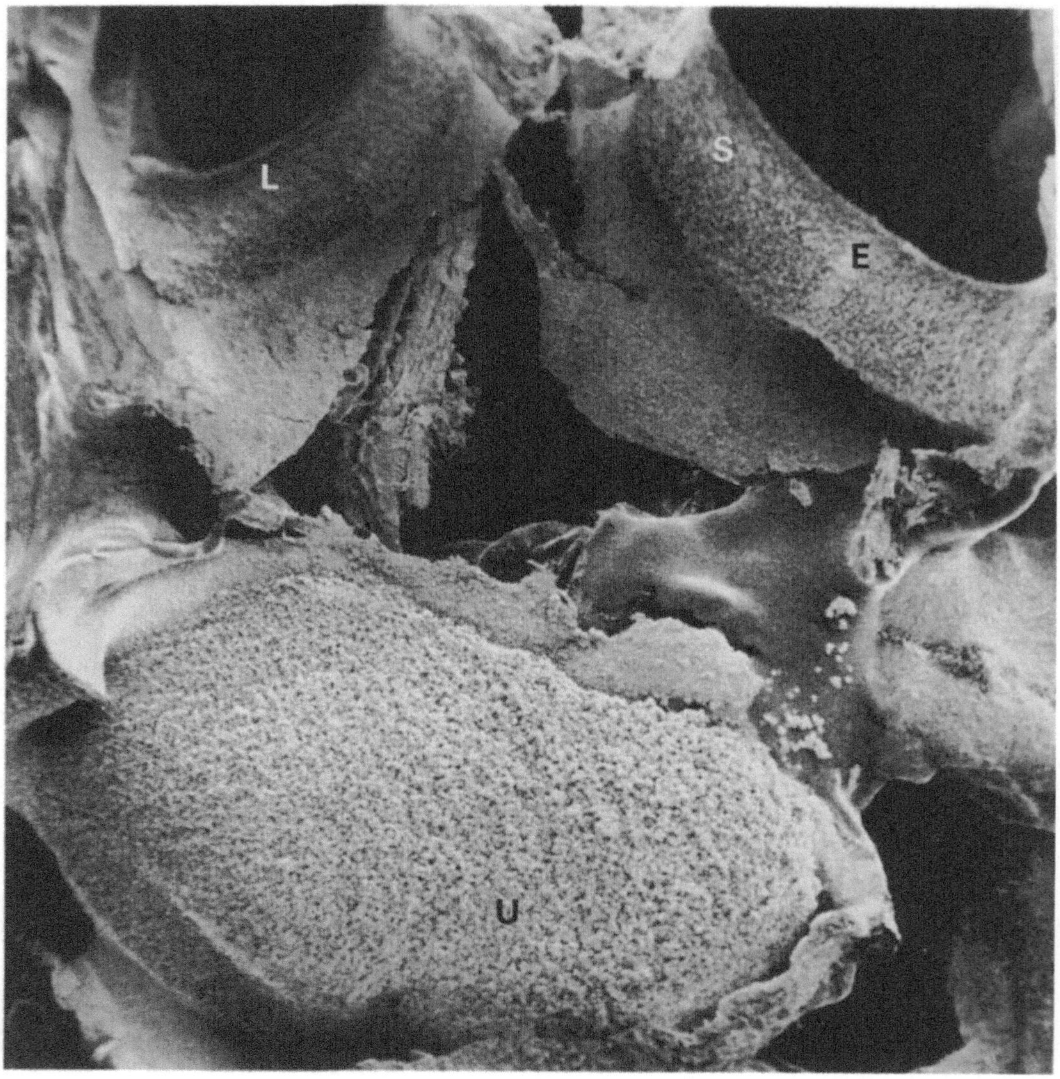

Figure 55 Utricular macula, cristae of the horizontal and anterior semicircular canal (dog). U: utricle; L: crista of the horizontal semicircular canal; S: crista of the anterior semicircular canal; E: eminentia cruciata. The ampulla of each semicircular canal opens into the utricle. The ampulla of the anterior semicircular canal is longer in diameter than that of the horizontal semicircular canal. E is the eminentia cruciata which appears as a narrow band in the centre of the anterior semicircular canal crista and has no sensory cilia (× 60)

a

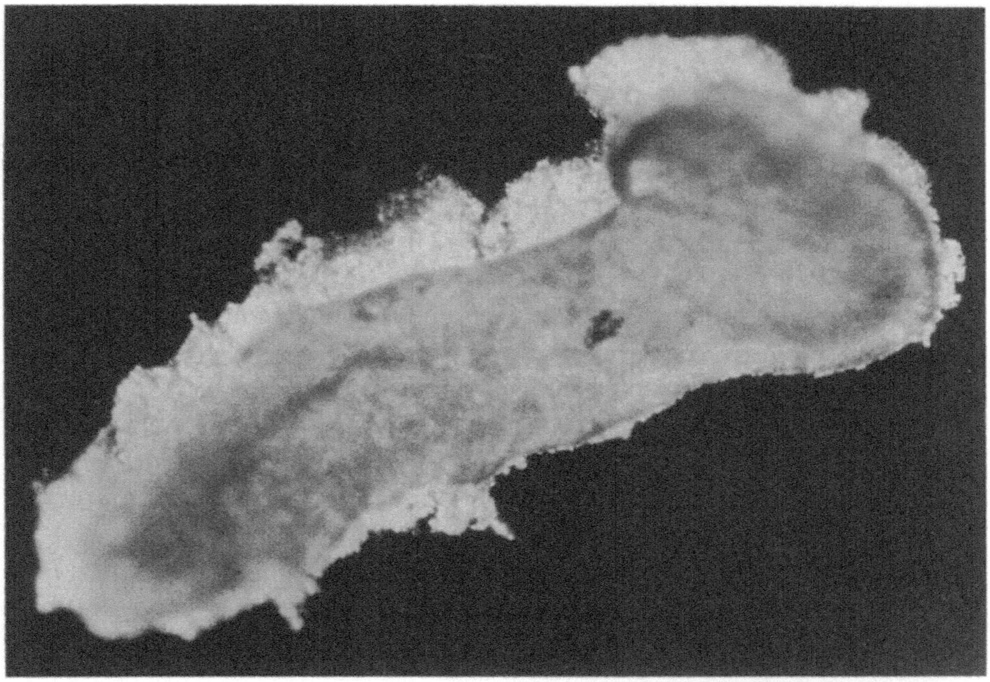

b

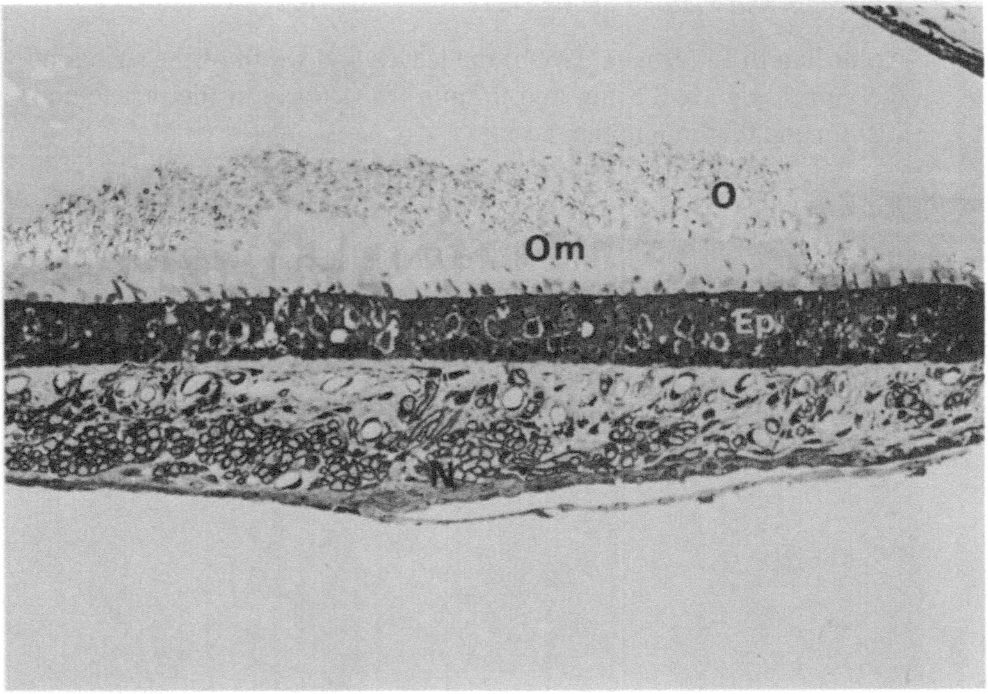

Figure 56 (**a**) Undersurface of the dissected saccular macula (guinea pig, light microscope) showing L-shape. (**b**) Sliced sections of the utricular macula (guinea pig, light microscope). In the striola, a big hole in the otolithic membrane is recognized. Otoconia are small in size in the striola portion. O: otolithic layer; Om: otolithic membrane; Ep: sensory epithelium; N: nerve

The striola

The striola was so named by Werner (1933), who found this as a linear portion on the utricular macula. In 1958, Engström and Wersäll reported that many type I cells were found in the striola and later the striola became interesting from both electrophysiological and histochemical stand points.

In the utricular macula the kinocilia of the sensory cells are located closer to the striola, while in the saccular macula kinocilia are closer to the lateral side. The striola has a high activity of succinic dehydrogenase (Suzuki, 1972) and among the structures of the macula is the first affected by ototoxic drugs (Lindeman, 1969a, Watanuki, 1972).

In the striola, the otolithic layer of the utricle is thinnest, and that of the saccule is the thickest (Watanuki, 1971).

The length and width of the striola

According to Lindeman (1969b) the length and width of the striola of the guinea pig are 2.6 mm and 0.2 mm respectively in the utricle and 2.0 mm and 0.15 mm in the saccule.

References

1. Lindeman, H. H. (1969a). Regional difference in sensitivity of the vestibular sensory epithelia to ototoxic antibotics. *Acta Otolaryngol.* (*Stockholm*), **67,** 177
2. Lindeman, H. H. (1969b). Regional differences in structure of the vestibular sensory regions. *J. Laryngol.* **83,** 1
3. Werner, C. F. (1933). Die Differenzierung der Maculae im Labyrinth insbesondere bei Säugetieren. *Z. Anat. Entwicklungsgesch.*, **99,** 696

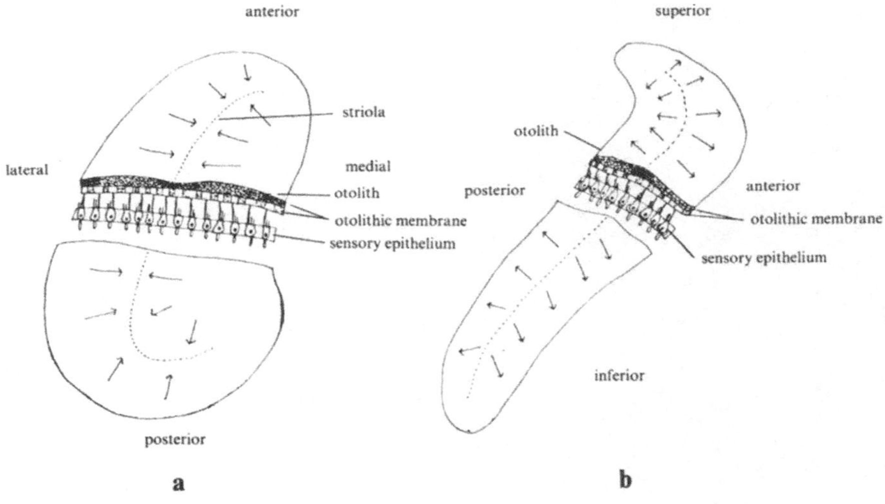

Figure 57 Schema of the utricular and saccular maculae (guinea pig). Dotted line is the striola. Arrows indicate the polarity. (**a**) utricular macula; (**b**) saccular macula

The sensory area of the macula

According to Watanuki (1976), the surface areas of the utricular and saccular maculae are $3.57\,mm^2$ and $2.20\,mm^2$ respectively. Rosenhall (1972) measured these areas as $4.29\,mm^2$ and $2.24\,mm^2$.

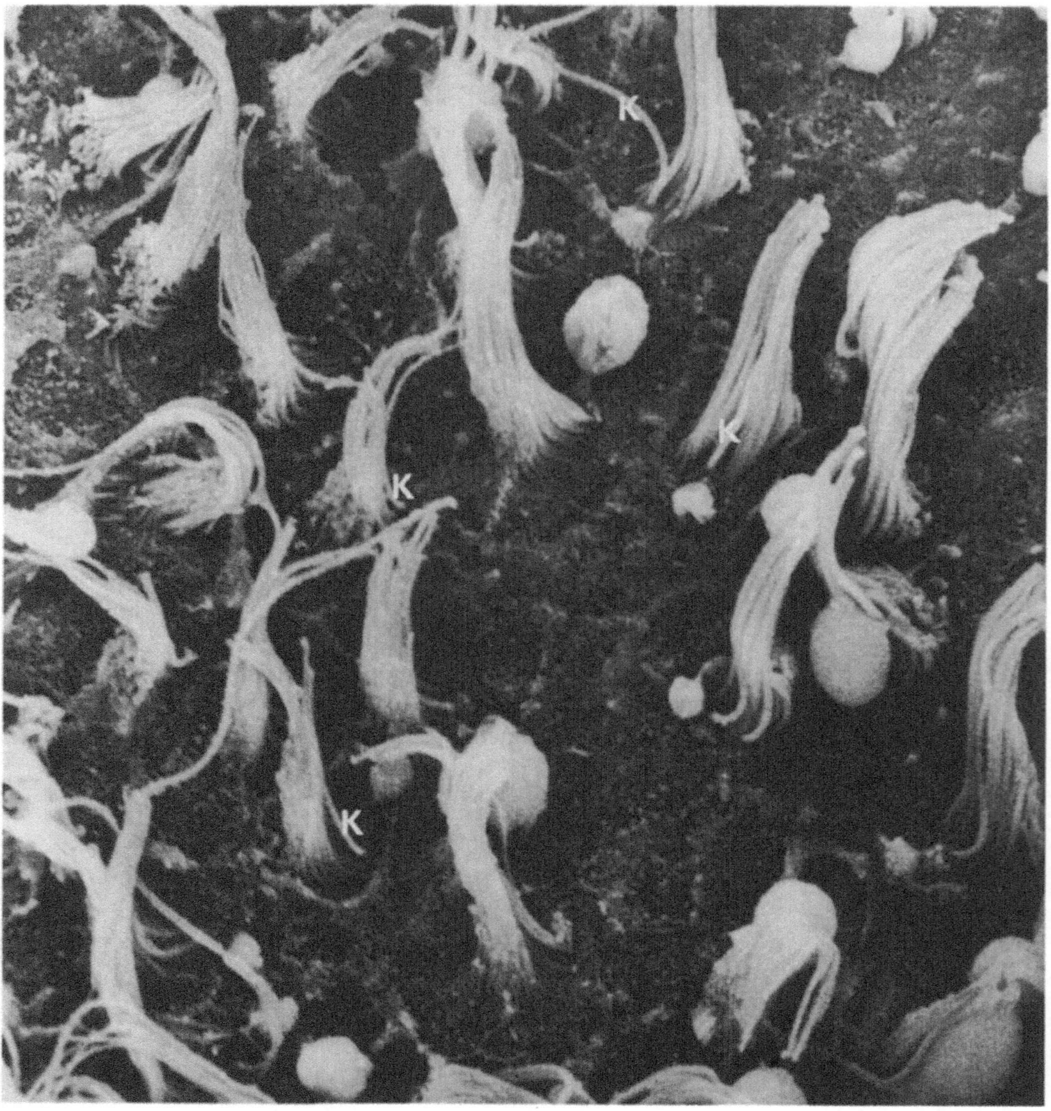

Figure 58 Striola of the utricle (kite). Kinocilia are facing each other on both sides of the striola (× 4500)

a

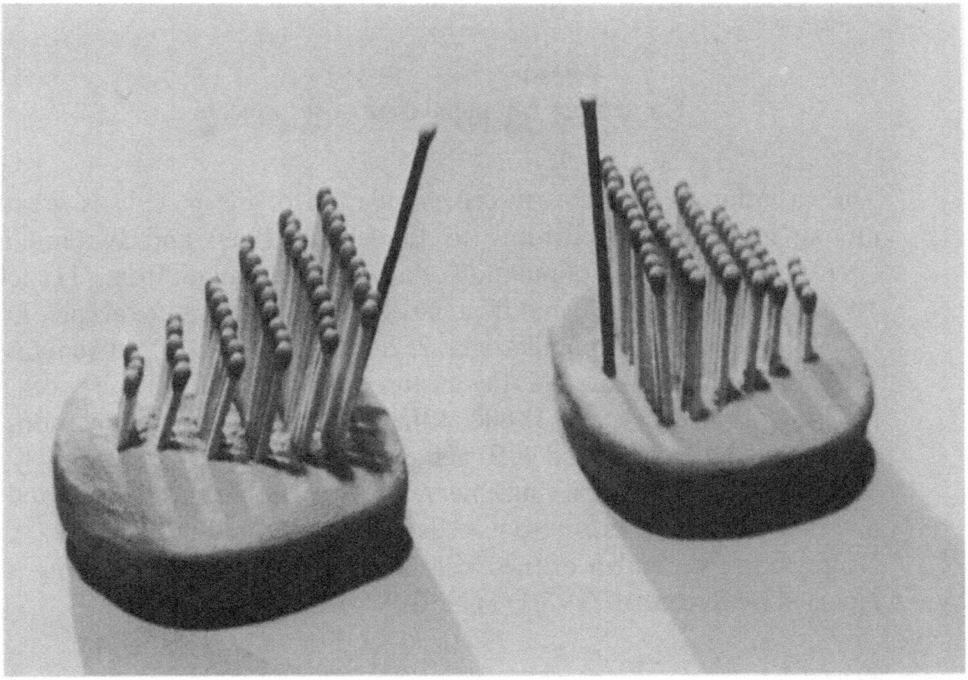

b

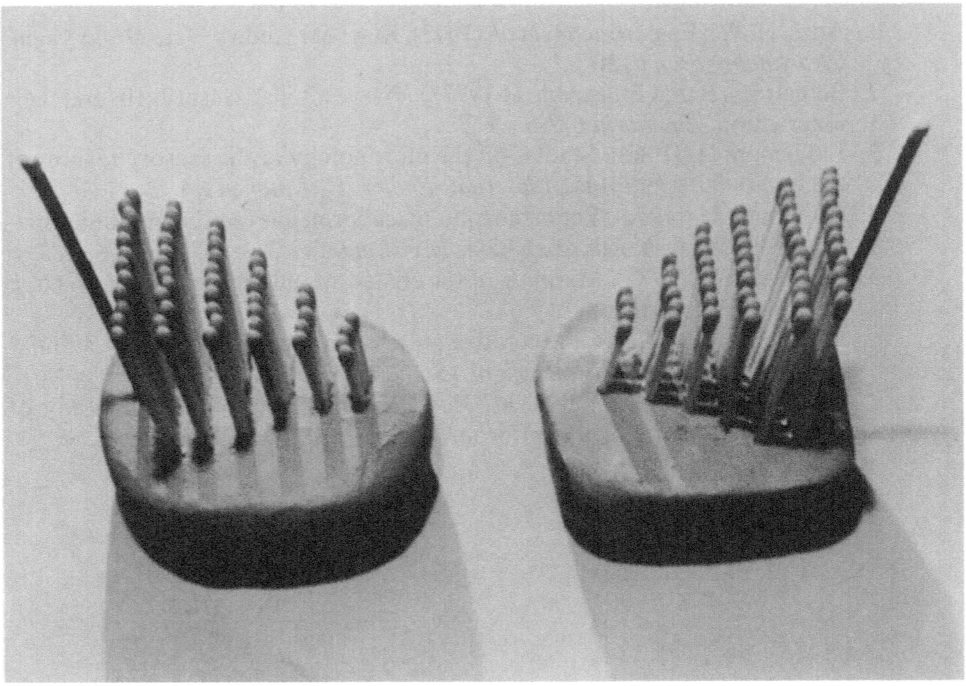

Figure 59 (**a**) A model of the utricular sensory cilia. The black stick indicates a kinocilium and the others stereocilia. The striola is a portion between the two kinocilia facing each other, (**b**) a model of the saccular sensory cilia. The striola lines between the two groups of the stereocilia

The sensory cell population of the macula

The variation in the sensory cell population of the macula is great among individuals. According to Lindeman (1969) and Watanuki (1970), the sensory cell population of a guinea pig ranges from 7118 to 10 760 cells in the utricle and from 6018 to 7983 cells in the saccule. In the pigeon's utricle the population is 2520 (Rosenhall, 1970). In humans between 20 and 40 years old, the mean population of the sensory cells is 33 100 in the utricle and 18 800 in the saccule, and these populations are innervated by 5952 and 4050 nerve fibres respectively (Ades, 1973). Therefore, in the utricle a single nerve fibre reaches five to six cells and in the saccule it reaches four to six cells (Bergström and Engström, 1973). Decrease in the number of these cells and nerve fibres due to ageing is reported by Rosenhall (1973) (Table 3).

References

1. Ades, H. W., Engström, H. *et al.* (1973). Inner ear studies. *Acta Otolaryngol. (Stockholm) Suppl.*, **30**
2. Bergström, B.and Engström, H. (1973). The vestibular sensory cells and their innervation. *Equilibrium Res.*, **3,** 27
3. Lindeman, H. (1969). Studies on the morphology of the sensory regions of the vestibular apparatus. *Adv. Anat. Embry. Cell Biol.*, **42,** 1
4. Rosenhall, U. (1970). Some morphological principles of the vestibular macula in birds. *Arch. Klin. Exp. Ohr. Nas. Kehlk. Heilk.*, **197,** 154
5. Rosenhall, U. (1972). Mapping of the cristae ampullares in man. *Ann. Otol. Rhinol. Laryngol.*, **81,** 882
6. Rosenhall, U. (1973). Degenerative patterns in the aging human vestibular neuro-epithelia. *Acta Otolaryngol. (Stockholm)*, **76,** 208
7. Watanuki, K. and Schuknecht, H. F. (1976). A morphological study of human vestibular sensory epithelia. *Arch. Otolaryngol.*, **102,** 583

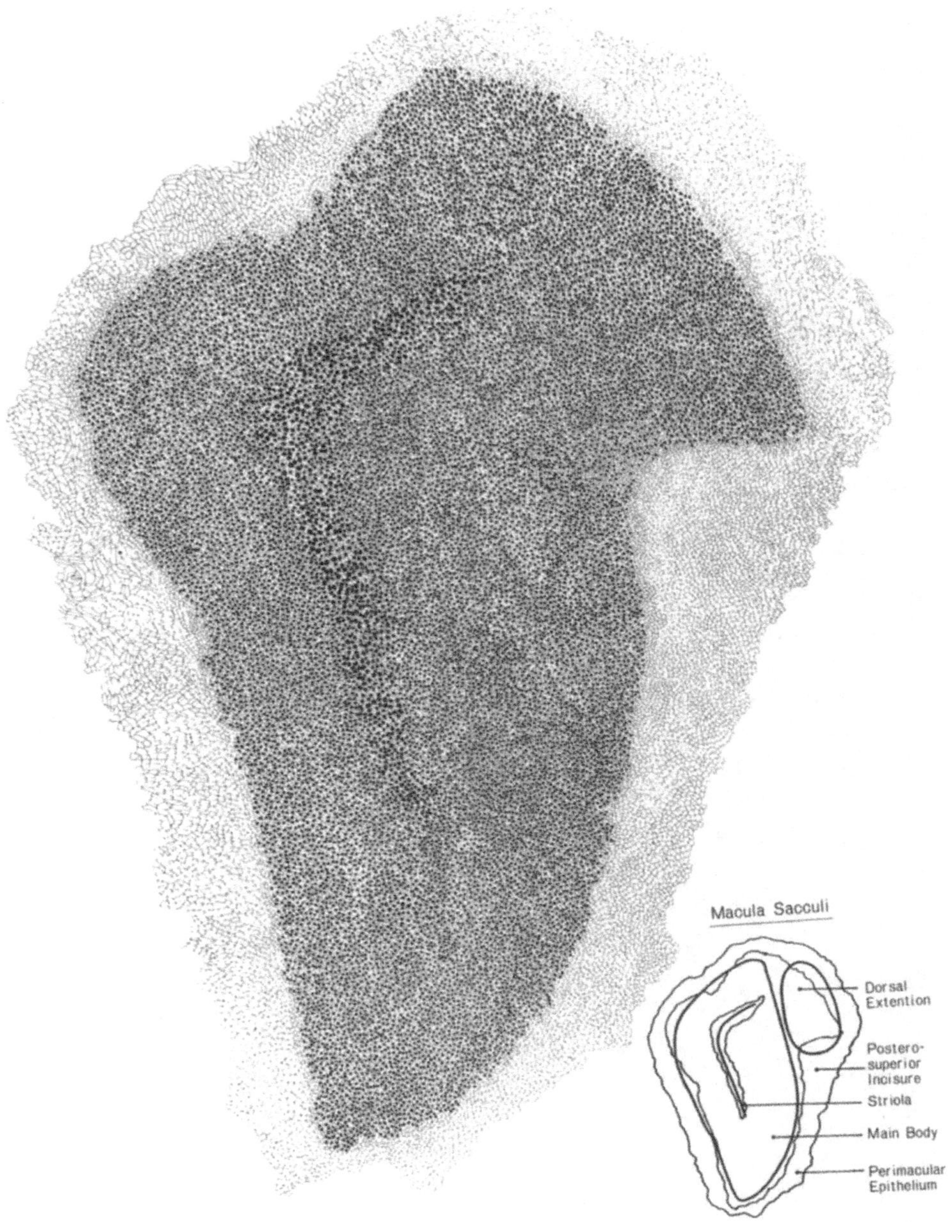

Figure 60 Graphic reconstruction of the right saccular macula from a 45-year-old man. The total number of sensory cells is 16933. (Courtesy Kozo Watanuki)

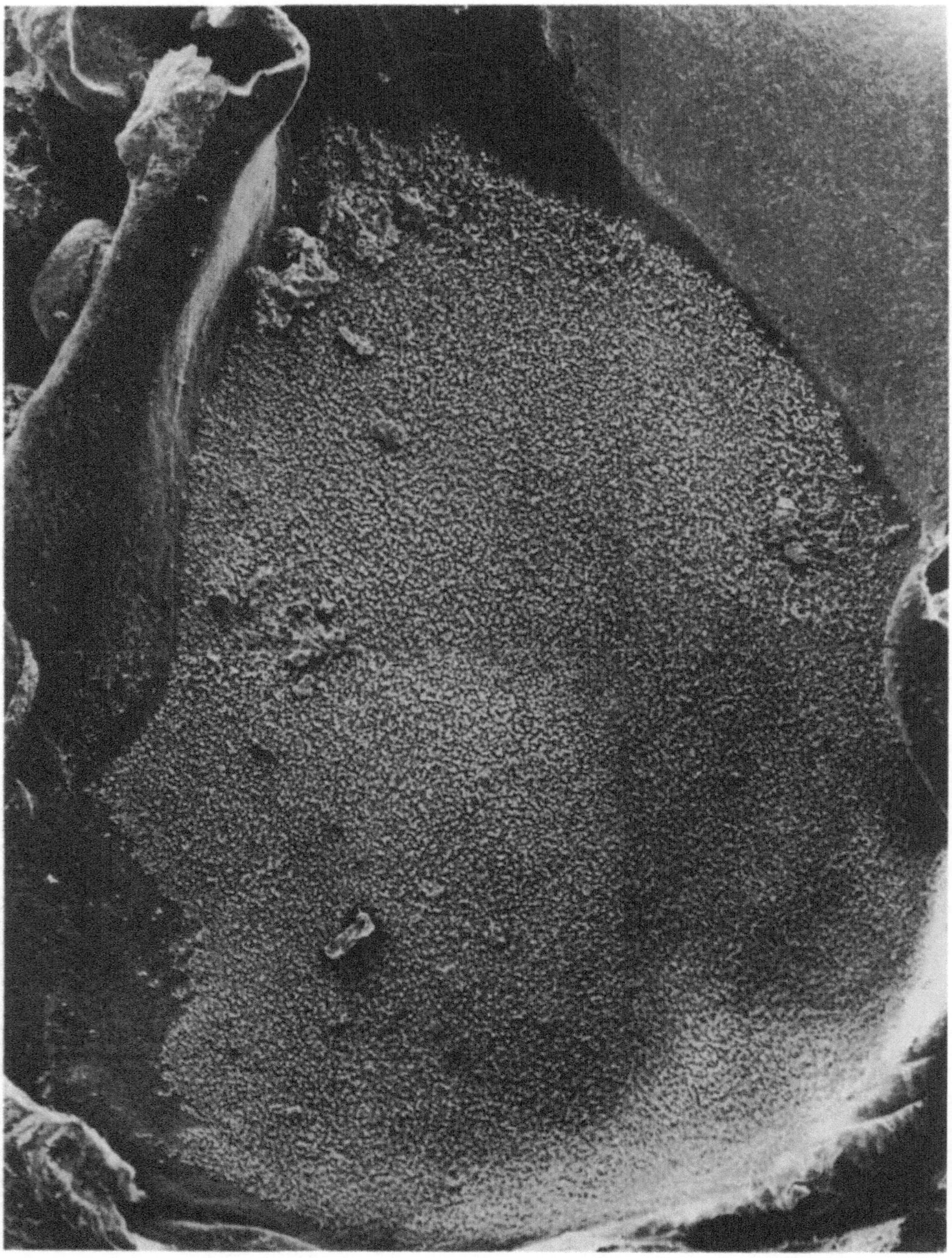

Figure 61 The surface of the left utricular macula (human) (× 95)

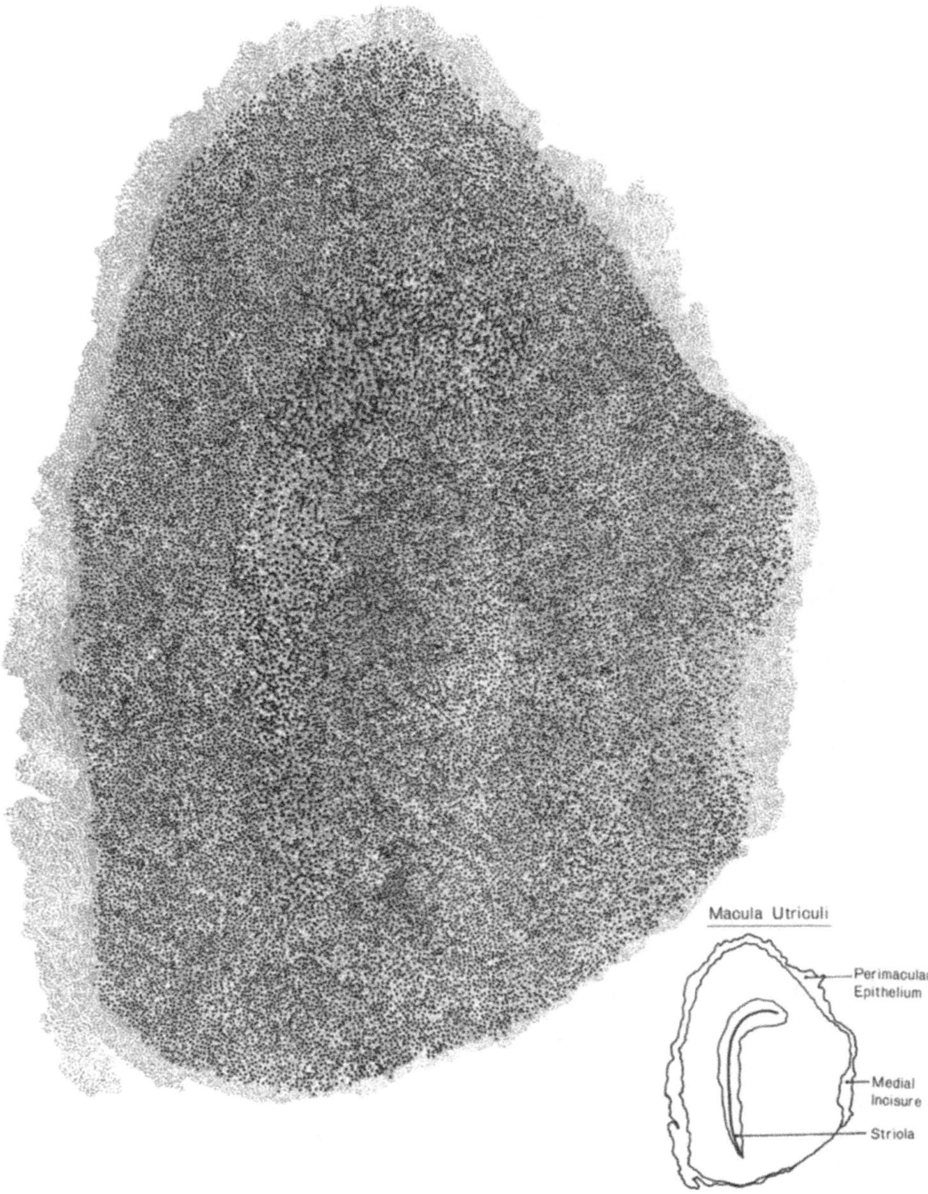

Figure 62 Graphic reconstruction of the right utricular macula (67-year-old man, number of the sensory cells 30 800) (courtesy Dr Kozo Watanuki)

The semicircular canals

The crista of the semicircular canal is a receptor of rotatory movement, which enables its perception in any plane of rotation. Three semicircular canals, horizontal, anterior and posterior, open into the utricle.

The anterior and posterior canals, which are also called vertical semicircular canals, respond to rotation in the vertical planes while the horizontal canal responds to rotation in the horizontal plane. Jellyfish and shellfish have only maculae, but the lamprey has two semicircular canals, anterior and posterior (de Burlet, 1934; Hoshino, 1975). Therefore, genetically anterior and posterior canals seem to be older than the horizontal canal.

References

1. de Burlet, H. M. (1934). Vergleichende Anatomie des statoacustischen Organs. In Bolk *et al.* (eds.) *Handbuch der vergleichenden Anatomie der Wirbeltiere.* Vol II, p. 1293. (Munich: Urban & Schwarzenberg)
2. Harada, Y. (1974). The shape of the vertical canal crista in various animals. *Equilibrium Res.*, **33,** 82
3. Hoshino, T. (1975). An electron microscopic study of the otolithic maculae of the lamprey (*Entosphenus japonicus*). *Acta Otolaryngol.* (*Stockholm*), **80,** 43

The function of the semicircular canals

The three semicircular canals lie at 90 degree angles to each other. The crista of each semicircular canal is stimulated by rotatory movement in its own plane. This enables perception of rotatory movement in any plane. These canals also respond to non-natural stimuli, such as cold or warm water applied in the ear canal, or electrical stimulation to the vestibule.

Study on the semicircular canals was initiated by Purkinje (1825) who reported vertigo and nystagmus induced by rotation. Flourens (1842) found disturbances of the postural maintenance and motor function in a pigeon after making a lesion to the semicircular canal. In 1860, Ménière demonstrated a lesion in the labyrinth of a patient with hearing loss and vertigo. Goltz (1870) first pointed out a close relationship between vestibular function and body balance. After these studies, vestibular research drew the attention of many researchers.

Electrophysiological study has revealed that, in the horizontal canal, ampullopetal flow of the endolymphatic fluid increases nerve discharge, while in the vertical canals it is increased by ampullofugal flow. This conclusion is based on Ewald's work (1892). He reported that when a semicircular canal is stimulated by a pneumatic hammer, the movement of a pigeon's head and eyes is specific to the plane of the stimulated canal. Further, he stated that in the horizontal canal, ampullopetal flow, which is directed toward the utricle, produced an excitatory effect, while ampullofugal flow produced an inhibitory effect. This relation was reversed in the vertical canals. Today, this is well known as Ewald's law. Later, in 1903, Bárány found a response of the semicircular canals to thermal change, which serves as an important vestibular function test (caloric test).

Ewald's law was electrophysiologically confirmed by the author (Harada, 1967, 1971, 1973, 1974). Endolymphatic flow was experimentally produced in a frog's semicircular canal and it was observed that the movement of the cupula produced an excitatory or inhibitory effect on nerve discharge.

References

1. Harada, Y. (1973). The scanning electron microscopic observation of the vestibular organ and electrical activity of isolated individual semicircular ampullae. *Adv. Oto. Rhino. Laryngol.* **19,** 49
2. Harada, Y. and Musso, E. (1971). Study of the action potential in the isolated posterior ampullar receptor. *Acta Otolaryngol.* (*Stockholm*), **72,** 274
3. Harada, Y., Musso, E. and Mira, E. (1967). Action of streptomycin, dihydrostreptomycin neomycin and kanamycin on the ampullar receptors of the frog. *Acta Otolaryngol.* (*Stockholm*), **64,** 372

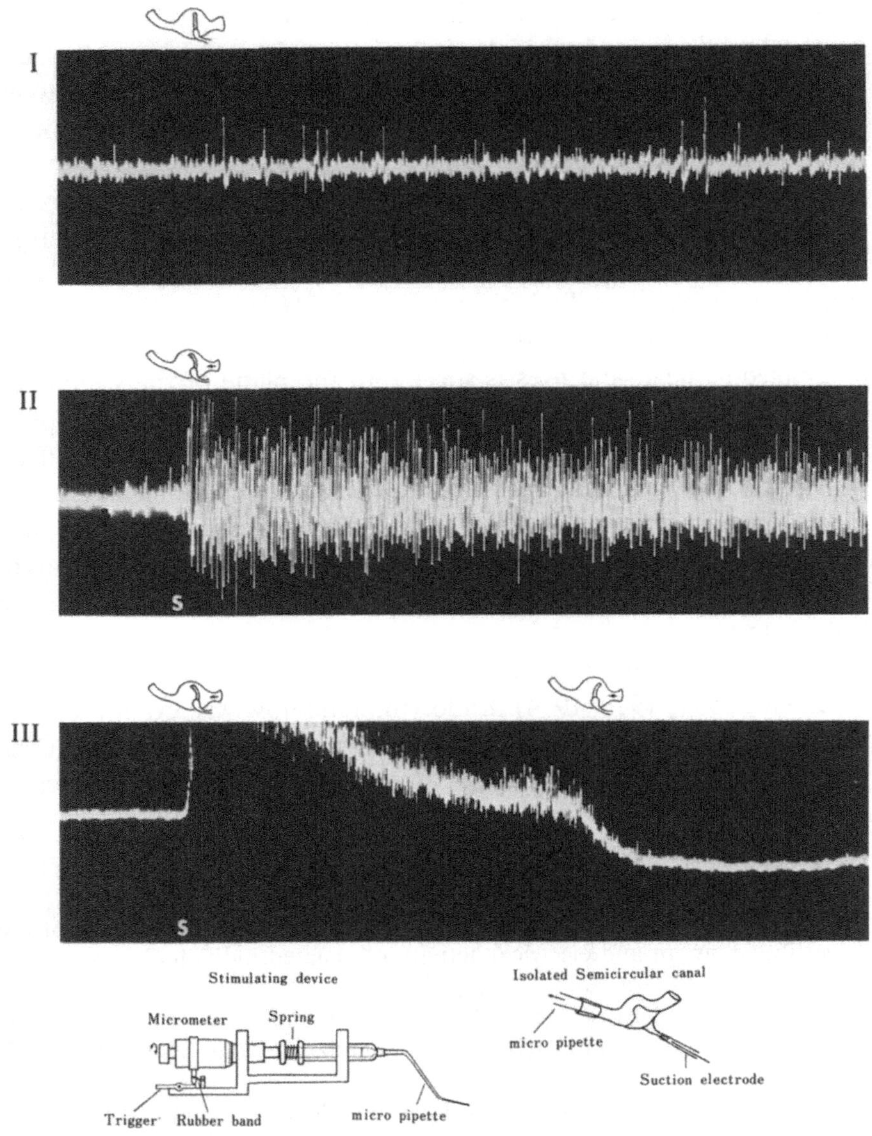

Figure 63 Action potential from the isolated semicircular canal of the frog. I: spontaneous discharge from the posterior semicircular canal, II: AC-amplified responses of the posterior semicircular canal evoked by ampullofugal stimulus, III: DC-amplified response of the posterior semicircular canal evoked by ampullofugal stimulus. Ampullofugal current evokes a positive slow potential with short rise time. A marked increase in discharge was also observed during the period of this potential. Ampullopetal current evokes a negative slow potential with a decrease in the spontaneous discharge

The polarity of the vestibular organs

The polarity of the otolithic organs and semicircular canals is already described. Here, these are schematically represented in Figures 60 and 61. It is found that depolarization takes place when the stereocilia lean towards the kinocilium.

References

1. Harada, Y. (1973). Structure and function of the vestibular sensory organs. *Otologia* (*Fukuoka*), **19,** 855
2. Lindeman, H.H. (1969). Regional differences in structure of the vestibular sensory regions. *J. Laryngol.*, **83,** 1

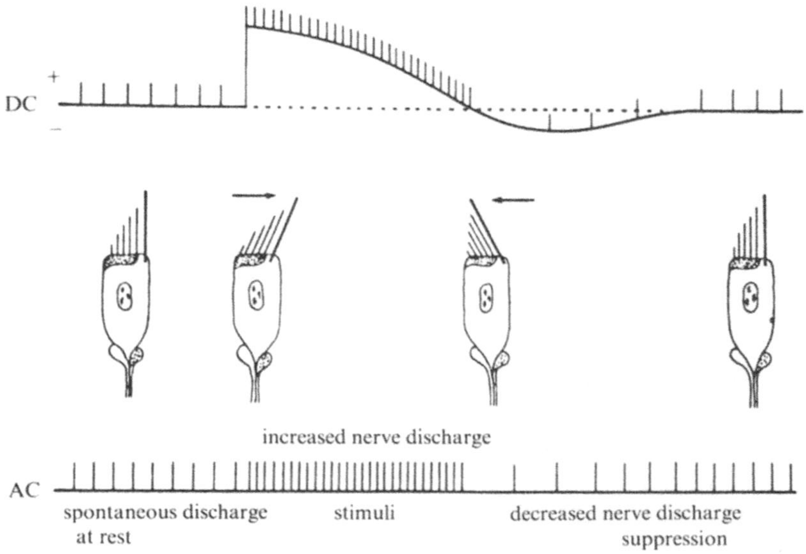

Figure 64 The mechanism of the depolarization and hyperpolarization in the semicircular canal receptor of the frog. Depolarization is observed when the endolymphatic flow shifts the stereocilia toward the kinocilium, thus increasing the discharge (excitation). The endolymphatic flow in the opposite direction evokes hyperpolarization and a decrease in the discharge (inhibition). Ampullopetal flow depolarizes the horizontal semicircular canal receptor, while ampullofugal flow depolarizes anterior and posterior canal receptors

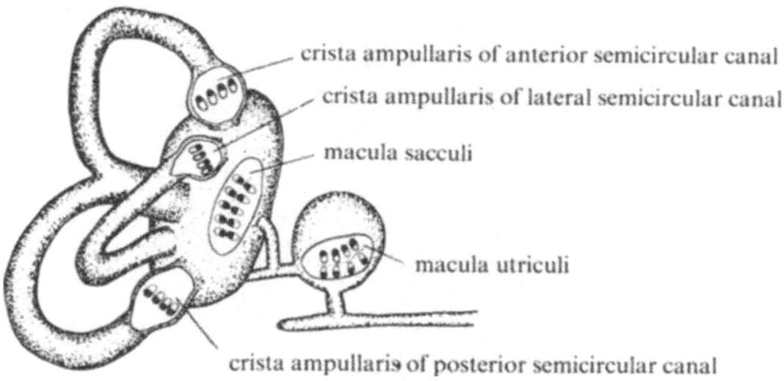

Figure 65 Polarity of the vestibular sensory organ. Black dots: the position of the kinocilium; dotted line: striola

The cupula

The cupula is gelatin-like substance with a fine tubular structure of diameter about 3–5 μm in the lateral face and with innumerable holes on top. This tubular structure was found to taper slightly toward the top (Harada, 1972; Lim, 1971). According to Igarashi *et al.* (1969) it contains mucopolysaccharide.

Morphological evaluation of the cupula is difficult because the gelatinous substance which forms the cupula frequently shrinks during the process of preparation (i.e. fixation and dehydration). The cupula is shaped like a cap and encapsulates the sensory epithelia.

The function of the cupula is to transmit the endolymphatic flow of the semicircular canal to the sensory hairs and to shift the sensory hairs in one direction.

In the human, monkey, guinea pig and rabbit, morphological features of the ampulla do not vary much between the horizontal and vertical semicircular canals. However, in birds, the eminentia cruciata in the ampulla of the vertical canal divides the sensory epithelia. Also the cupula is divided in half in the middle of the crista (Harada, 1972, 1974).

References

1. Harada, Y. (1972). Surface structure of semicircular ampullae. *Equilibrium Res. Suppl.* **4,** 53
2. Harada, Y. (1974). The shape of the vertical canal crista in various animals. *Equilibrium Res.*, **33,** 82
3. Igarashi, M. and Alford, B. R. (1969). Cupula, cupular zone of otolith membrane and tectorial membrane in the squirrel monkey. *Acta Otolaryngol.* (*Stockholm*), **68,** 420
4. Lim, D. J. (1971). Vestibular sensory organs. *Arch. Otolaryngol.*, **94,** 69

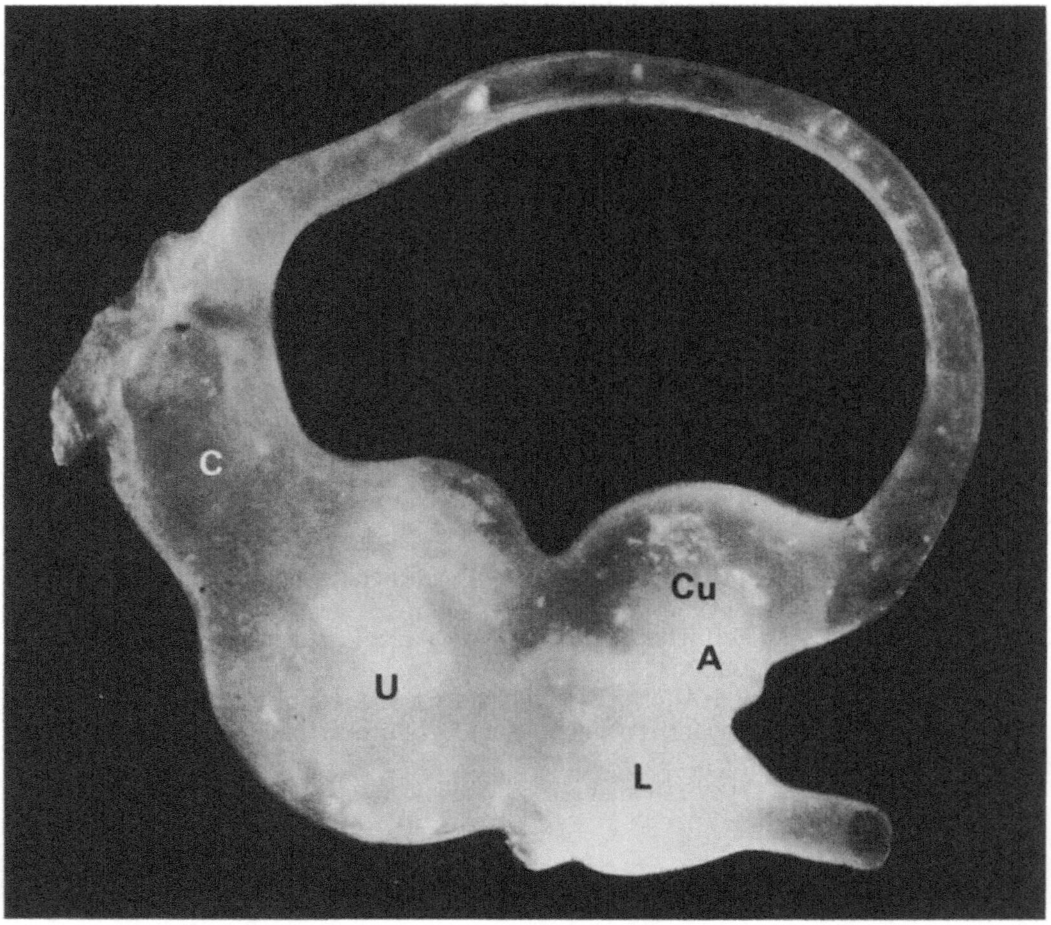

Figure 66 The utricle and the ampulla of the anterior and lateral semicircular canal (human). U: utricle; L: ampulla of the lateral semicircular canal; A: ampulla of the anterior semicircular canal; C: crus commune; C: cupula (× 30)

a

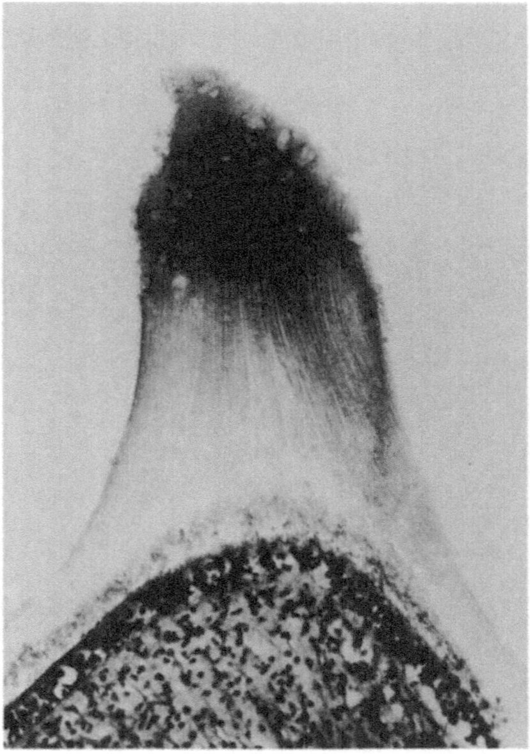

b

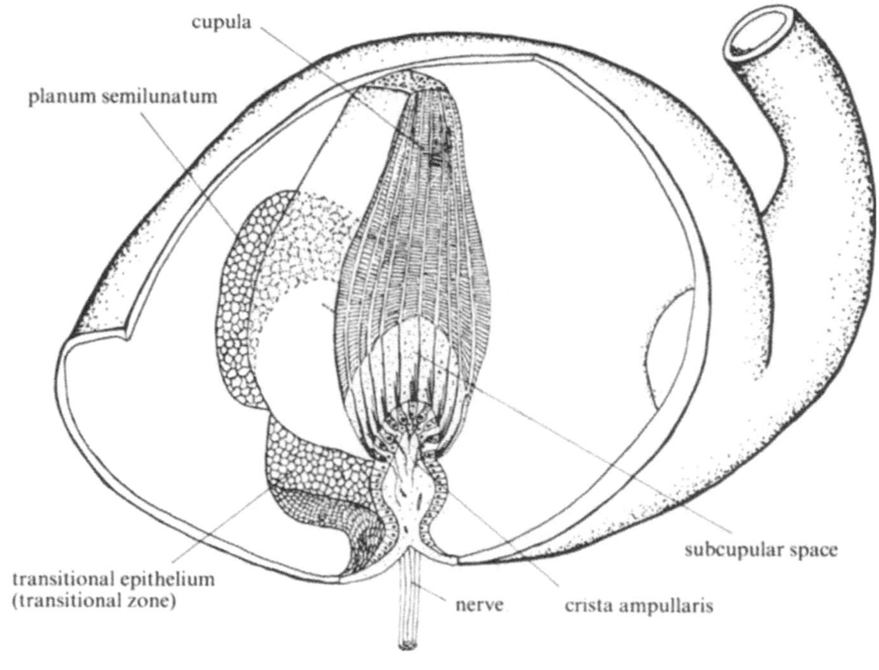

Figure 67 (**a**) Crista of the semicircular canal ampulla (human), (**b**) schema of the ampulla

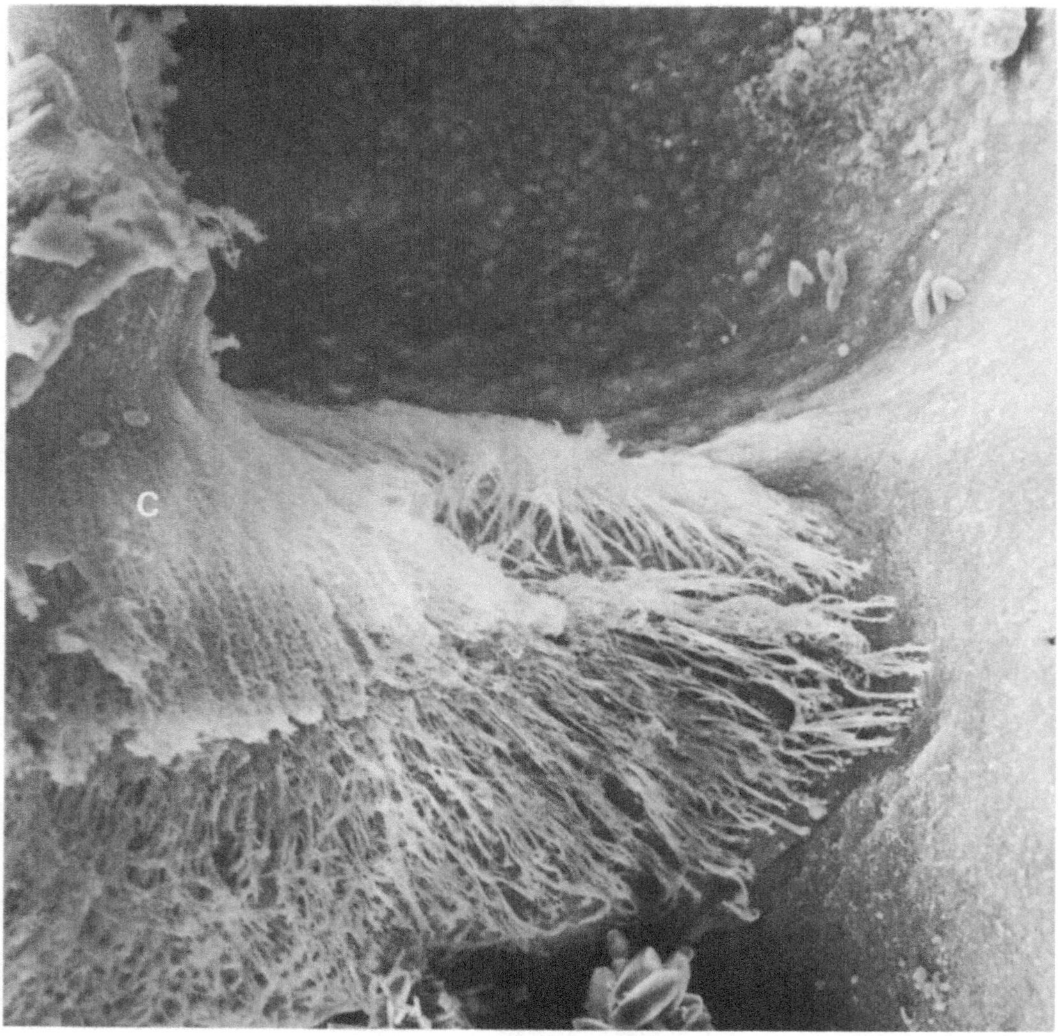

Figure 68 Cupula (lateral semicircular canal of the chicken). Cupula (C) is shrunken due to fixation and dehydration. Sensory cilia are leaning toward the cupula (C) (× 1500)

a

b

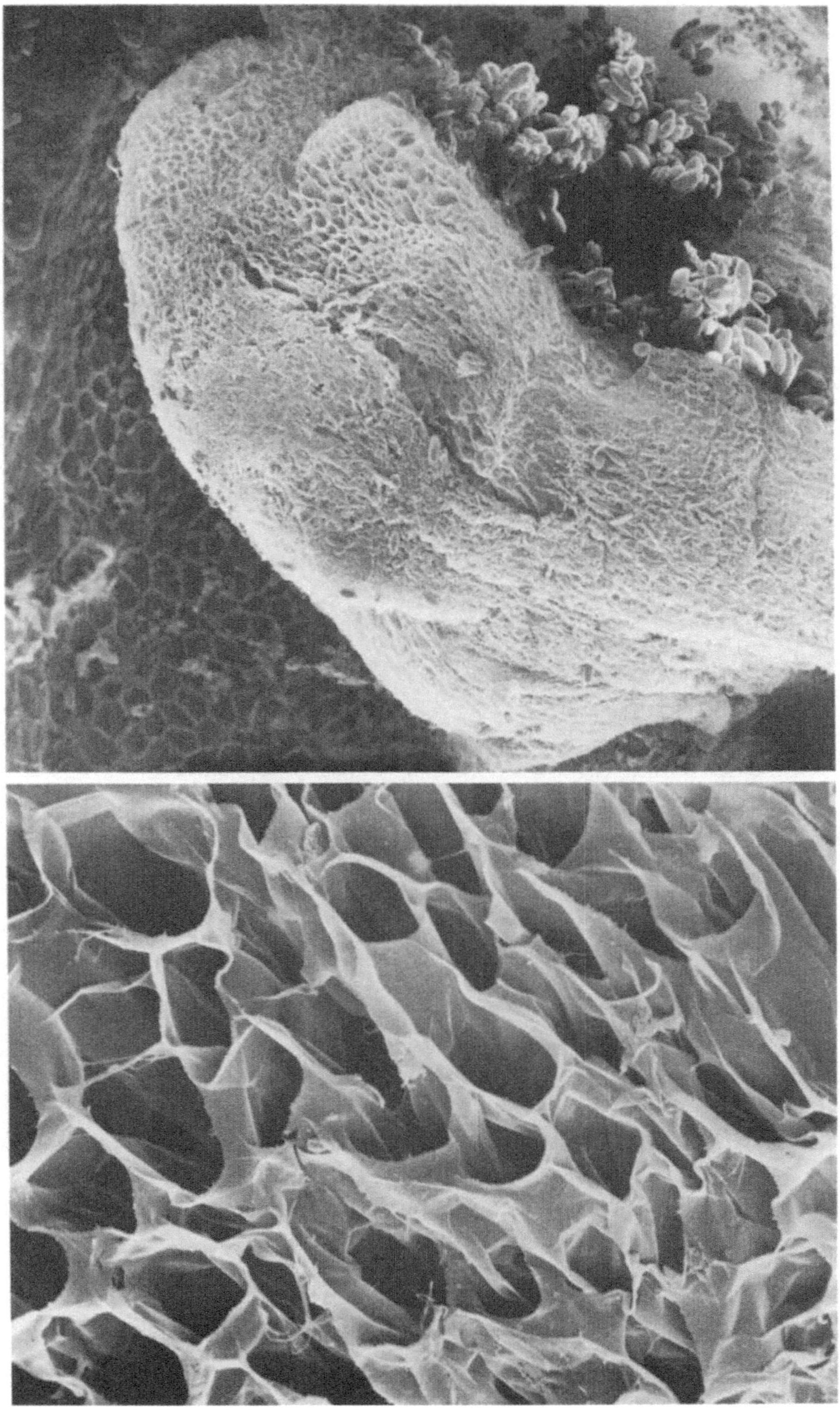

Figure 69 Cupula (pigeon). (**a**) The top surface of the cupula. Numerous holes are observed (× 400), (**b**) high magnification of (a) (× 3600)

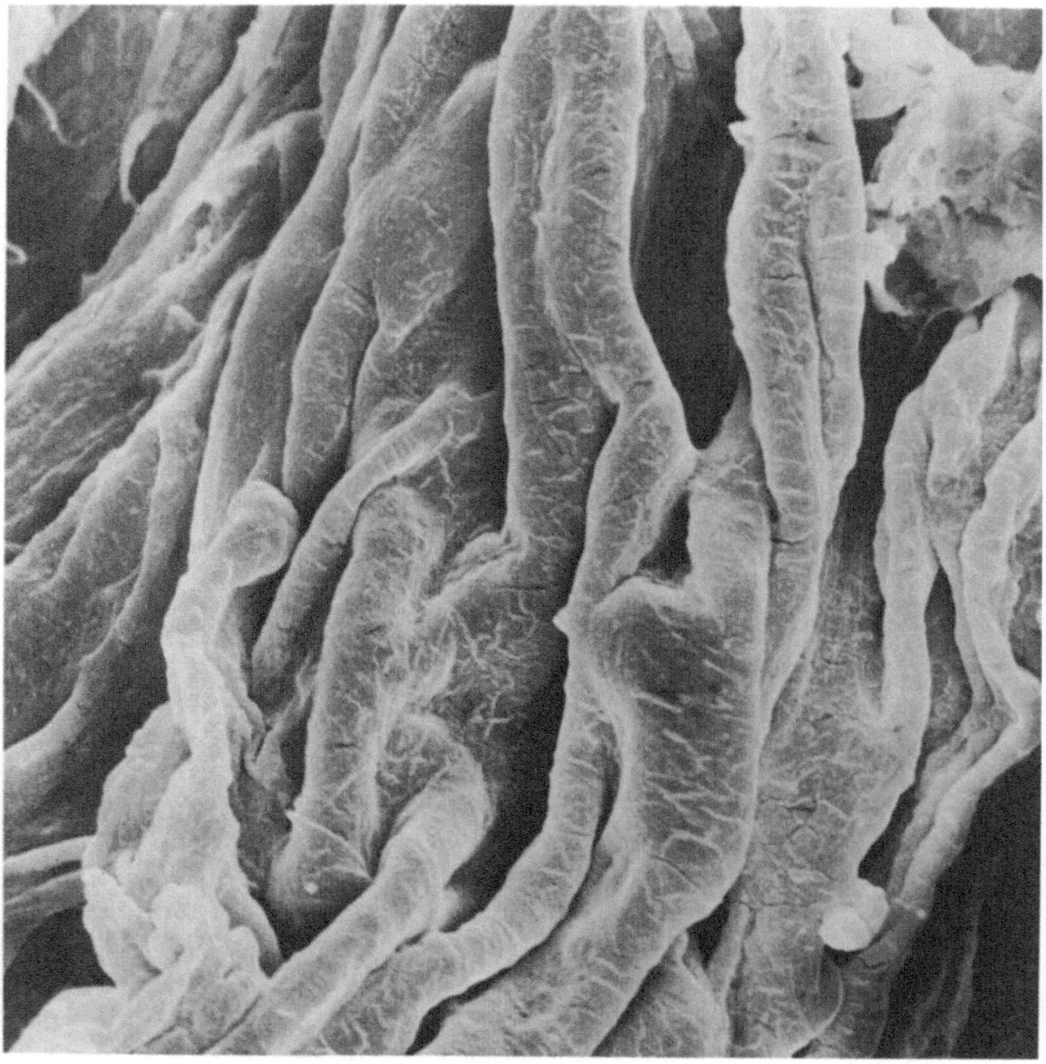

Figure 70 Cupula (pigeon). The side of the cupula, which shows a tubular structure (× 4200)

The sensory epithelium of the crista

The sensory cells of the crista are classified into hair cell type I and II (Wersäll, 1956). Hair cell type I is abundant in the central part of the crista, while hair cell type II is mainly seen in the circumferential part (Wersäll, 1956; Lindeman, 1969). Functional difference between type I and II cells is not yet clear, but it is known that the type II cell is old genetically and the type I cell is more developed (Wersäll, 1962) and is more vulnerable. The hair cells of either type have one kinocilium and many stereocilia. The stereocilia show a stair-like arrangement in a cell (Lim, 1969; Lim and Lane, 1969; Harada, 1971, 1972).

Being different from kinocilia, stereocilia have a cuticular plate and become narrow at the base. Stereocilia are smaller in diameter than kinocilia (Harada, 1972). The arrangement of the stereocilia is in five to eight steps, each with seven to eight cilia.

The kinocilium is located next to the longest stereocilia and determines the polarity of the cell (Lindeman, 1969; Flock and Wersäll, 1962). The importance of polarity is mentioned above. Also it is found that in the anterior and posterior semicircular canals, the kinocilium is located closer to the crus, while in the horizontal semicircular canal, it is located closer to the utricle (Wersäll, 1956; Flock and Wersäll, 1962; Harada, 1972).

In the sensory epithelium there are also supporting cells. The cells have a central cilium on the surface and secrete mucopolysaccharide. Mucopolysaccharide is probably enclosed in the granular substance frequently found on the sensory epithelium. The function of the granular substance is not yet clarified; however, it is assumed that it protects cilia by filling the interciliary space, or it takes part in supplying nutrition to the cupula.

References

1. Flock, Å. and Wersäll, J. (1962). A study of the orientation of the sensory hairs of the receptor cells in the lateral line organ of fish, with special reference to the function of the receptor. *J. Cell Biol.*, **15**, 19
2. Harada, Y. (1972). Surface structure of semicircular ampullae. *Equilibrium Res. Suppl.*, **4**, 53

3. Lim, D. J. (1969). Three-dimensional observation with the scanning electron microscope. *Acta Otolaryngol.* (*Stockholm*) *Suppl.*, **255,** 1
4. Lim, D. J. and Lane, W. C. (1969). Vestibular sensory epithelia. *Acta Otolaryngol.* (*Stockholm*), **90,** 283
5. Lindeman, H. H. (1969). Regional differences in structure of the vestibular sensory regions. *J. Laryngol.*, **83,** 1
6. Wersäll, J. (1956). Studies on the structure and innervation of the sensory epithelium of the cristae ampullares in the guinea pig as revealed by the electron microscope. *Acta Otolaryngol.* (*Stockholm*) *Suppl.*, **126,** 1

Figure 71 Sensory cilia of the semicircular canal crista (rabbit). K: kinocilium; S: stereocilia; arrow: polarity (× 10 000)

a

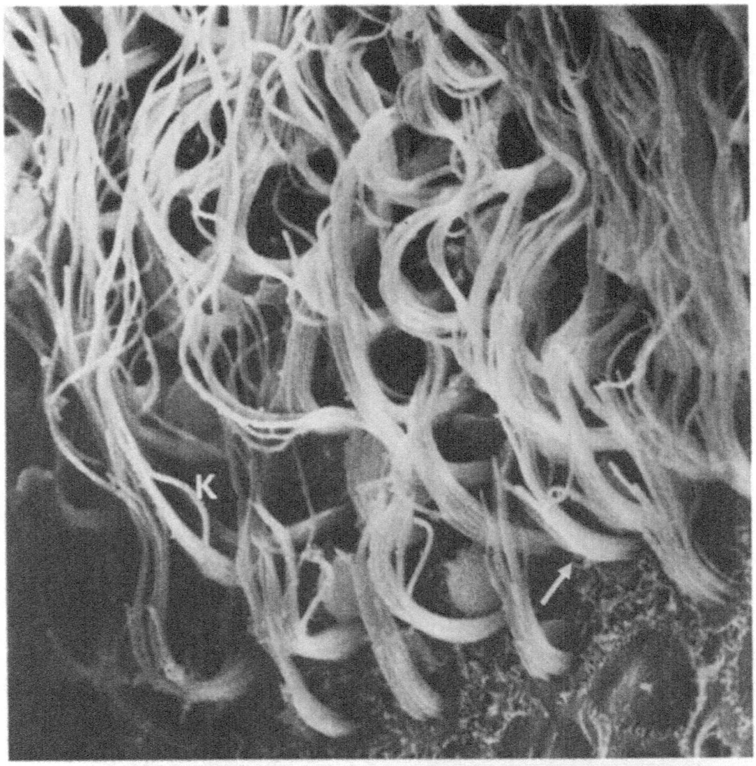

b

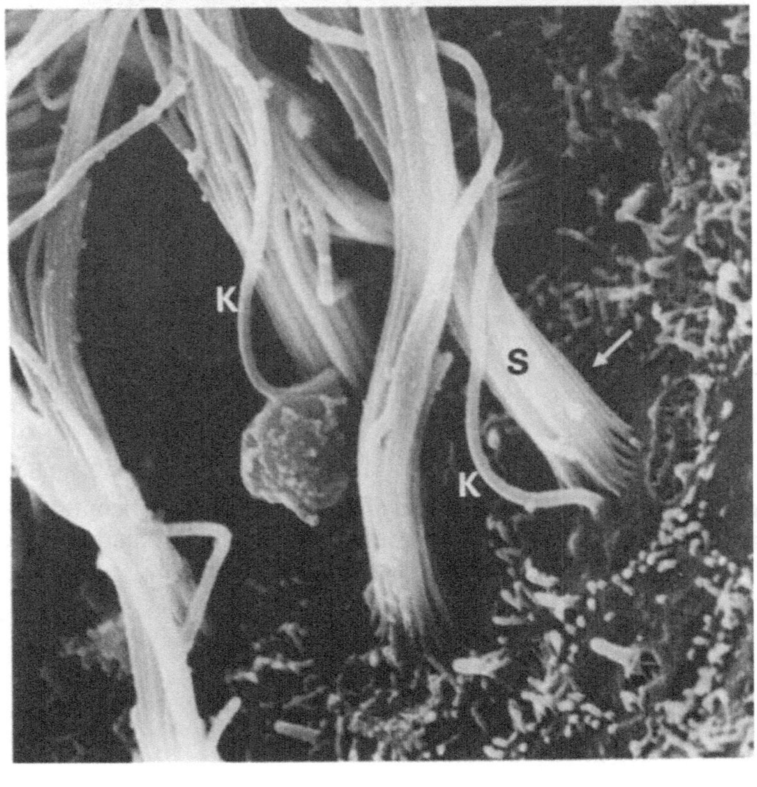

Figure 71

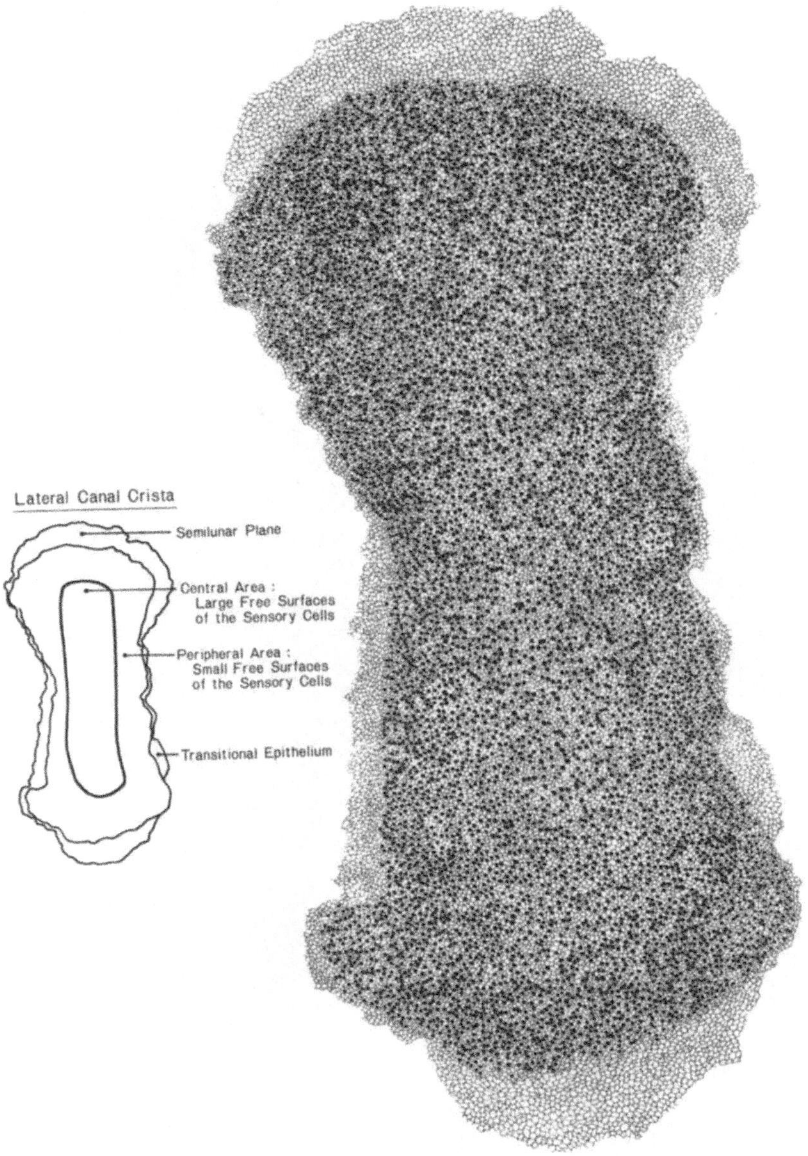

Figure 72 Graphic reconstruction of the surface of the horizontal semicircular canal crista (right side), removed from 42-year-old male. Number of the sensory cells: 6902 (courtesy Dr K. Watanuki)

The shape of the cristae ampullares

The crista ampullaris of the horizontal semicircular canal differs in shape from the cristae of the vertical canals in each species. The shape of the cristae, especially of the vertical canals, varies among the species. Some animals, such as cat, dog, mouse, bat, bird, tortoise and frog have a process called the eminentia cruciata in the vertical semicircular canal (Harada, 1974). This is most prominent in birds, which show a protrusion like a cross and have the cupula divided into two by the eminentia cruciata (Harada, 1972).

There seems to be a functional difference between animals with and without eminentia cruciata. Apparently animals with eminentia have better postural reflex to rotatory movement in the vertical plane.

References

1. Harada, Y. (1972). Surface structure of semicircular ampullae. *Equilibrium Res. Suppl.*, **4,** 53
2. Harada, Y. (1974). The shape of the vertical canal crista in various animals. *Equilibrium Res.*, **33,** 82
3. Igarashi, M. and Yoshinobu, T. (1969). Comparative observation of the eminentia cruciata in birds and mammals. *Anat. Rec.*, **155,** 269

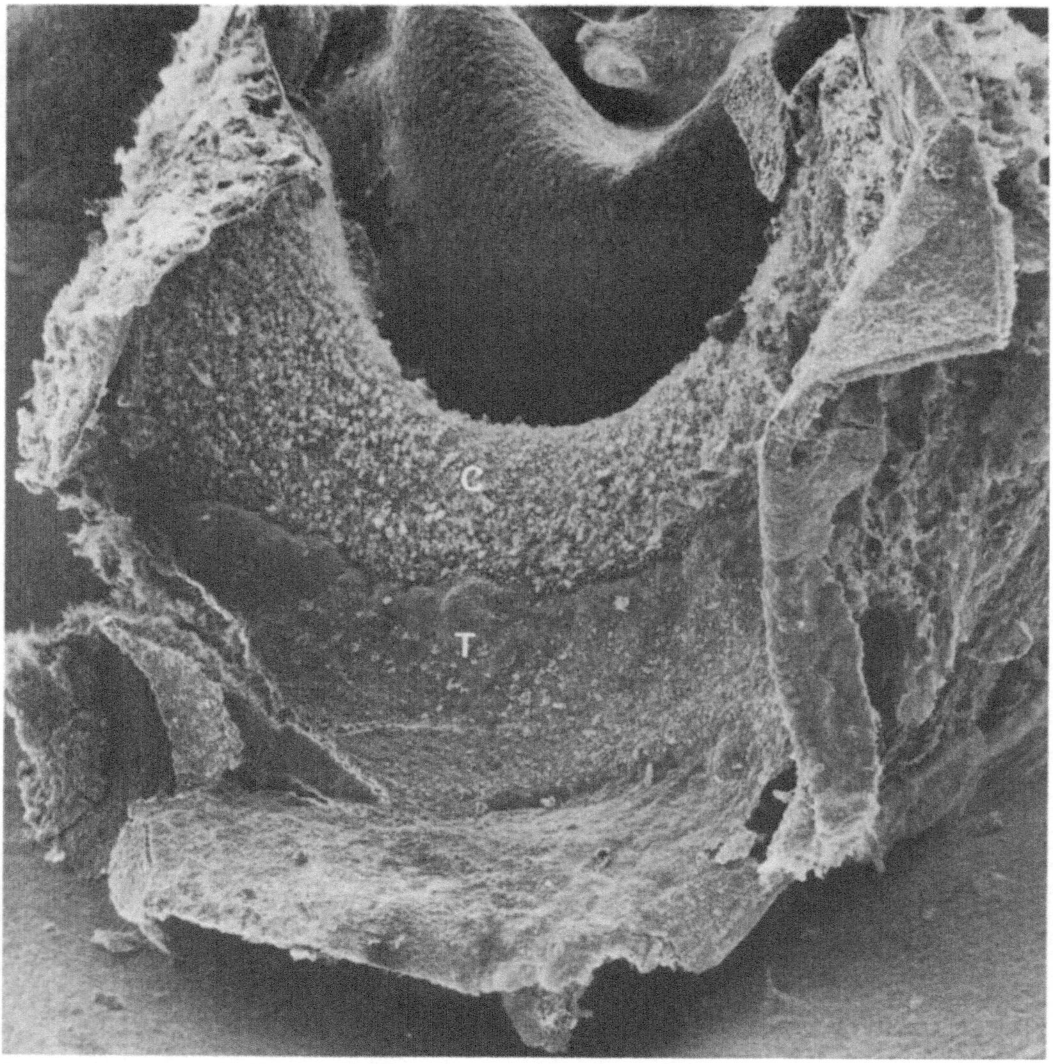

Figure 73 Ampulla of the horizontal semicircular canal (human). C: crista; T: transitional cell epithelium (× 100)

Animals without eminentia cruciata

In many animals of this category, such as the human, monkey, rabbit and guinea pig, the horizontal semicircular canal develops very well. However, a newt has a poorly-developed canal, although it lacks the eminentia cruciata.

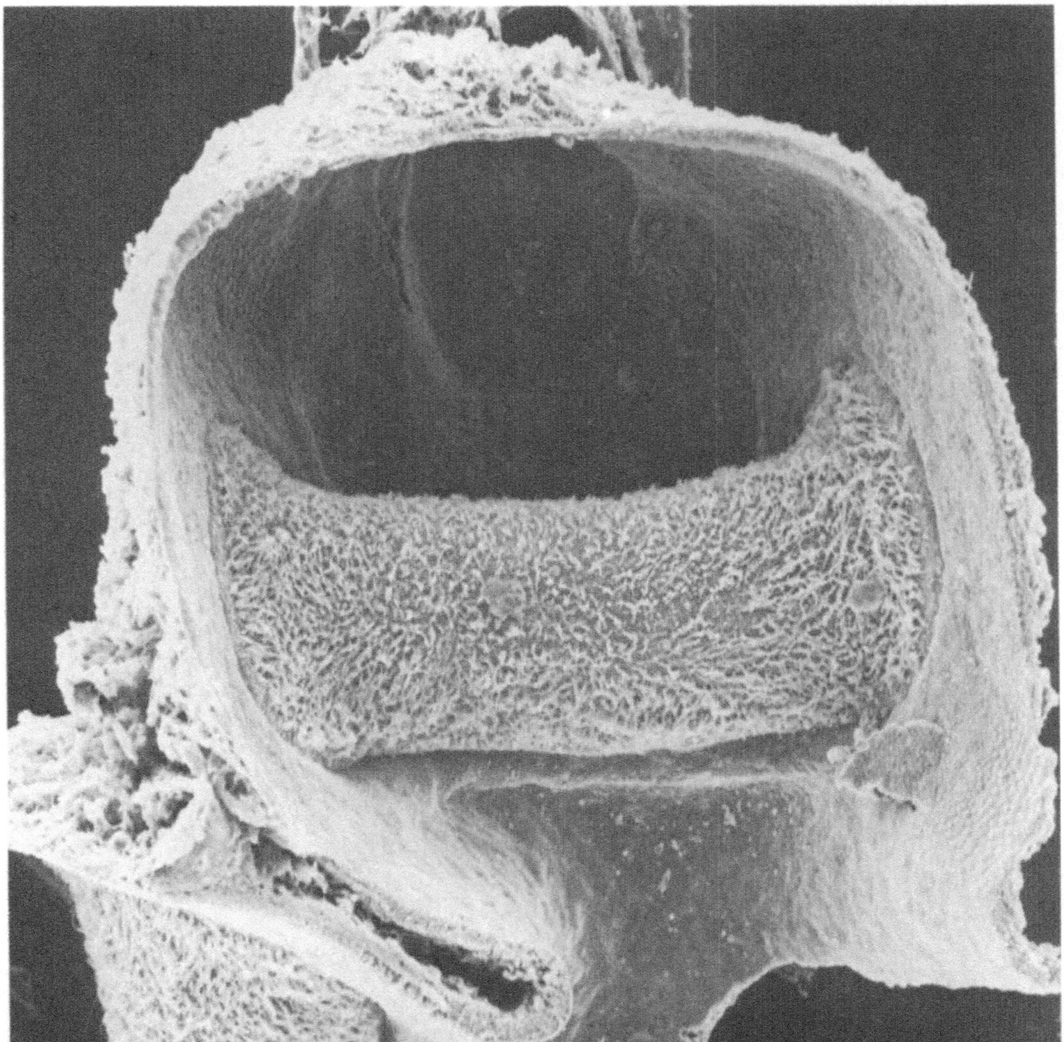

Figure 74 Horizontal semicircular canal (guinea pig). The lateral portion of the horizontal semicircular canal crista does not develop well in birds and amphibians. However, in the guinea pig, both ends of the crista show good development with abundant sensory cilia (× 1500)

The shape of the crista of the vertical semicircular canal in birds

The crista of the horizontal semicircular canal was studied in a kite, pigeon and hen. The eminentia cruciata protrudes in the centre of the crista giving an impression of a cross. The term, eminentia cruciata probably derives from this shape.

The central part of the eminentia lacks sensory hairs and this zone divides the sensory epithelia into two identical portions. Presumably the subcupular space is separated too. It is not clear if each section of the separated cupula moves differently in the endolymphatic flow or not. This type of cupula may have some significance in a bird's motor function.

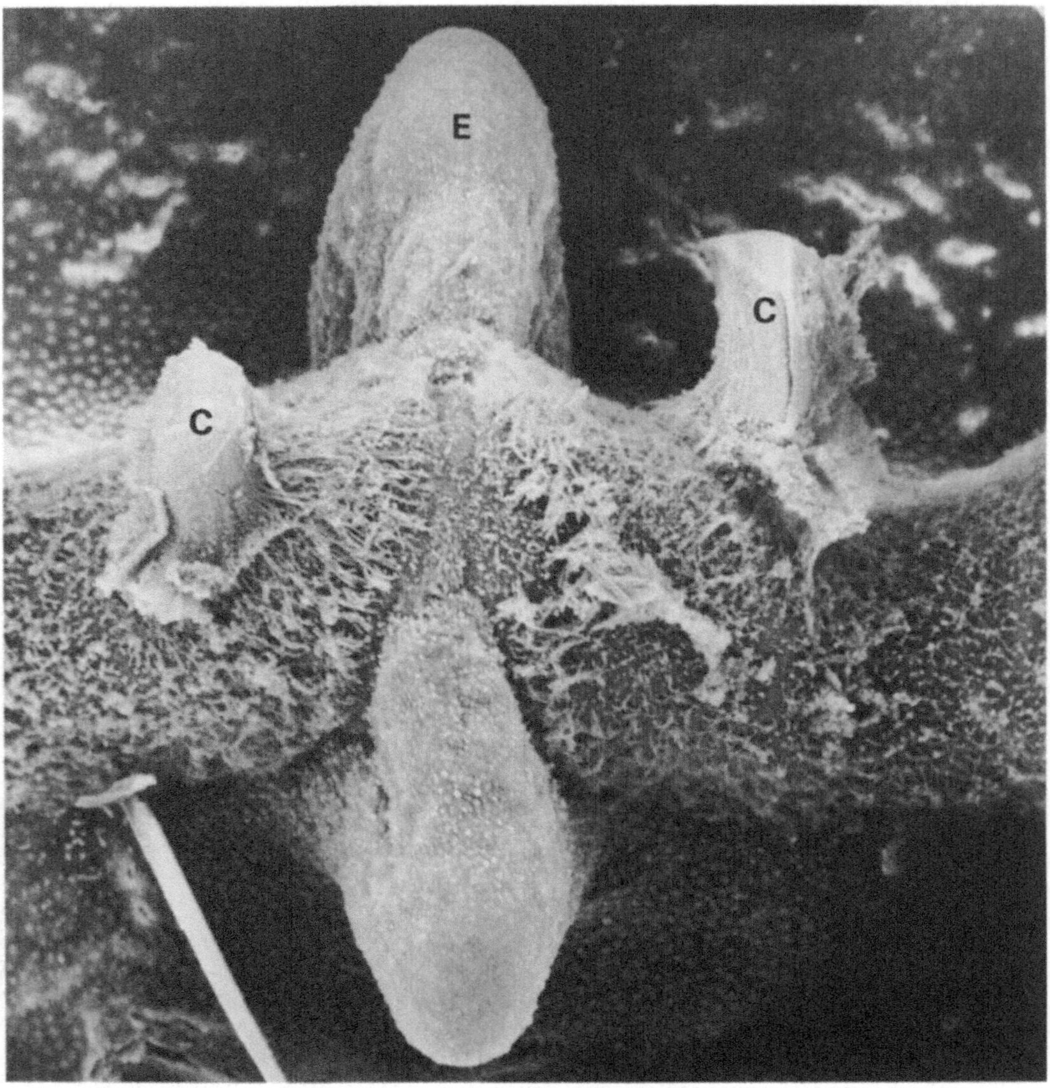

Figure 75 Crista of bird (chicken). The cupula (C) is divided by the eminentia cruciata (E). The central part of the crista lacks sensory cilia (× 200)

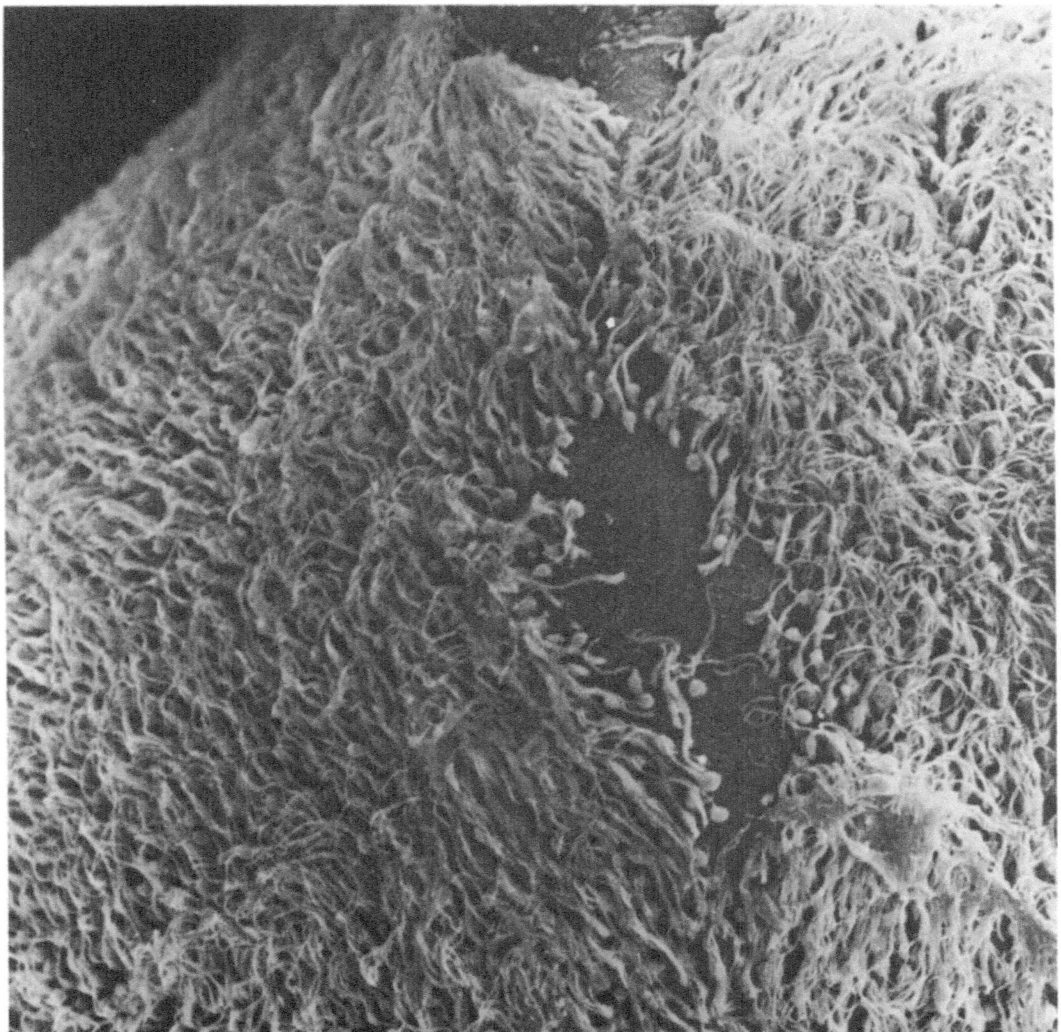

Figure 76 Crista of a bird (kite). The central part which lacks the sensory cilia is clearly seen (× 4500)

a

b

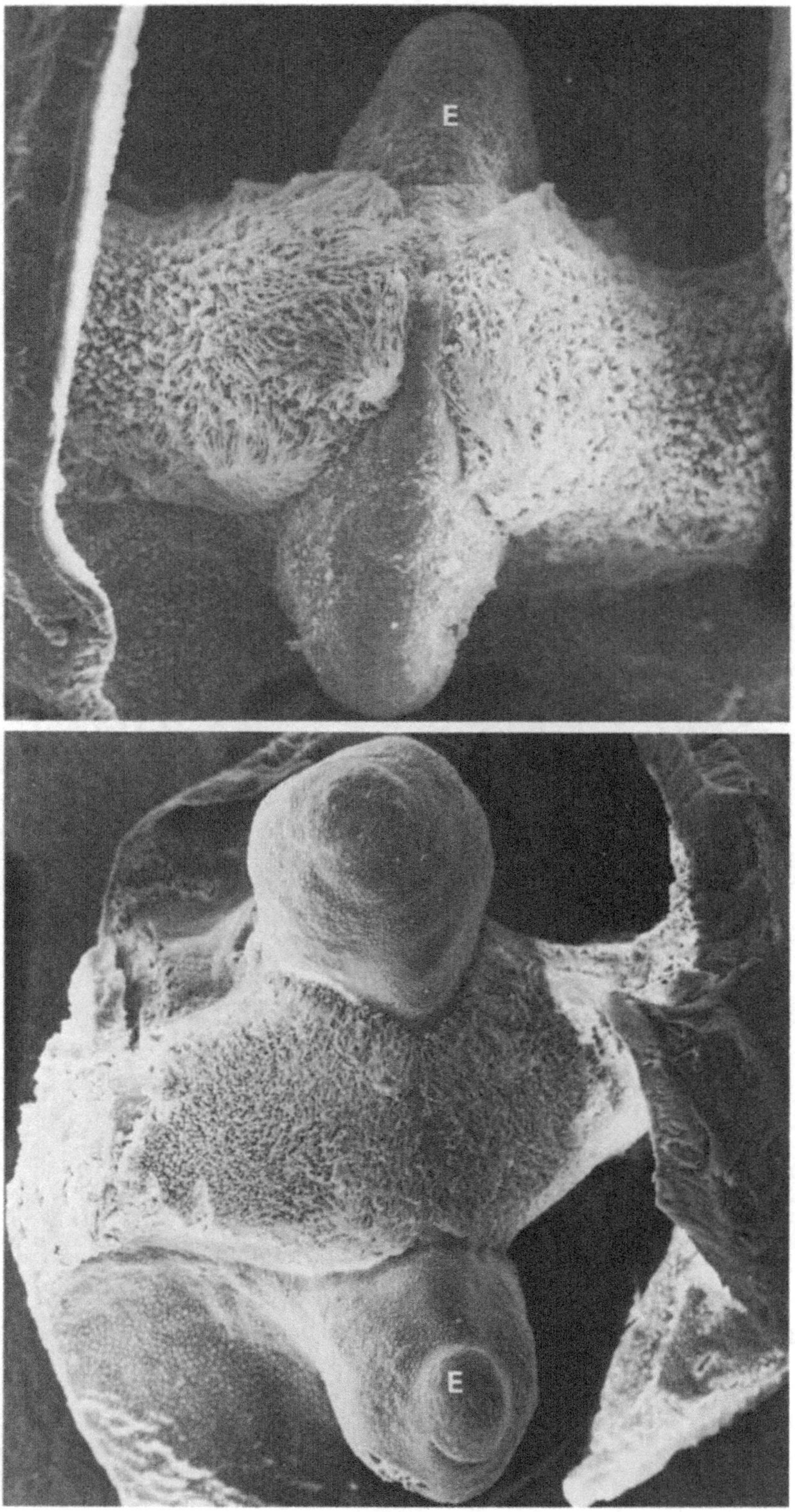

Figure 77 Crista of a bird. (**a**) Anterior semicircular canal crista (chicken), (**b**) anterior semicircular canal crista (kite). Eminentia cruciata (E) is observed as a protrusion on both sides of the crista (× 100)

Mountain-shaped eminentia cruciata

In the cat and mouse, the eminentia is a mountain-like process in the middle of the anterior semicircular canal (Figure 74). Like the bird, on the eminentia no sensory hairs are present and the sensory epithelium is divided in two by the eminentia. Also in the frog, a similar, but small eminentia was identified; however, sensory hairs were present. In the bat, the shape of the eminentia was not a cross as seen in the bird, but mountain-shaped. This shows that animals which fly do not necessarily have a cross-shaped eminentia.

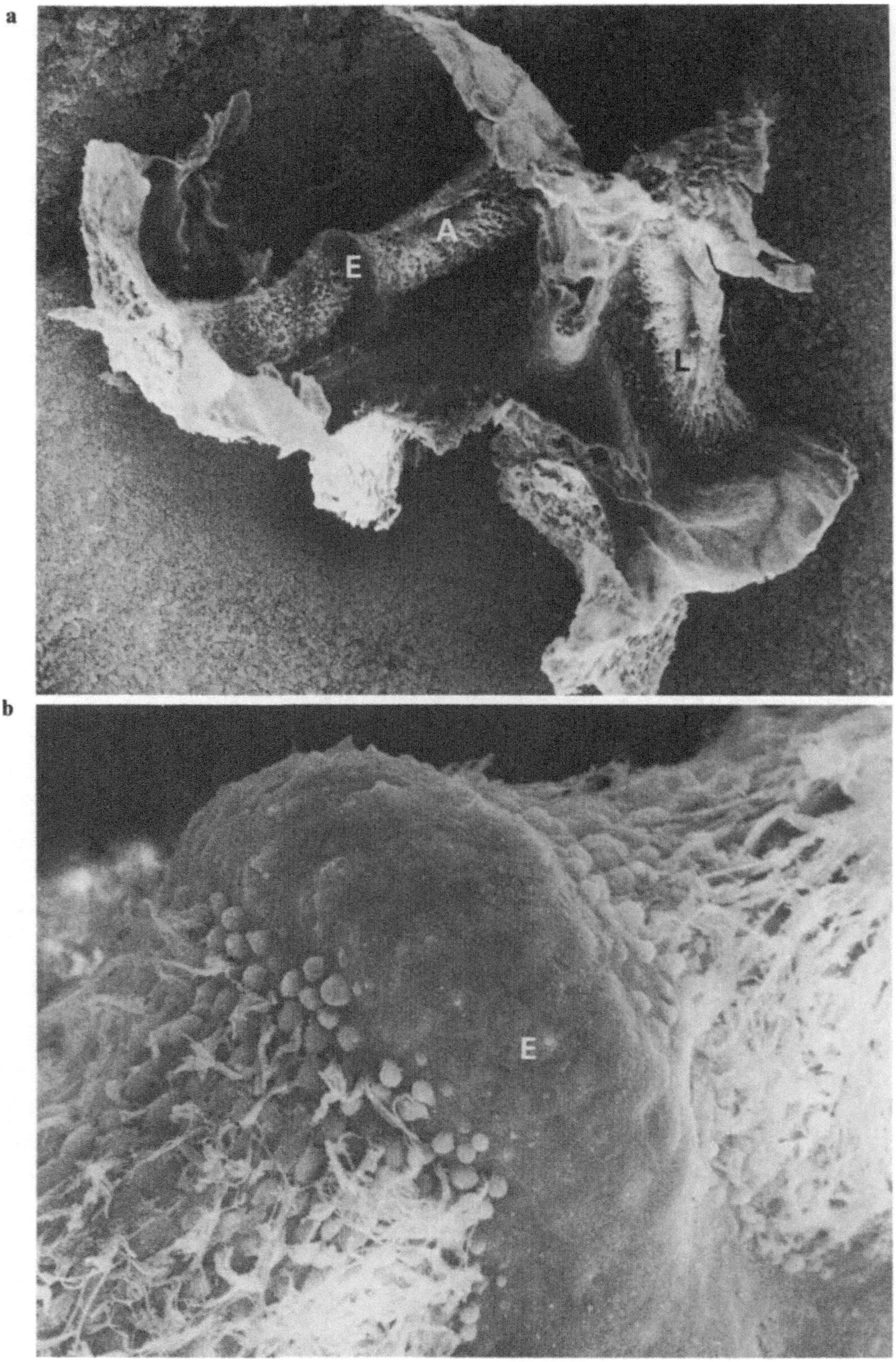

Figure 78 Mountain-shaped eminentia cruciata (mouse). (**a**) E: eminentia crista; A: anterior semicircular canal crista; L: lateral semicircular canal crista (× 150). (**b**) Eminentia (E) of the anterior semicircular canal crista. The eminentia lack sensory cilia (× 1300)

a

b

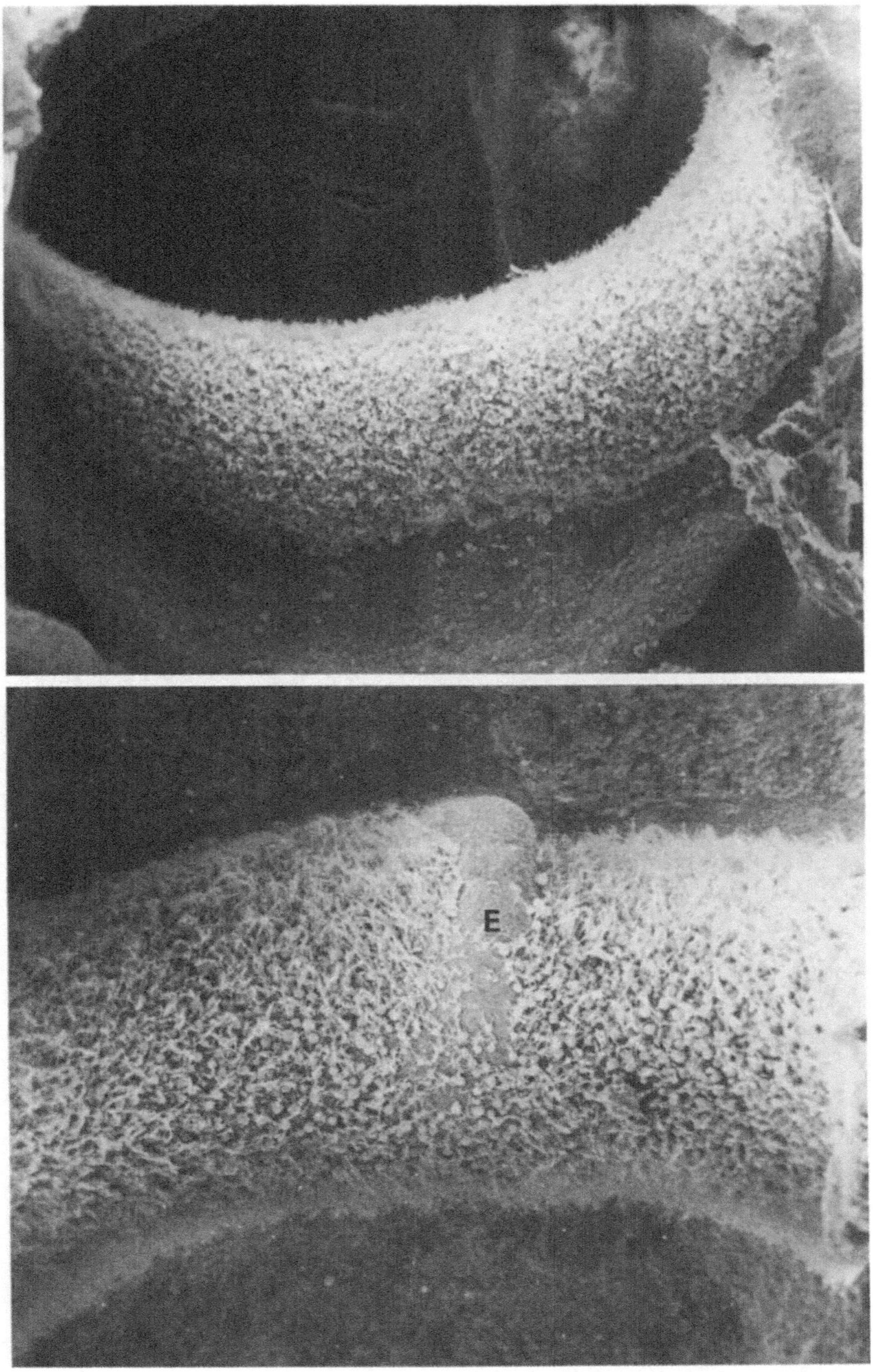

Figure 79 (**a**) Lateral semicircular canal crista (dog) (× 150), (**b**) posterior semicircular canal crista (dog) (× 250)

a

b

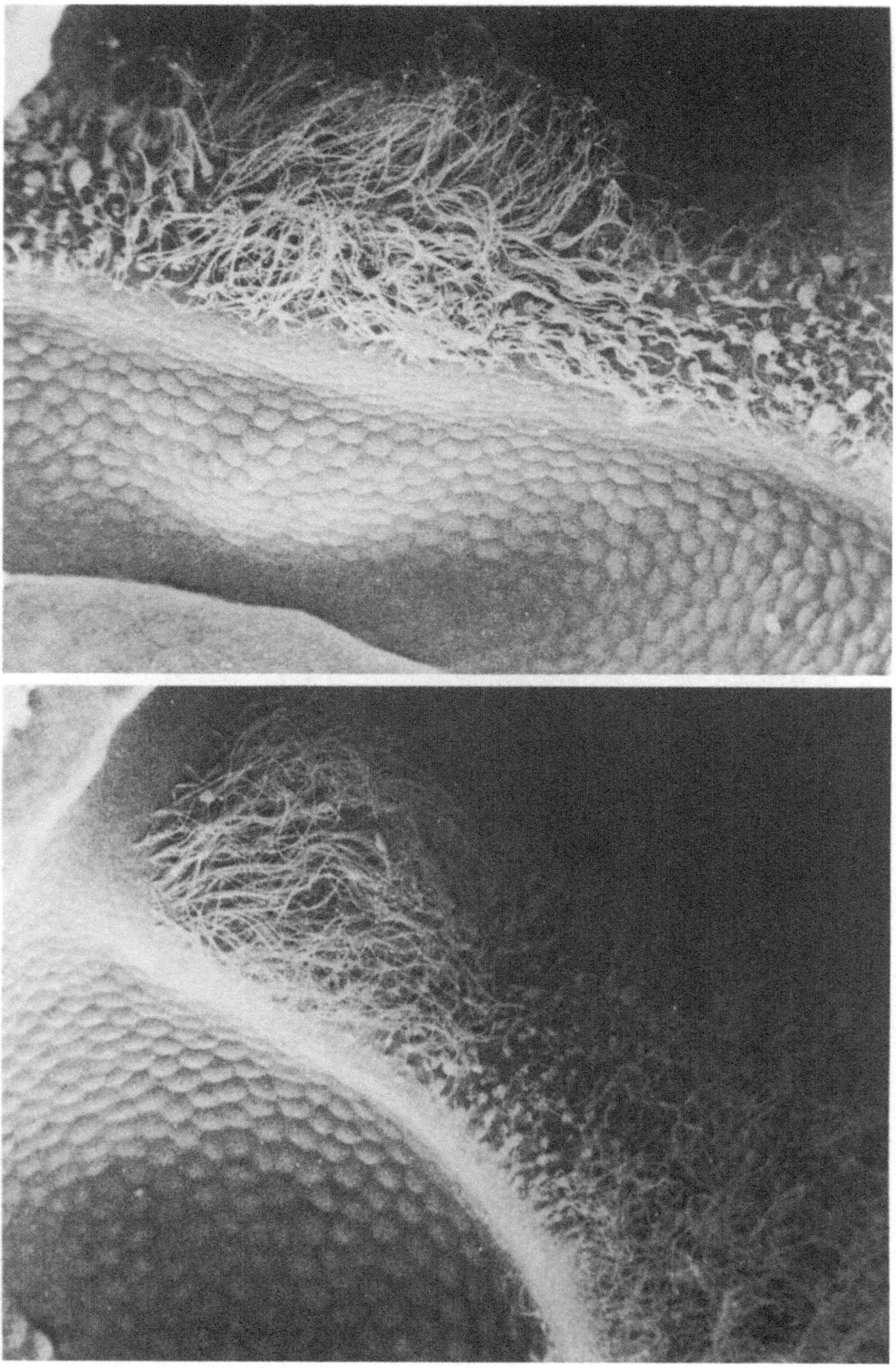

Figure 80 (**a**) Posterior semicircular canal crista (frog) (× 500), (**b**) lateral semicircular canal crista (frog) (× 500)

The crista neglecta

The crista neglecta is originally one of the peripheral vestibular organs seen in lower animals (Gacek, 1961). However, there are some reports of a crista neglecta being found in humans (Montandon *et al.* 1970; Schuknecht, 1974). According to Schuknecht, a crista neglecta was found in five ears out of 500 human temporal bone specimens. The crista neglecta is found between the utricular macula and the crista of the posterior semicircular canal. Its morphological structure is similar to that of the cristae ampullares; for example, hair cell type I and II have both afferent and efferent nerve endings (Montandon *et al.* 1970).

References

1. Gacek, R. (1961). The macula neglecta in the feline species. *J. Comp. Neurol.*, **116,** 317
2. Montandon, P., Gacek, R. and Kimura, R. (1970). Crista neglecta in the cat and human. *Ann Otol. Rhinol. Laryngol.*, **79,** 105
3. Schuknecht, H. F. (1974). *Pathology of the Ear.* (Harvard University Press)

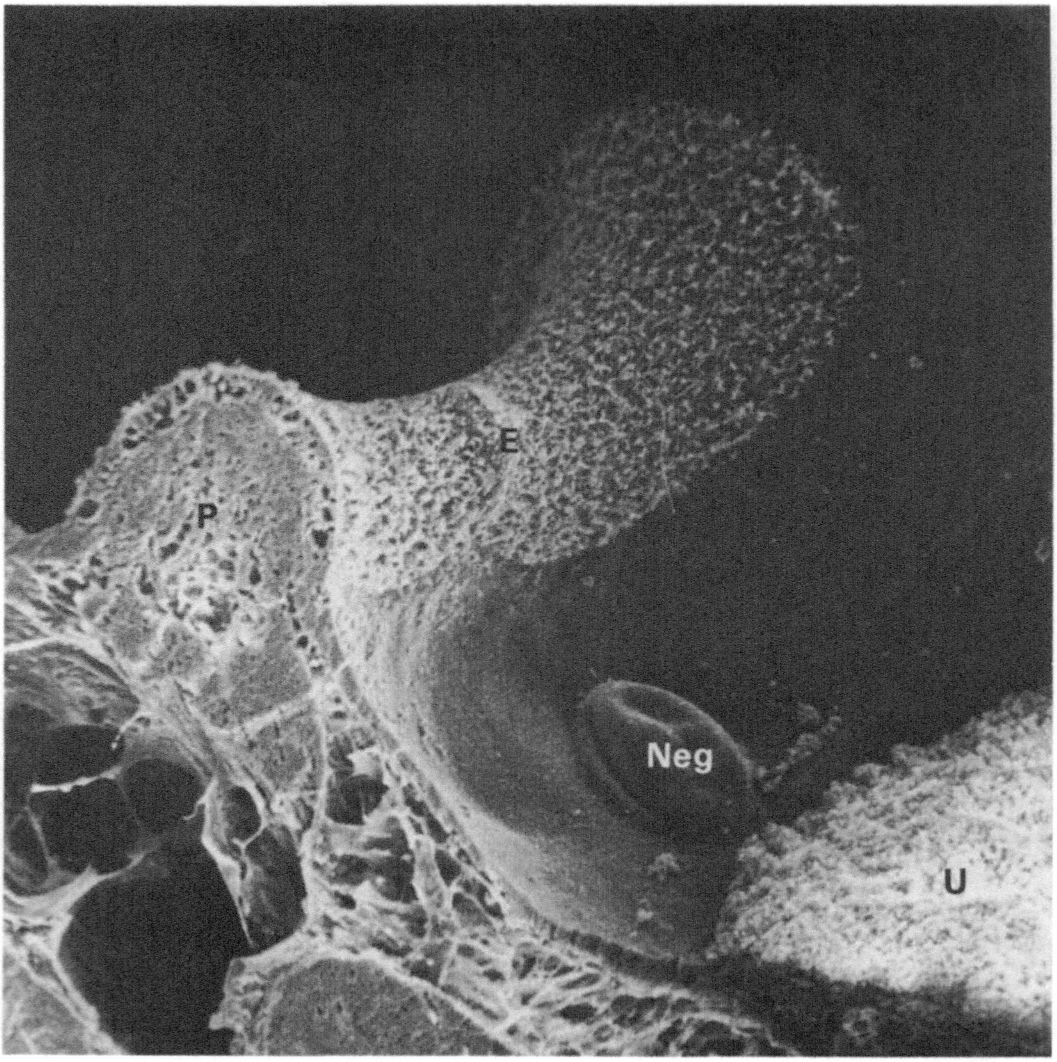

Figure 81 Crista neglecta (dog). Dome-like crista neglecta (Neg) is seen between the cracked posterior semicircular canal crista (P) and the utricular macula (U). No sensory cilia are seen in this area. E: eminentia cruciata (× 120)

The planum semilunatum

The planum semilunatum is a semilunar portion of the lateral wall of the crista ampullaris, where different types of epithelia are found. Since 1835 when Steifensand called it the planum semilunatum, many studies have been done (Dohlman, 1965; Harada, 1971, 1972, 1973). All these studies are on the secretory function of the cells; for instance, the isotope study by Dohlman. In the bottom of the cells in this area are found basal infolding and abundant capillaries, probably indicating a function related to the exchange of the endolymphatic fluid.

The cell body of the planum semilunatum is like a long cylinder, the length of which decreases approaching the top of the ampulla and also toward the utricular and canal side. In the centre of the cell body, a centriole is sometimes identified. In the basal part of the cell, innumerable processes reach the cytoplasm. The nucleus is round and many vesicles are found in the upper part of the cell body. There is structural similarity between these cells and cells of kidney, pancreas, choroid plexus and stria vascularis, all of which have either secretory or filtering functions. Apocrine-like secretion is found on the surface of the planum semilunatum and this is probably secretion of endolymphatic fluid.

References

1. Dohlman, G. F. (1965). The mechanism of secretion and absorption of endolymph in the vestibular apparatus. *Acta Otolaryngol. (Stockholm)*, **59,** 295
2. Harada, Y. (1971). In vivo and scanning electron microscopic observation of semicircular canal ampullae. *Equilibrium Res. Suppl.*, **1,** 81
3. Harada, Y. (1972). Observation of the vestibular sensory organ with the scanning electron microscope. *Practica Otol. (Kyoto)*, **65,** 1335
4. Harada, Y. (1973). Scanning electron microscopic observation of vestibular specific cells. *Practica Otol. (Kyoto)*, **66,** 1293

a

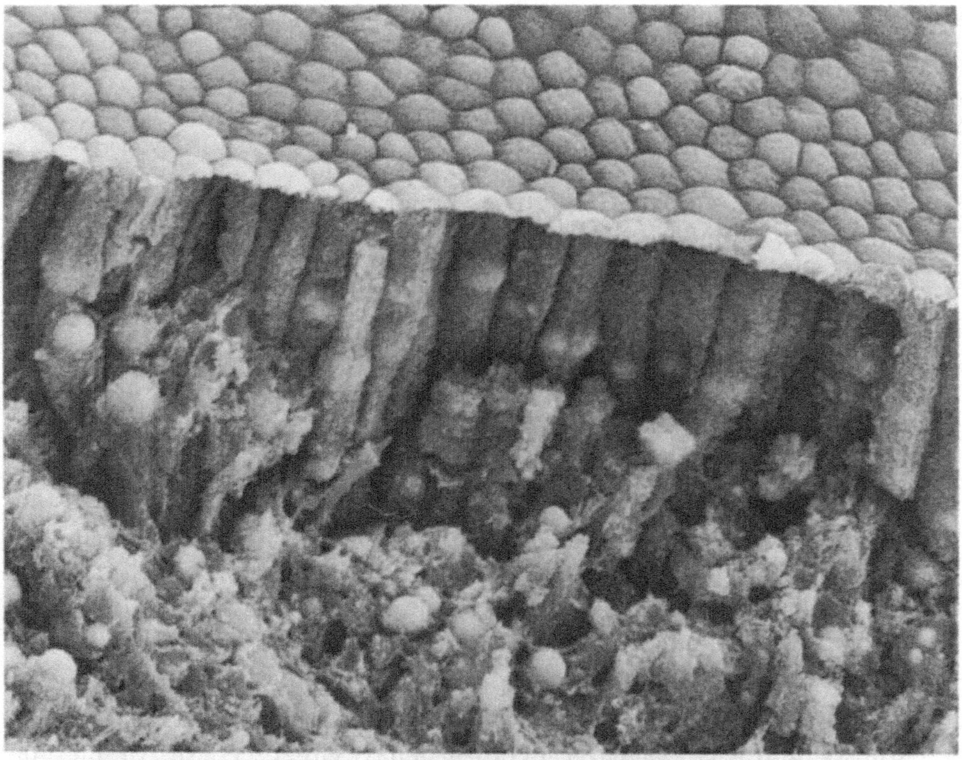

b

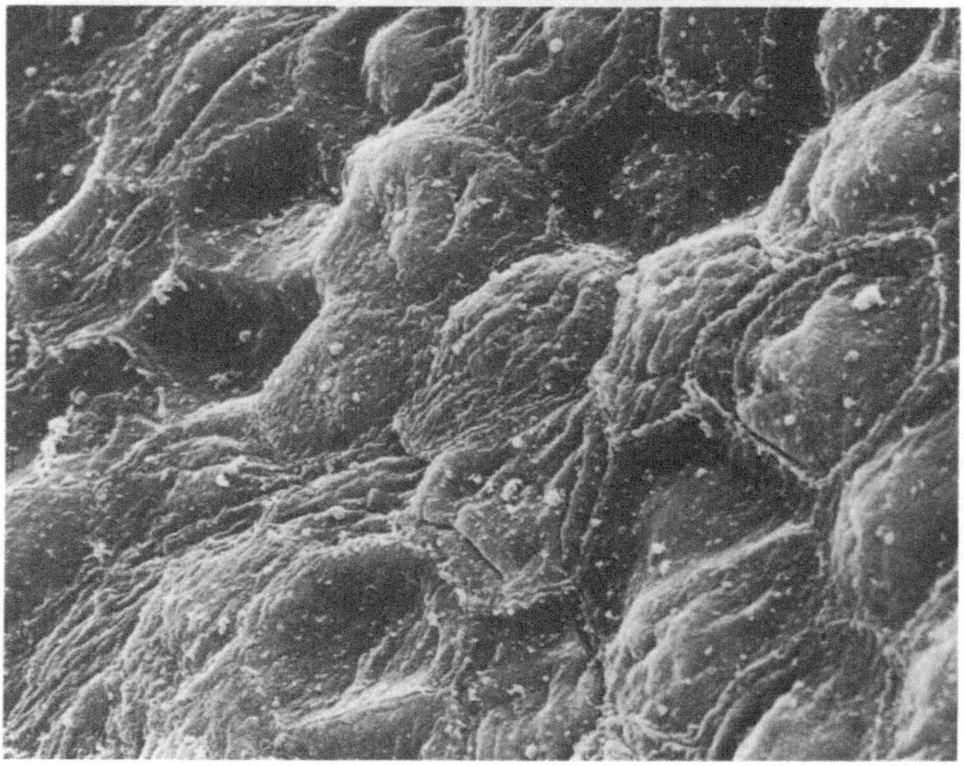

Figure 82 Cells of the planum semilunatum (kite). (**a**) Cell surface of the planum semilunatum is convex like a dome. Each tall cylindrical cell has clear cell border (× 1300). (**b**) A few microvilli are seen on the surface (× 8000)

The transitional epithelium

The transitional epithelium, of which the cell surface is slightly convex, surrounds the sensory epithelia of the cristae ampullares (Steifensand, 1835). The cells are cylindrical and the cell bottoms interdigitate. There is a single centriole on the cell surface, which a few animals lack (Harada, 1973). This epithelium extends to the dark cell area at the bottom of the ampulla. Dark cells are sometimes found mixed with the transitional cells. The transitional epithelium is composed of secretory cells and has structural similarity with cells of the planum semilunatum and the eminentia cruciata.

References

1. Harada, Y. (1973). Scanning electron microscopic observation of vestibular specific cells. *Practica Otol.* (*Kyoto*), **66,** 1293
2. Steifensand, K. K. (1835). Untersuchungen über die Ampullen des Gehörorganes. *Arch. Anat. Phys. Wiss.*, **2,** 171

a

b

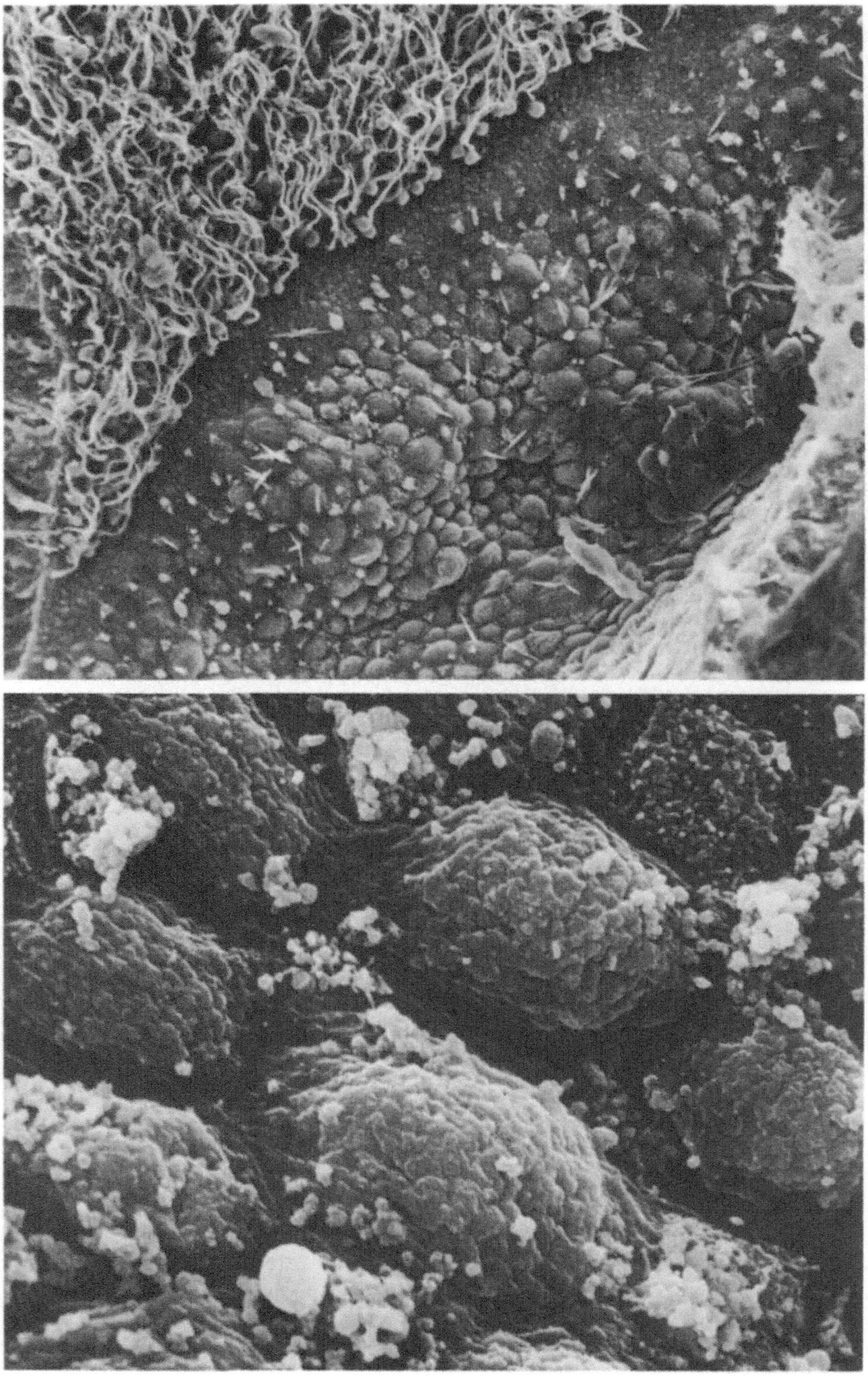

Figure 83 Transitional epithelium (chicken). (**a**) Transitional epithelium has the same morphological features regardless of the species. Each cell is relatively big and dome-like (× 430), (**b**) high magnification of (a). Microvilli are scarce in number. Small cells with long microvilli are seen between the large dome-like cells (× 4300)

Vestibular supporting cells

The supporting cells are found between the sensory epithelial layer and the basement membrane and they vary in their shape. On the cell surface, there are many microvilli and a single centriole. Sometimes a global substance protrudes on this surface (Harada, 1971, 1973). The supporting cell has an oval nucleus and well developed Golgi apparatus and mitochondria. In the upper portion of the cell, there are many round or oval granules. A fine fibrous structure is also identified in the cell body, which is considered to enhance the cell function (Nakai, 1973).

References

1. Harada, Y. (1973). Scanning electron microscopic observation of vestibular specific cells. *Practica Otol.* (*Kyoto*), **66,** 1293
2. Nakai, Y. (1973). Electronmicroscopic study of the vestibular sensory epithelium and epithelial linings. *Otolaryngology* (*Tokyo*), **19,** 845

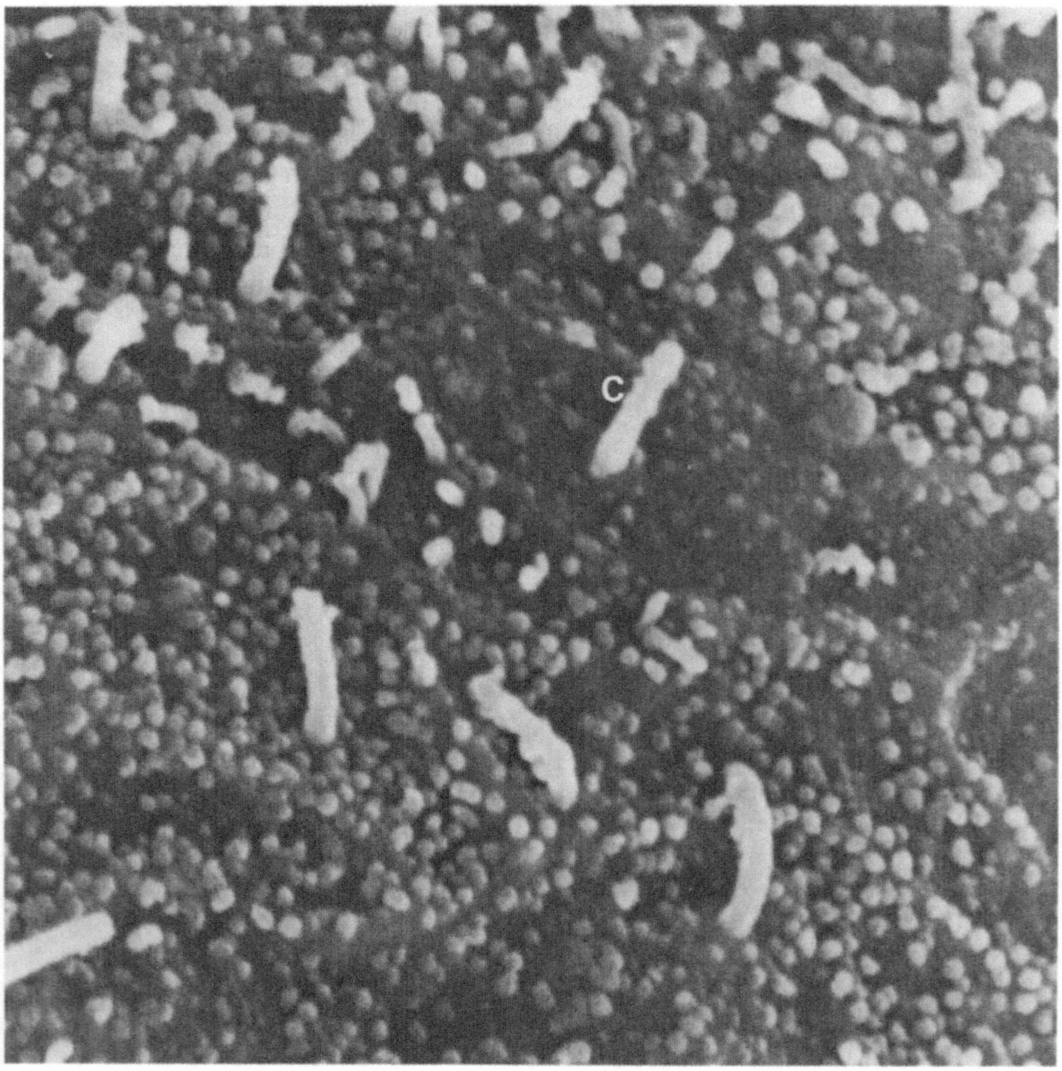

Figure 84 Vestibular supporting cell (kite). Suporting cells of the crista. Some of them have a centriole (C) (× 15000)

Vestibular dark cells

The distribution of the dark cells in the guinea pig is described in detail by Kimura (1969). In the pigmented guinea pig, localization of the dark cells coincides with that of the melanin and a similar localization is found also in the albino. In coloured races of humans, melanin is found in the bottom of the ampulla and utricular wall cells. This is recognized as a blackish dark cell area in the surface preparation.

The surface of the dark cell is relatively flat and there are a few microvilli on the cell borders. The interdigitation into the cell cytoplasm is seen in the basal part of the cell body. The dark cell is morphologically similar to the cell of the planum semilunatum. Functionally, absorption and secretion of the fluid takes place in this area. Otoconia are absorbed in this area as mentioned in the chapter on the otolithic organ (Harada, 1973, 1976).

References

1. Harada, Y. (1973). Scanning electron microscopic observation of vestibular specific cells. *Practica Otol. (Kyoto)*, **66,** 1293
2. Harada, Y. *et al.* (1976). The effect of ototoxic drugs on metabolic disorder of statoconia. *Ear Res.* **7,** 60
3. Kimura, R. (1969). Distribution, structure and function of dark cells in the vestibular labyrinth. *Ann. Otol. Rhinol. Laryngol.*, **78,** 542

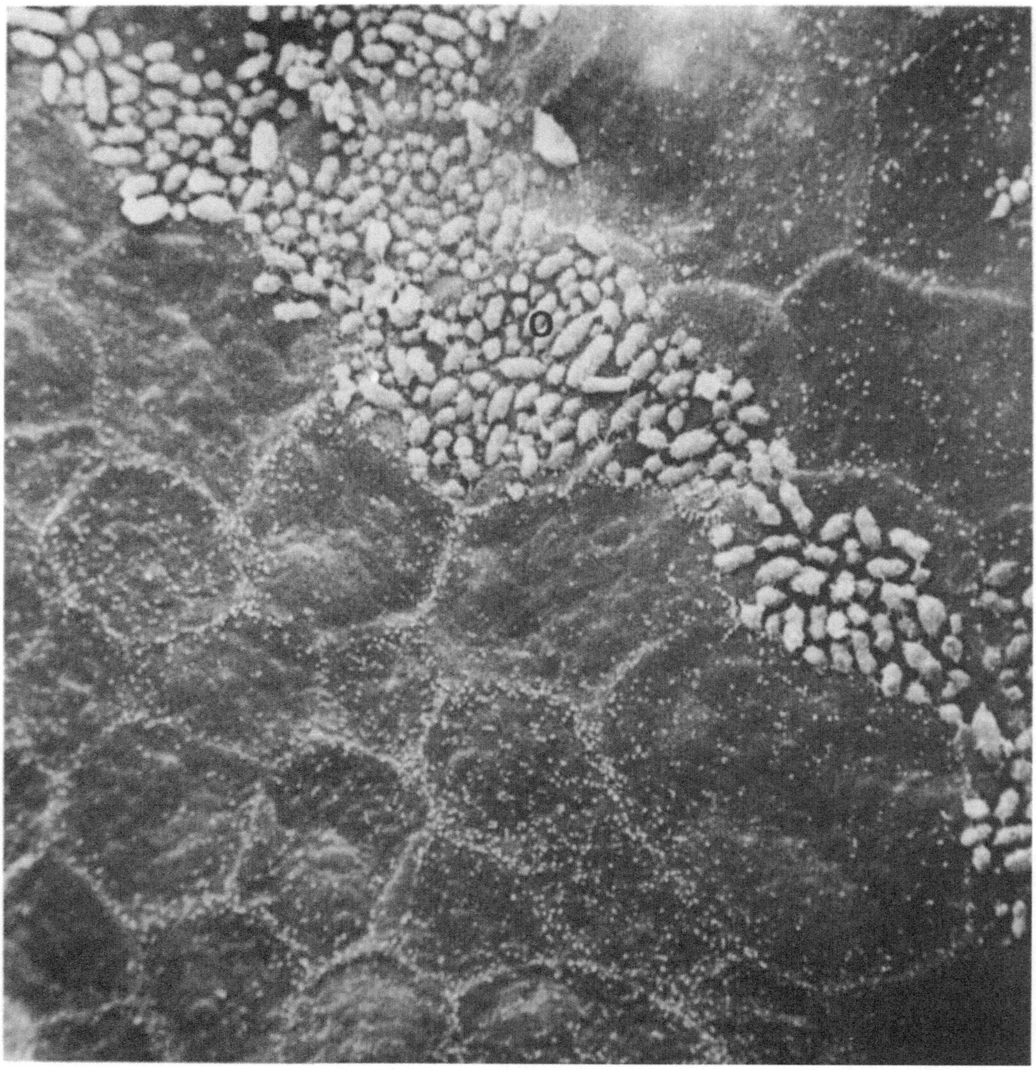

Figure 85 Dark cell area of the utricle (guinea pig). Cells with and without centriole are observed in the vestibular dark cell area. These cells, which are either hexagonal or pentagonal, are arranged like a pavement. Fragmented otoconia are sometimes attached to the utricular dark cell even in the normal animal. Numbers of fragmented otoconia were found attached to the dark cell surface in case of a streptomycin-injected guinea pig. O: fragmented otoconia (× 4500)

Vestibular wall cells

The wall cells of the utricle, saccule, semicircular canal, ductus reuniens and transitional portion of the endolymphatic sac are included in this category. All of the above do not have the same morphological structure.

The wall cells of the semicircular canal present a polygonal surface, varying from pentagons to octagons with a smooth surface and a small number of microvilli. In the wall cells of the ductus reuniens, however, abundant microvilli are sometimes observed. Some wall cells seen in the utricular wall distal to the macula have a centriole. The function of the centriole is still unknown.

a

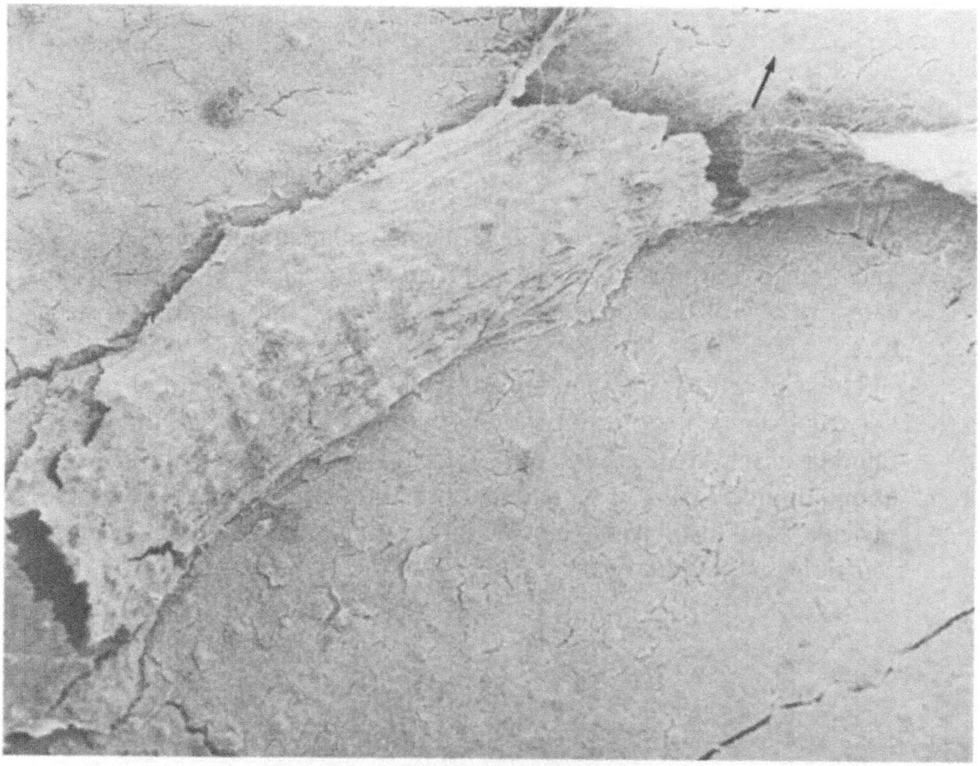

b

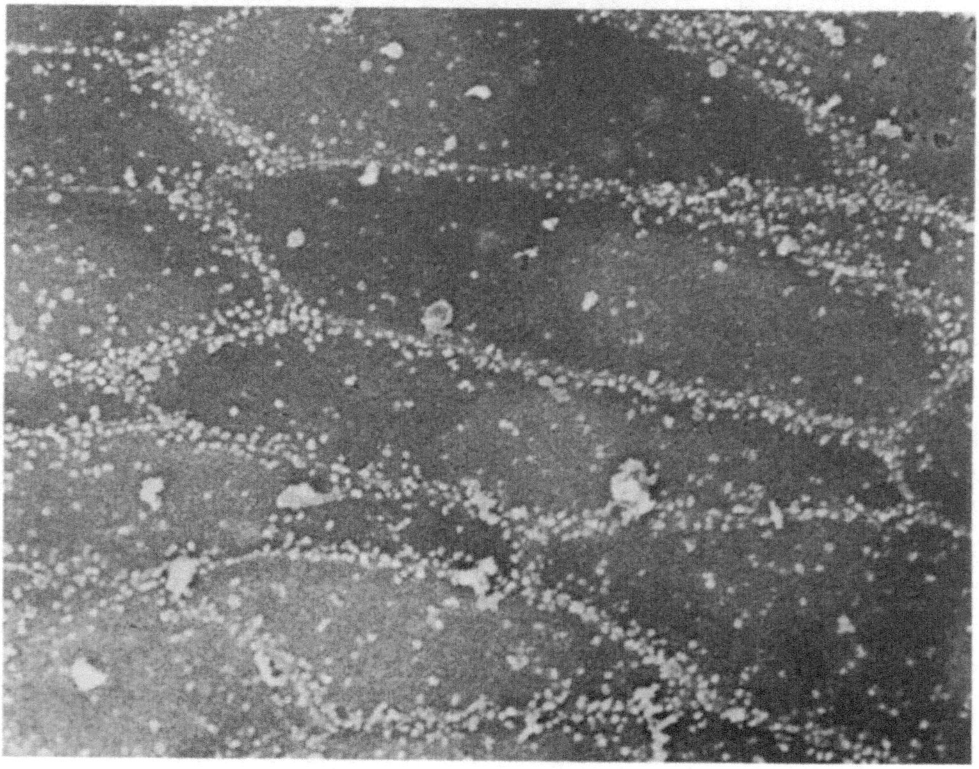

Figure 86 Ductus reuniens (guinea pig). (**a**) A nucleus appears protruding from the outside wall (× 260), (**b**) high magnification of the arrowed part of (a). This is the luminal surface of the ductus reuniens which is closed to the cochlear hook portion. Long polygonal cells with short microvilli are seen (× 5200)

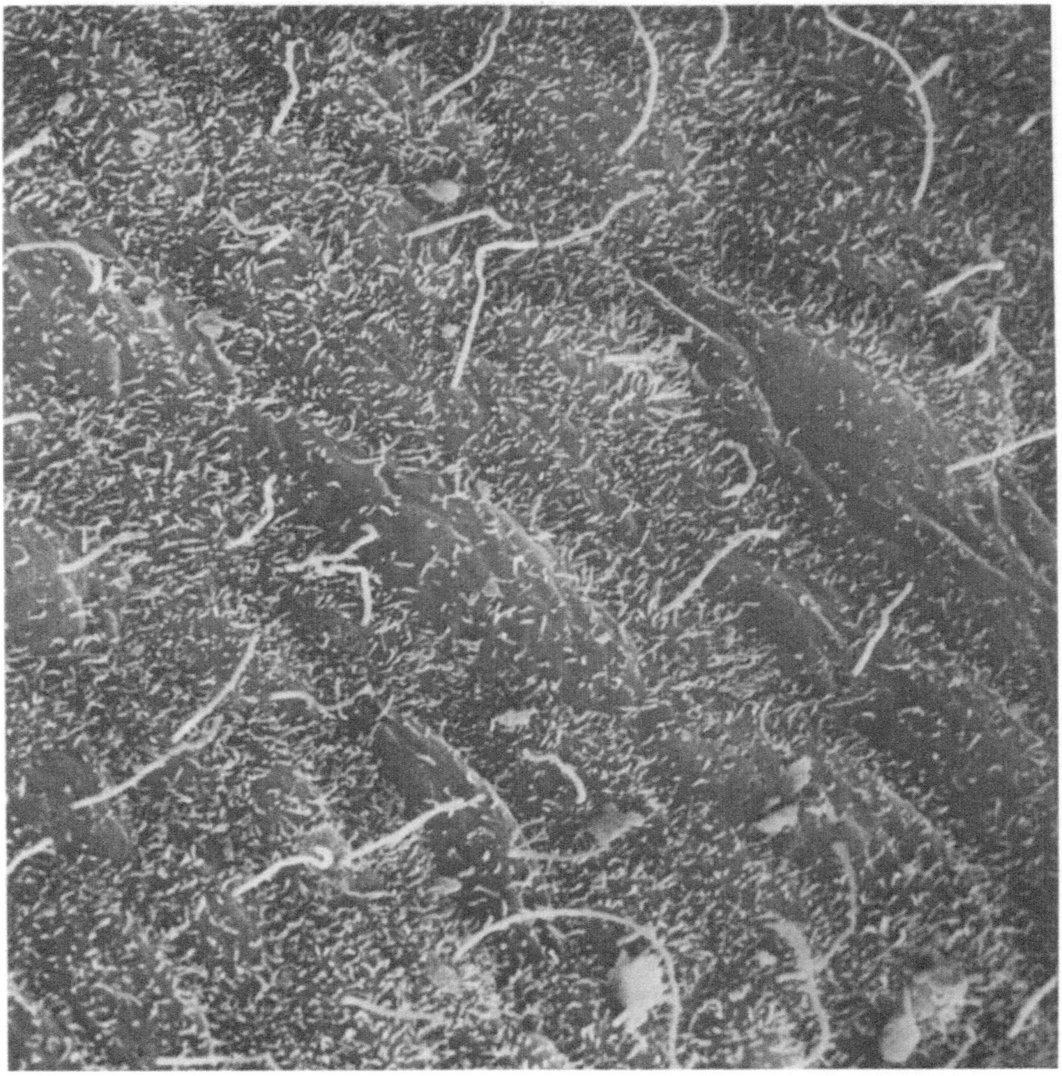

Figure 87 Luminal surface of the ductus reuniens (guinea pig). Cells with long microvilli and a central cilium are observed on the luminal surface close to the saccular macula (× 15 000)

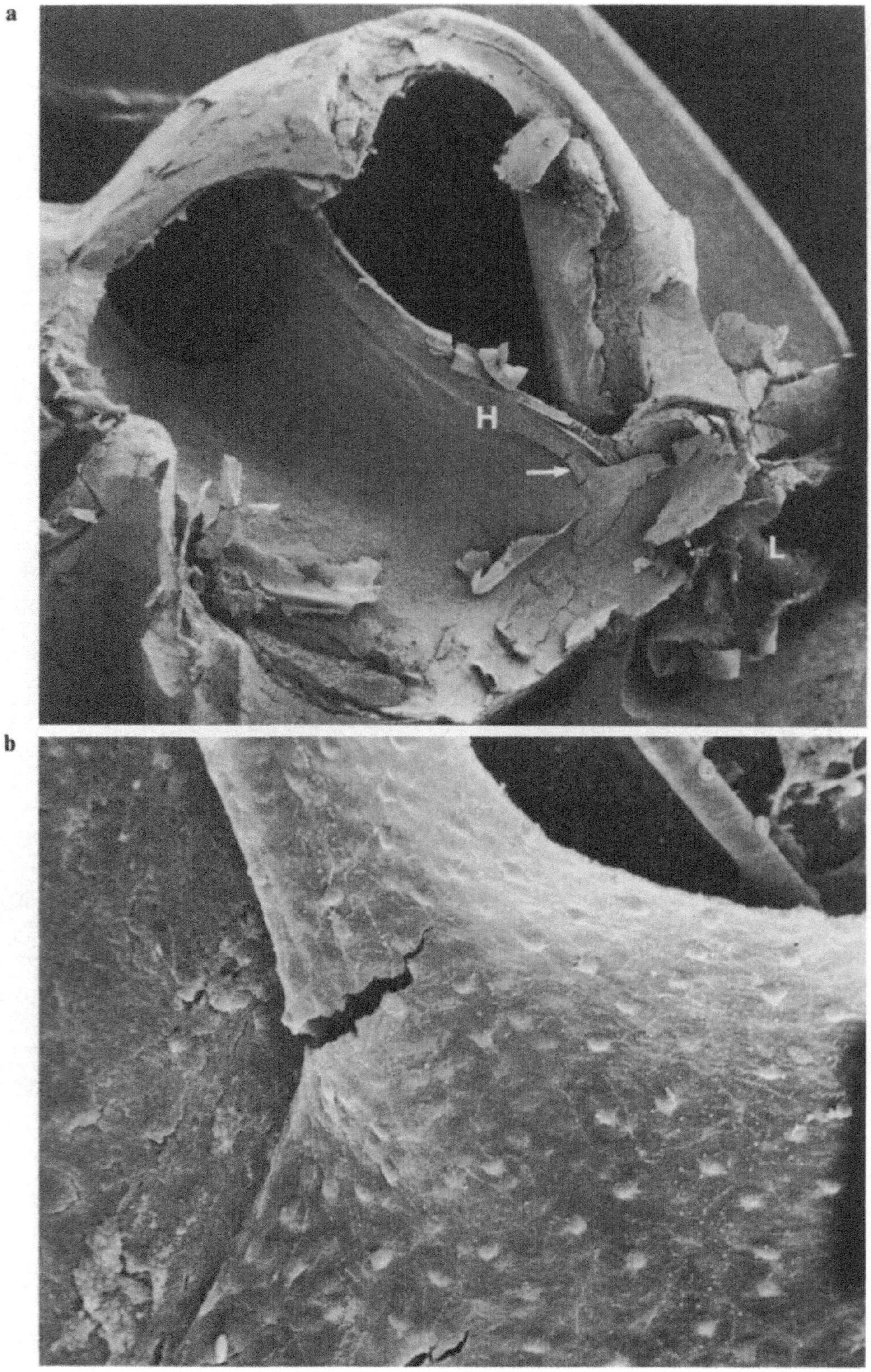

Figure 88 Cochlear hook portion. (**a**) Branching portion (arrow) from cochlear hook (H) to ductus reuniens. L: lateral semicircular canal crista (× 30). (**b**) High magnification of the part indicated by arrow in (a) (× 500)

The calibre and number of the vestibular nerve fibres

The vestibular nerve consists of myelinated fibres with a diameter of about 1–10 μm and unmyelinated fibres with a diameter below 1 μm. The myelinated fibres include both afferent and efferent fibres, while the unmyelinated fibres include afferent and sympathetic nerve fibres (Wersäll, 1956; Gacek and Rasmussen, 1961).

In the guinea pig, 60% of the fibres which innervate the posterior canal ampulla are 3–5 μm in diameter, 23% are 1–2 μm and 9% are 6–9 μm. Thick fibres distribute to the hair cell type I and fine fibres distribute mainly to the hair cell type II (Wersäll, 1967).

The average number of vestibular nerve fibres in a human aged from 2 to 26 years is 18 900 and is 18 000 in those 46 to 60 years old (Rasmussen, 1940). According to Naufal and Schuknecht (1972), the ganglion cells in normal subjects number 18 439, but they reduce to 12 430 in elderly subjects with diabetes mellitus. In these subjects, nerve fibres also reduced to 10 910. There is a detailed study on the number of the vestibular nerve fibres to each vestibular organ in subjects aged 0 to 85 years (Bergström, 1973). Age-related decrease in the number of the vestibular sensory epithelial cells and nerve fibres is reported by Rosenhall (1972a, b, 1973).

When a nerve fibre is cut, degeneration proceeds to its periphery (Wallerian degeneration), but degeneration also develops toward the nerve cell (retrograde degeneration). This retrograde degeneration is found in the cochlear nerve, but not in the vestibular nerve.

Hilding and House (1964) and Harada (1973) reported the sensory hairs missing on the vestibular sensory epithelia in cases of Ménière's and other vertiginous disease. In these cases, however, the nerve endings remained intact even though some vesicles were formed in the sensory cell body (Harada, 1973).

References

1. Bergström, B. (1973). Morphology of the vestibular nerve. II. The number of myelinated vestibular nerve fibers in man at various ages. *Acta Otolaryngol.* (*Stockholm*), **76,** 173

2. Gacek, R. R. and Rasmussen, G. L. (1961). Fiber analysis of the stato-acoustic nerve of guinea pig, cat and monkey. *Anat. Res.*, 139L455
3. Harada, Y. (1973). Observation of morphological changes in the vestibular sensory epithelia. *Equilibrium Res.*, **3,** 1
4. Hilding, D. A. and House, W. F. (1964). An evaluation of the ultrastructural findings in the utricle in Ménière's disease. *Laryngoscope*, **74,** 1135
5. Naufal, P. and Schuknecht, H. (1972). Vestibular facial and oculomotor neuropathy in diabetes mellitus. *Arch. Otolaryngol.*, **96,** 468
6. Rasmussen, A. T. (1940). Studies of the VIIIth cranial nerve of man. *Laryngoscope*, **50,** 67
7. Rosenhall, U. (1972a). Vestibular macular mapping in man. *Ann Otol.*, **81,** 339
8. Rosenhall, U. (1972b). Mapping of the cristae ampullares in man. *Ann. Otol.*, **81,** 882
9. Rosenhall, U. (1973). Degenerative patterns in the aging human vestibular apparatus. In manuscript
10. Wersäll, J. (1956). Studies on the structure and innervation of the sensory epithelium of the cristae ampullares in the guinea pig as revealed by the electron miscroscope. *Acta Otolaryngol.* (*Stockholm*) Suppl., **126,** 1
11. Wersäll, J. (1967). Vestibular nerve. *Submicroscopic Structure of the Inner Ear*. p. 245. (London: Pergamon)

a

b

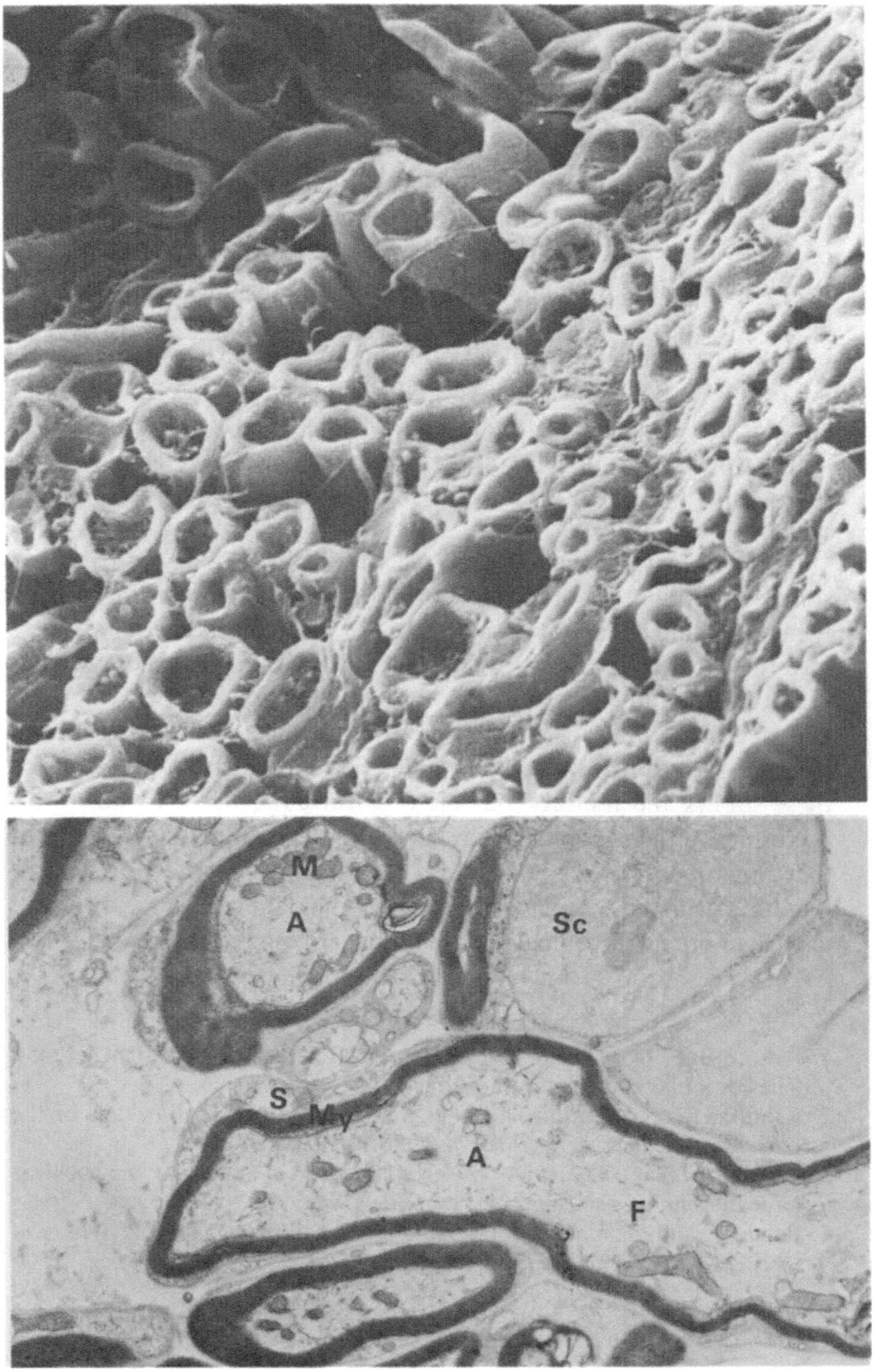

Figure 89 (**a**) Cracked surface of the vestibular nerve (guinea pig) (× 4200), (**b**) transmission electronmicrograph of the vestibular nerve (guinea pig). M: mitochondria; S: Schwann's sheath; Sc: Schwann's cell; My: myelin sheath; A: axon; F: neurofilaments (× 5500)

The cochlear aqueduct

The cochlear aqueduct is a fine duct connecting the scala tympani with the subarachnoid space. Intraductal space is occupied by mesh-like connective tissue. The internal aperture which has a separating membrane opens at the inner ridge of the round window. The external aperture opens in the subarachnoid space at the inferior surface of the petrous pyramid. There is variation in its size among the reports. According to Palva and Dammert (1969) the diameters of the internal and external aperture are 0.1 mm and 1.0 mm respectively and the length is approximately 6 mm in both apertures. Newborns have a thicker duct than adults (Palva, 1970) and the lower animals also have a thicker duct.

Its physiological function is not yet clarified. Years ago, there were some assumptions, such as transportation of the cerebrospinal or perilymphatic fluid, or prevention of entry of a foreign body or infection into the cochlea. However, Ritter (1965) concluded that there was no cerebrospinal fluid flow into the cochlea after experiments using dye and isotopes. Kimura (1974) found no histological change in the inner ear after occlusion of the cochlear aqueduct. Judging from the results of these studies and the fact that the cochlear aqueduct tends to shrink according to the progress of development of an animal, it is doubtful that this organ plays any role in a human. For the present, Ritter's hypothesis, that the cochlear aqueduct may moderate the pressure change in the cerebrospinal fluid and the perilymph, is agreeable.

References

1. Anson, B. J., Donaldson, J. A., Warpeha, R. L. and Winch, T. R. (1965). The vestibular and cochlear aqueducts. *Laryngoscope*, **75,** 1203
2. Kimura, R., Schuknecht, H. and Carol, Y. Ota (1974). Blockage of the cochlear aqueduct. *Acta Otolaryngol.* (*Stockholm*), **77,** 1
3. Ku Won Suh and Thane D. (1974). Obliteration of vestibular and cochlear aqueducts in the guinea pig. *Laryngoscope*, **84,** 1352
4. Palva, T. and Dammert, K. (1969). Human cochlear aqueduct. *Acta Otolaryngol.* (*Stockholm*) *Suppl.*, **246,** 1

5. Palva, T. (1970). Cochlear aqueduct in infants. *Acta Otolaryngol.* (*Stockholm*), **70,** 83
6. Ritter, F. N. and Lawrence, M. (1965). A histological and experimental study of cochlear aqueduct patency in adult human. *Laryngoscope*, **75,** 1224

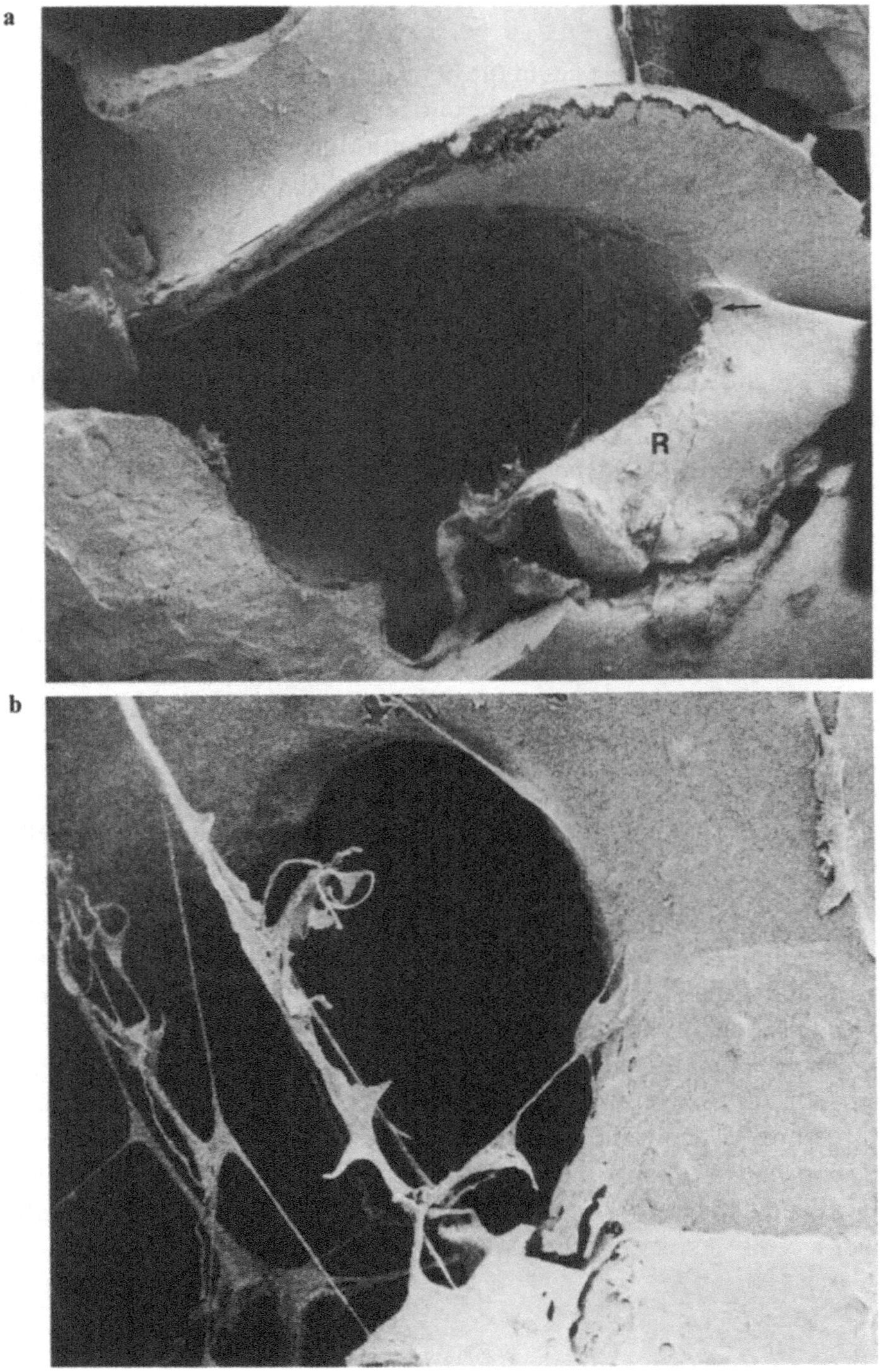

Figure 90 (**a**) Internal aperture of the cochlear aqueduct (monkey). The internal aperture opens at the internal edge of the round window (arrow). R: round window membrane (× 30). (**b**) High magnification of internal aperture (× 450)

The endolymphatic sac

The endolymphatic sac lies in the bony niche of the posterior surface of the pyramid. It partly touches the dura mater of the posterior fossa. The endolymphatic sac communicates with the endolymphatic system through the endolymphatic duct. The epithelia of the sac are either squamous cell or cuboidal cell.

Lundquist (1964) classified the endolymphatic sac into the following portions.

(1) *The proximal portion* This is in the bony niche and consists of slightly longer epithelial cells than the cells of the endolymphatic duct.

(2) *The intermediate portion* This is a portion from the bony niche to the dura mater. The epithelium consists of long cylindrical cells. Two kinds of cells, the light cell and the dark cell are found.

- (a) The light cell. This cell has a light cytoplasm, many pinocytotic vesicles and inclusion bodies. There are many microvilli on the cell surface.
- (b) The dark cell. This cell has dense cytoplasm, with a small number of the pinocytotic vesicles and microvilli.

(3) *The distal portion* This portion touches the dura mater above the transverse sinus. The cells are cuboidal and the light cells prevail.

These three portions of the endolymphatic sac are differently termed. For example, Anson and Bast (1949) called the distal portion pars intraduralis and the intermediate portion pars rugosa from the fact that the inner wall of the intermediate portion forms many folds.

The cells of the endolymphatic sac, especially of the intermediate portion, are not easily classified simply from their size and surface structure. This morphological complexity draws the attention of many scientists. Up till now the function of the endolymphatic sac has been considered to be absorption of the endolymphatic fluid and pinocytosis, but recently a secretory function has been speculated.

References

1. Adlington, P. (1967). The ultrastructure and the functions of the saccus endolymphaticus and its decompression in Ménière's disease. *J. Laryng.*, **81,** 759
2. Anson, B. J. and Bast, T. H. (1949). The temporal bone and the ear. III. (Springfield, Illinois: Charles C. Thomas)
3. Harada, Y. and Gaafar, H. (1976). Scanning electron microscopy of the endolymphatic sac epithelium. *ORL*, **38,** 257
4. Lundquist, P. G., Kimura, R. S. and Wersäll, J. (1964). Ultrastructure organization of the epithelial lining in the endolymphatic duct and sac in the guinea pig. *Acta Otolaryng. (Stockholm)*, **57,** 65
5. Lundquist, P. G. (1965). The endolymphatic duct and sac in the guinea pig. An electron microscopic and experimental investigation. *Acta Otolaryng. (Stockholm), Suppl.* **201,** 1
6. Mitsuya, K. Observation of the luminal surface of endolymphatic sac in the guinea pig under the scanning electron microscope. *Otolaryngology (Tokyo)*, **45,** 345

a

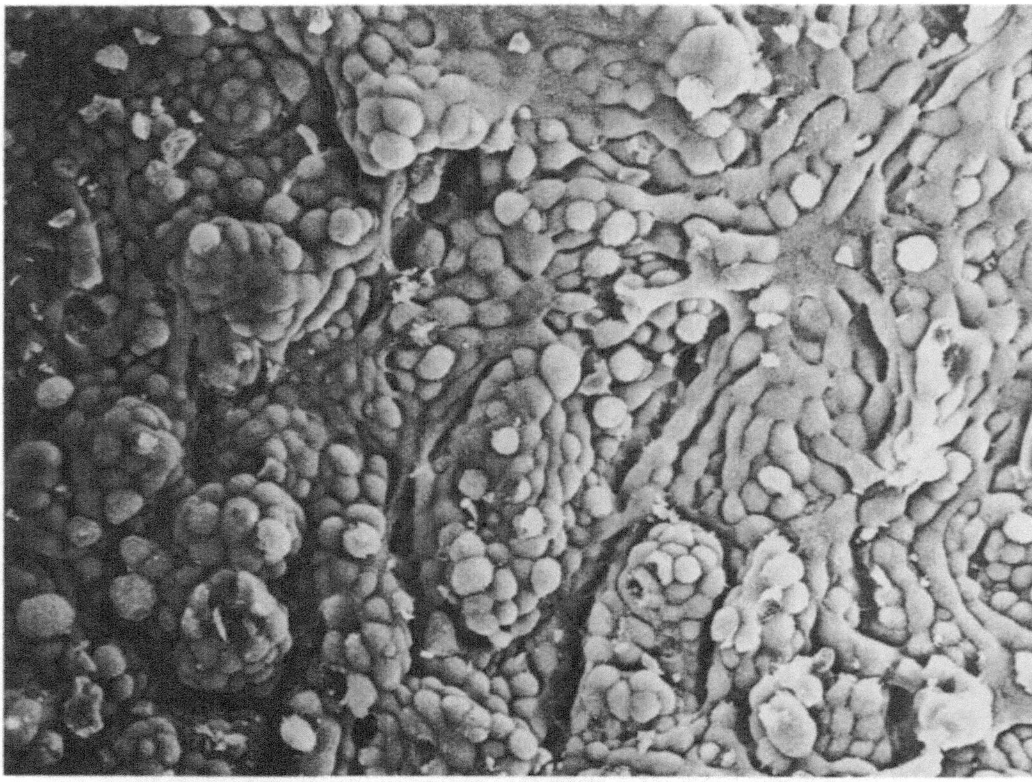

b

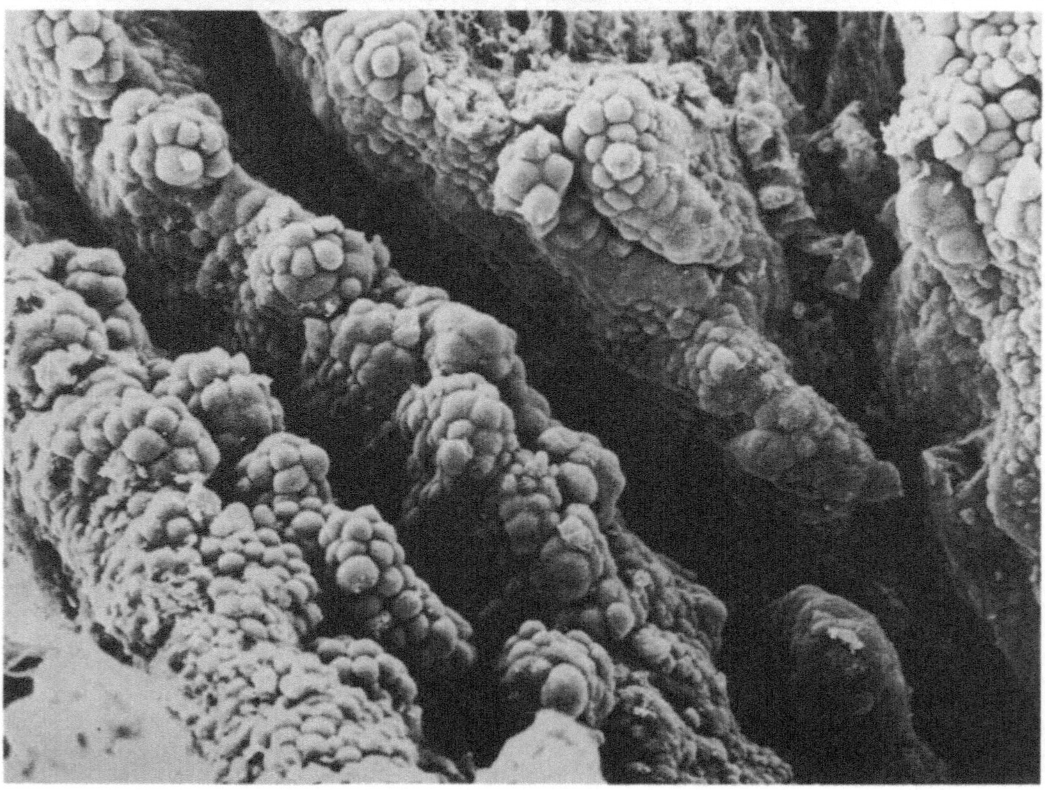

Figure 91 Cell surface of the intermediate portion (dog). (**a**) Whole area is covered with dome-like cells which form a few papillae (× 800), (**b**) folds are formed in some portions (× 330)

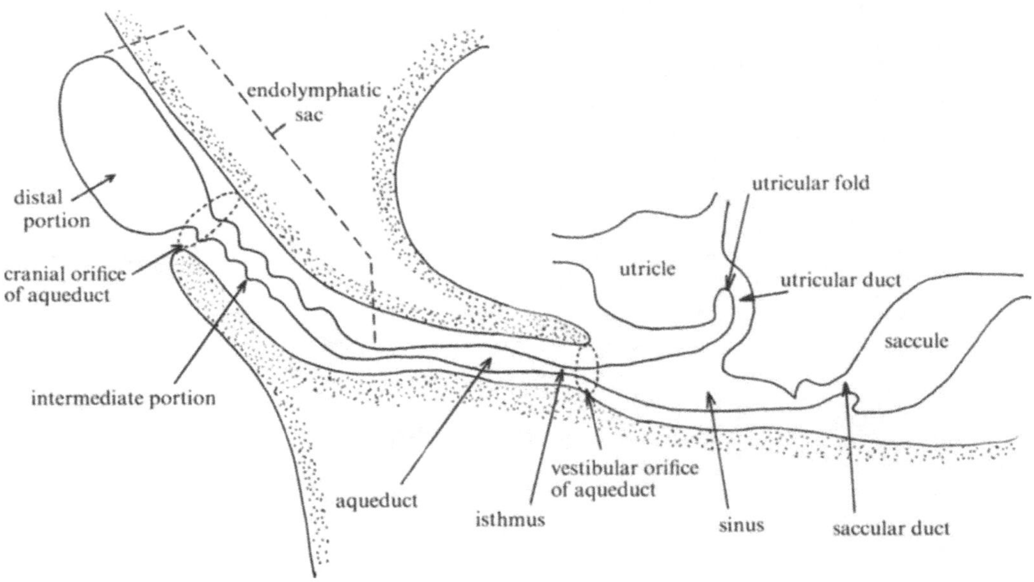

Figure 92 Schema of the endolymphatic sac (courtesy Drs Anson and Donaldson)

a

b

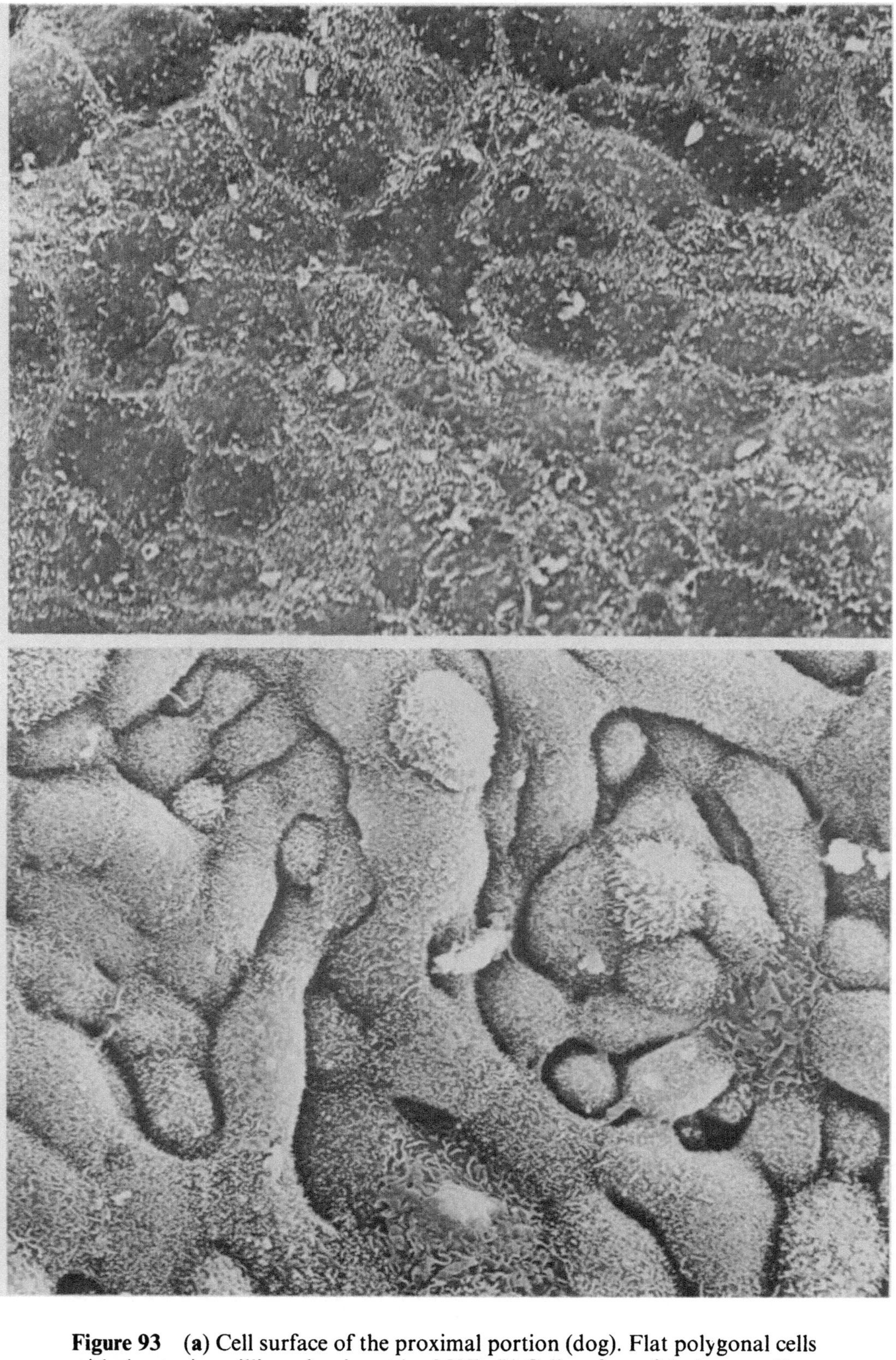

Figure 93 (**a**) Cell surface of the proximal portion (dog). Flat polygonal cells with short microvilli are dominant (× 2500). (**b**) Cell surface of the intermediate portion (dog). Two types of cells; light cells with a number of long microvilli and dark cells with short microvilli are observed (× 3000)

a

b

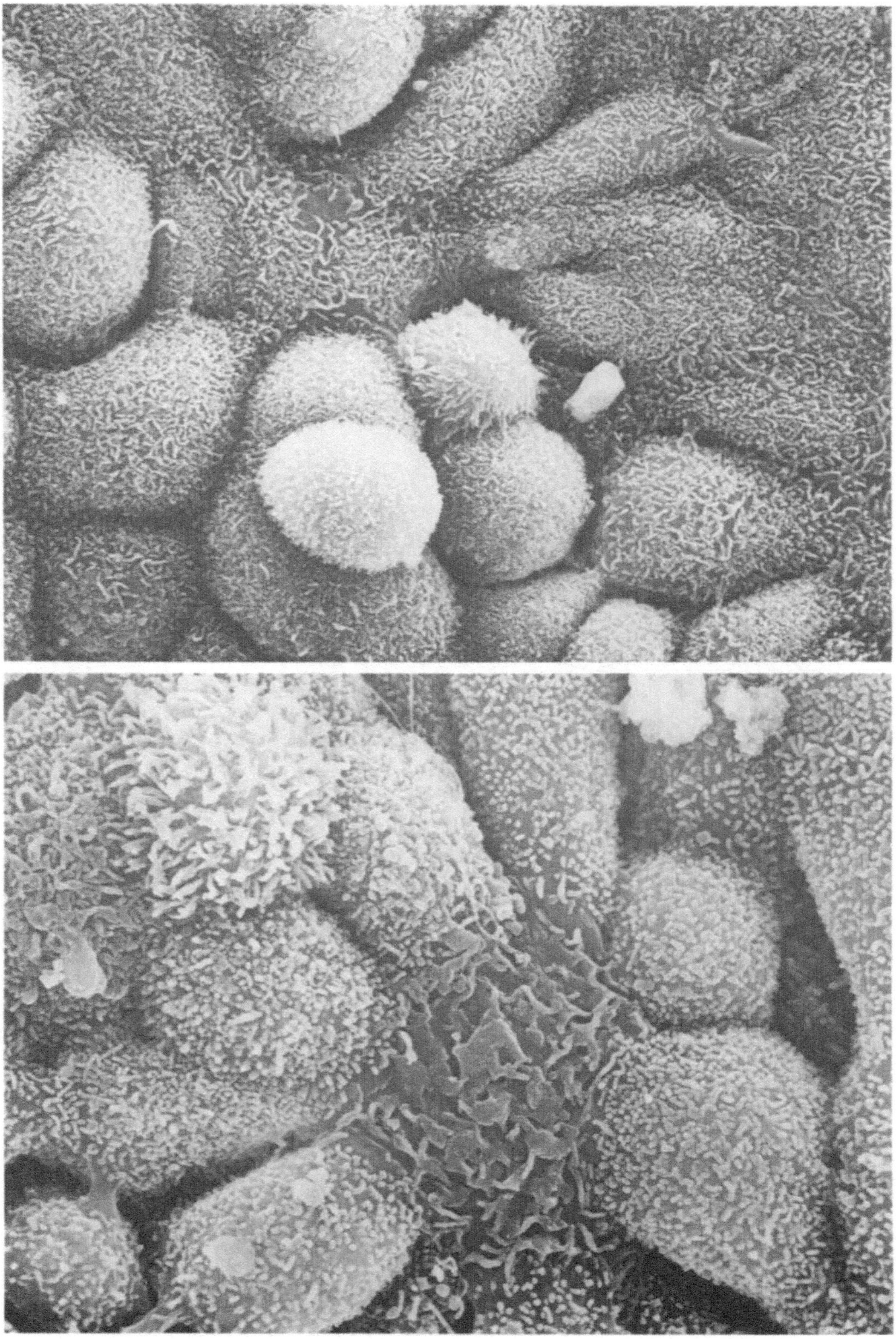

Figure 94 Cell surface of the intermediate portion (dog). (**a**) Light cells and dark cells are present (× 4500), (**b**) cells with bent microvilli are also found among the light and dark cells (× 8000)

a

b

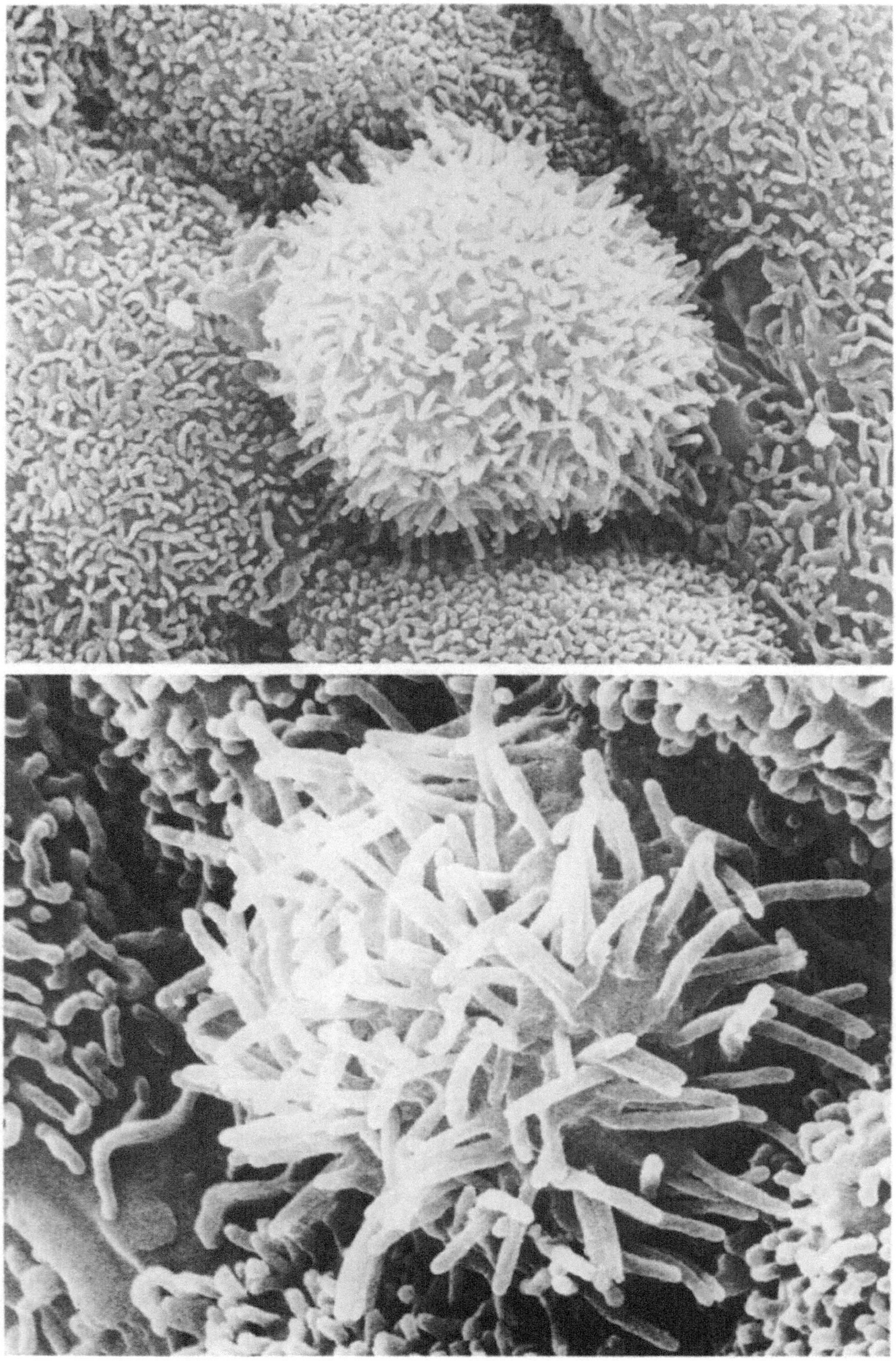

Figure 95 (**a**) Long microvilli on the light cell (× 12 000), (**b**) high magnification of light cell with long microvilli (× 30 000)

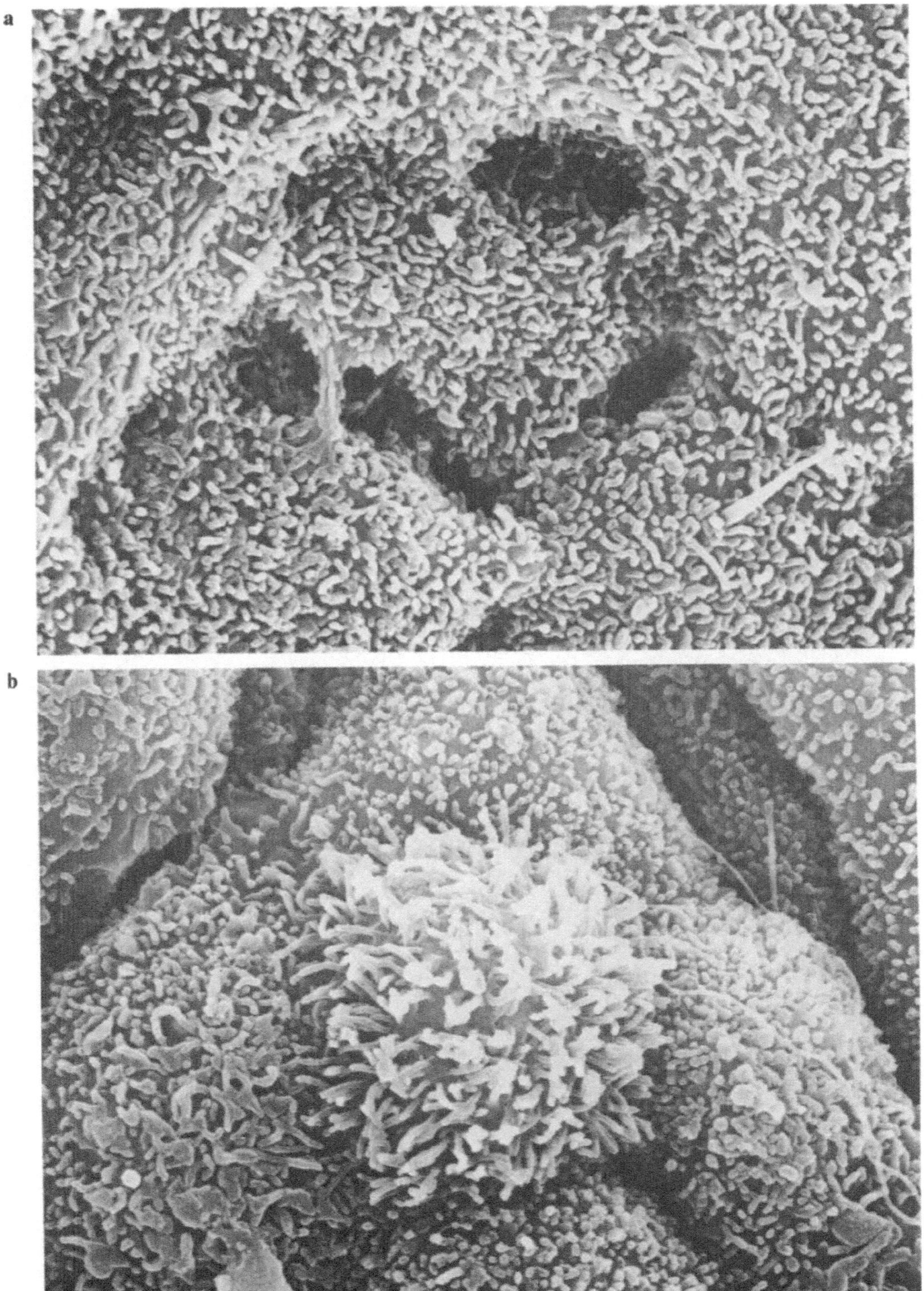

Figure 96 Cell surface of the intermediate portion (dog). (**a**) Clefts are occasionally observed (× 12 000), (**b**) some cells have microvilli with polypous bulging on top of them (× 12 000)

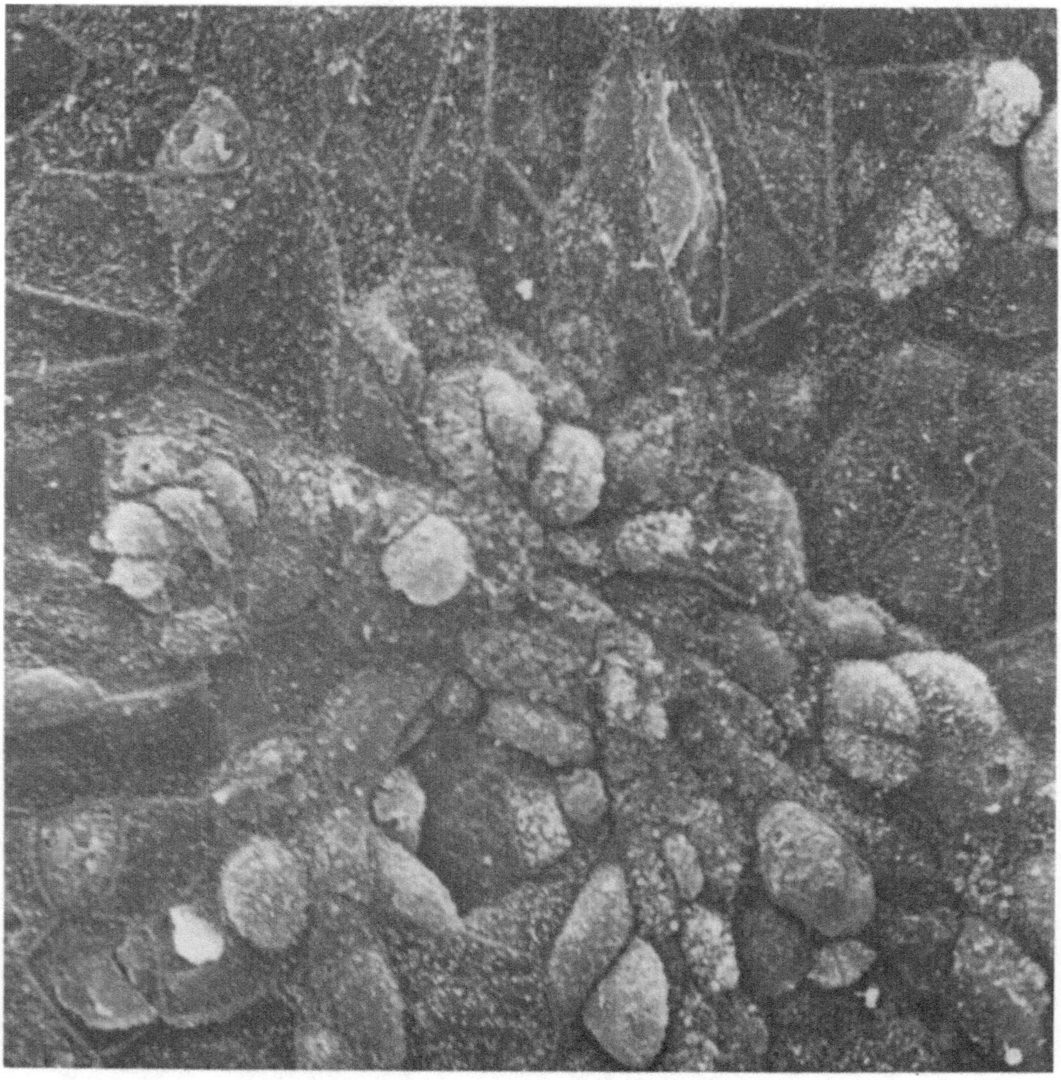

Figure 97 Endolymphatic sac (human). Borderline of the intermediate and distal portion. Dome-like cells form a papilla (× 1500)

a

b

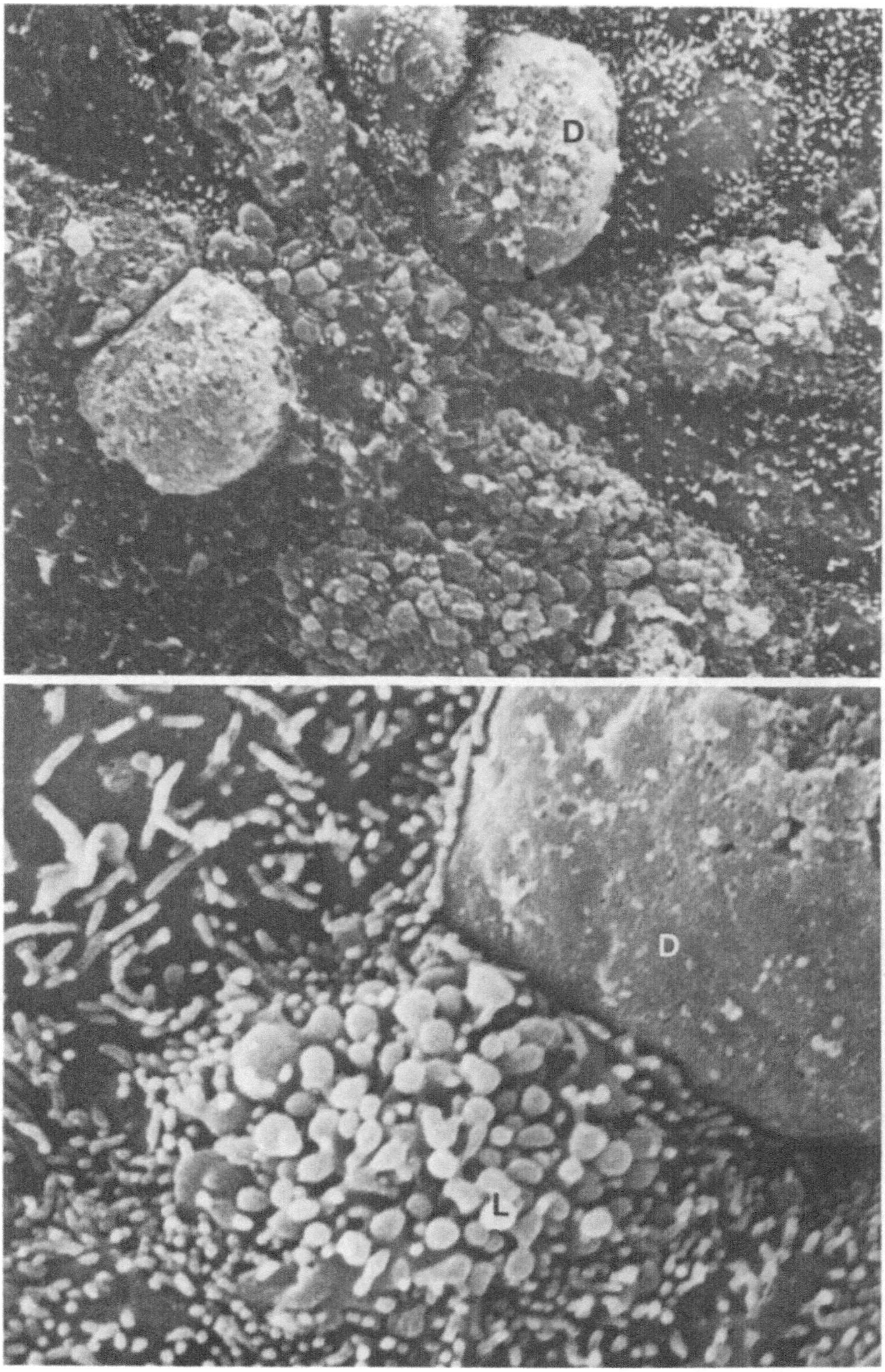

Figure 98 Endolymphatic sac (human). (**a**) Polyp-shaped microvilli and dome-like dark cells (D) are seen (× 4000), (**b**) high magnification of (a). The cell with polypous microvilli is a light cell (L) (× 13 000).

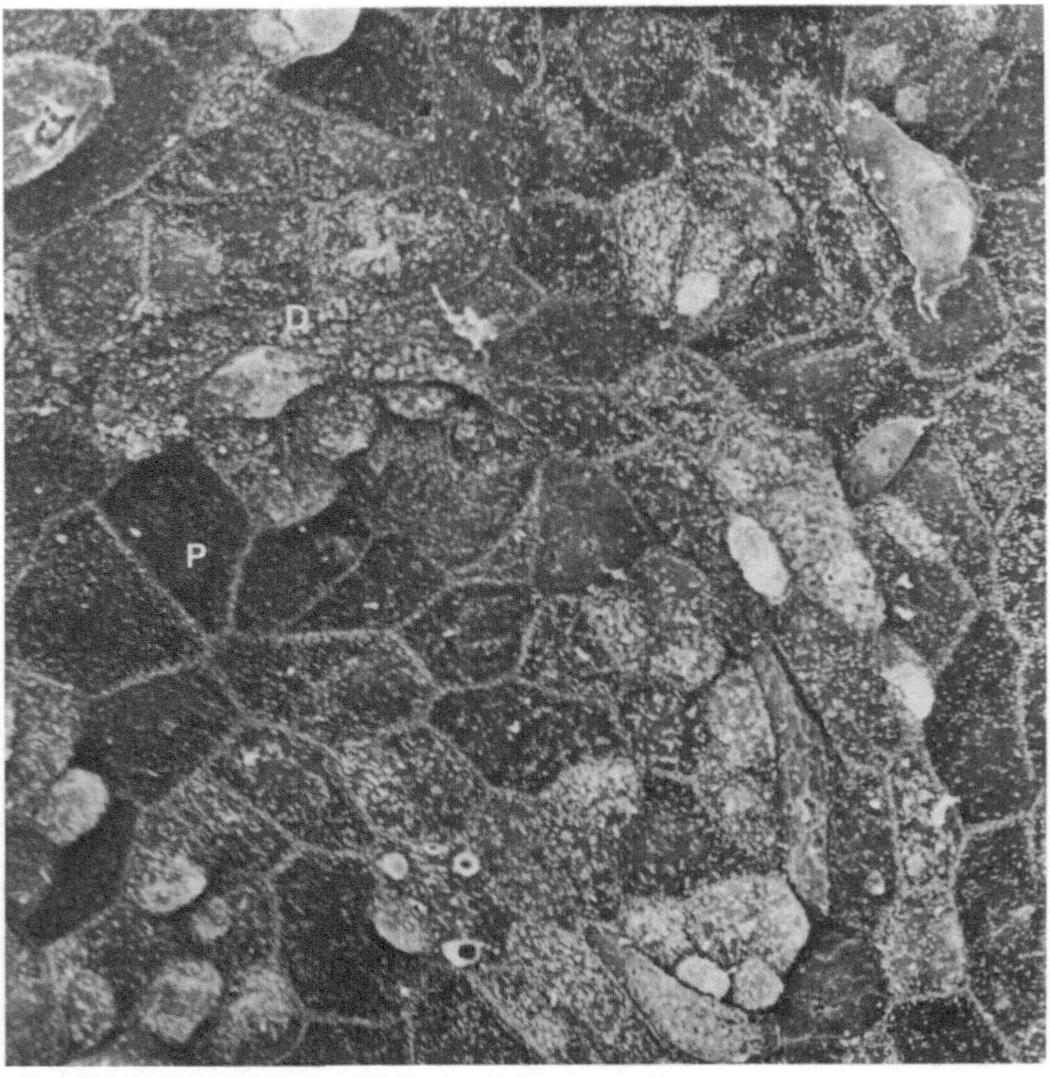

Figure 99 Endolymphatic sac (human). Cells found in the distal portion. Two kinds of cells, flat ones (P) with a few microvilli and dome-shaped ones (D) with more microvilli, are observed (× 1500)

The Cochlea

The organ of Corti

The sensory cells of the organ of Corti are outer hair cells of three to four rows and inner hair cells of a single row, which are fixed on the basal lamina by the supporting cells. The tectorial membrane extends to cover the hair cells and the Hensen's cell. At the bottom of the sensory cells, there are nerve endings.

The first order neurons of the cochlear nerve, which are the afferent fibres, run through the habenula perforata and two bony spiral laminae to reach the spiral ganglion cells. It is known that there are also efferent nerve fibres distributing to the sensory cells.

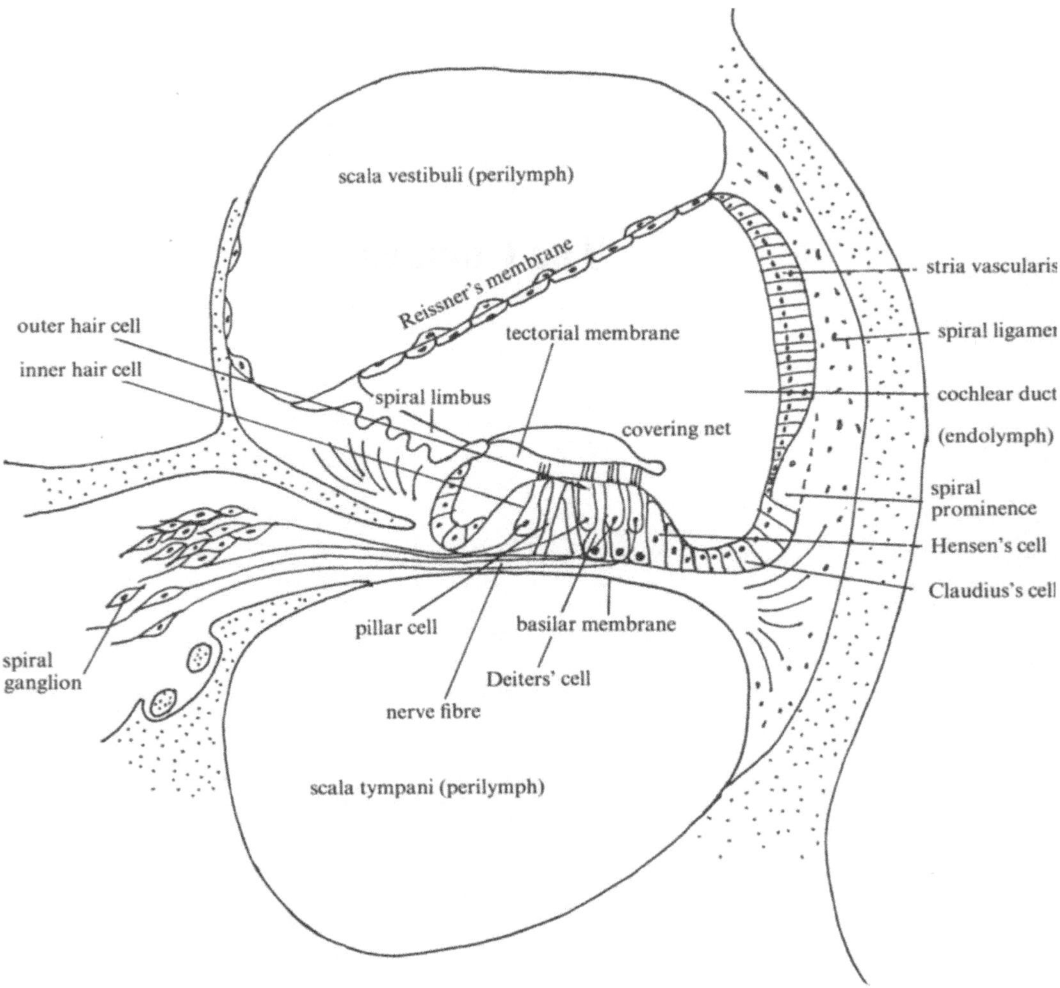

Figure 100 Schema of the cochlear duct

(1) *The outer hair cell*

The structure of the outer hair cells is considerably different from that of the inner hair cells. The outer hair cell is long and cylindrical in shape with a round or nearly pentagonal upper surface and a semiglobal lower portion. The space between the outer pillar cell and the first row of the outer hair cells is called Nuel's space. The space between Hensen's cell and the third row of the outer hair cells is the outer tunnel. The top layer of the outer hair cell is called the cuticular plate, or lamina. This part stains well, suggesting a dense structural substance (Iurato, 1961). On this cuticular plate, the auditory hairs are arranged in a W shape (Kolmer, 1927; Iurato, 1961; Engström *et al.*, 1962; Kimura, 1966). In the human or monkey, the W pattern is composed of four rows of the hairs. The hairs are longest in the outermost row, the cell bodies are shortest and the intracellular spaces are narrowest. Approaching the apex, the cell bodies become longer and the intracellular spaces wider. Also Hensen's cell bodies and the auditory hairs are longer in the more apical turn.

The rows of the outer hair cells usually number three at the basal turn; however, more than three rows are sometimes found in the upper turn. In the human cochlea, it is often seen that the upper middle portion of the basal turn already has the fourth row and the apical turn has even a fifth row (Hoshino, 1975, Kawabata, 1976).

(2) *The inner hair cell*

The inner hair cells are separated from the outer hair cells by Corti's tunnel which is formed by the inner and outer pillar cells. The cell body is shorter and thicker than the outer hair cells, taking a barrel shape. Unlike the outer hair cells, there is no intracellular space. The upper part of the cell touches the inner phalangeal process and the rest of the cell body is surrounded by the inner phalangeal cells. The inner hair cells have a cuticular plate and hairs like the outer cells; however, the hairs are shorter and are arranged in flat W shape. The cell body is light and its height does not vary as much according to the turn of the cochlea as the outer hair cell does. An extra hair cell row is very seldom seen.

References

1. Engström, H. *et al.* (1962). Structure and functions of the sensory hairs of the inner ear. *J. Acoust. Soc. Am.*, **34,** 1356

2. Hoshino, T. (1975). The structure of the cochlea. *Otolaryngology (Tokyo)*, **47,** 951
3. Iurato, S. (1961). Submicroscopic structure of the membranous labyrinth. II. The epithelium of Corti's organ. *Z. Zellforsch.*, **53,** 259
4. Kimura, R. S. (1966). Hairs of the cochlear sensory cells and their attachment to the tectorial membrane. *Acta Otolaryngol. (Stockholm)* **61,** 55
5. Kolmer, W. (1927). Gehörorgan. In Möllendorff, W. (ed.). *Handbuch der Mikroskopischen Anatomie des Menschen.* p. 250

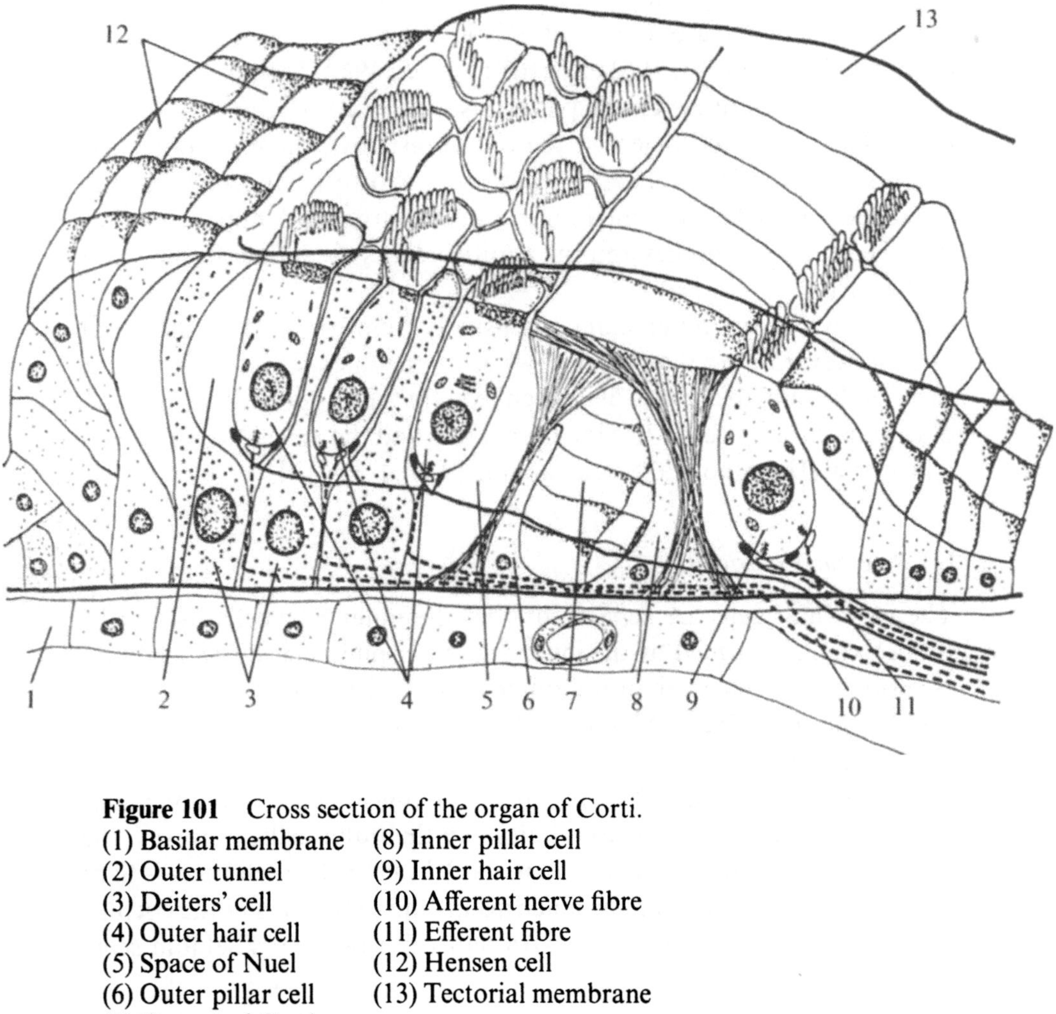

Figure 101 Cross section of the organ of Corti.

(1) Basilar membrane	(8) Inner pillar cell
(2) Outer tunnel	(9) Inner hair cell
(3) Deiters' cell	(10) Afferent nerve fibre
(4) Outer hair cell	(11) Efferent fibre
(5) Space of Nuel	(12) Hensen cell
(6) Outer pillar cell	(13) Tectorial membrane
(7) Tunnel of Corti	

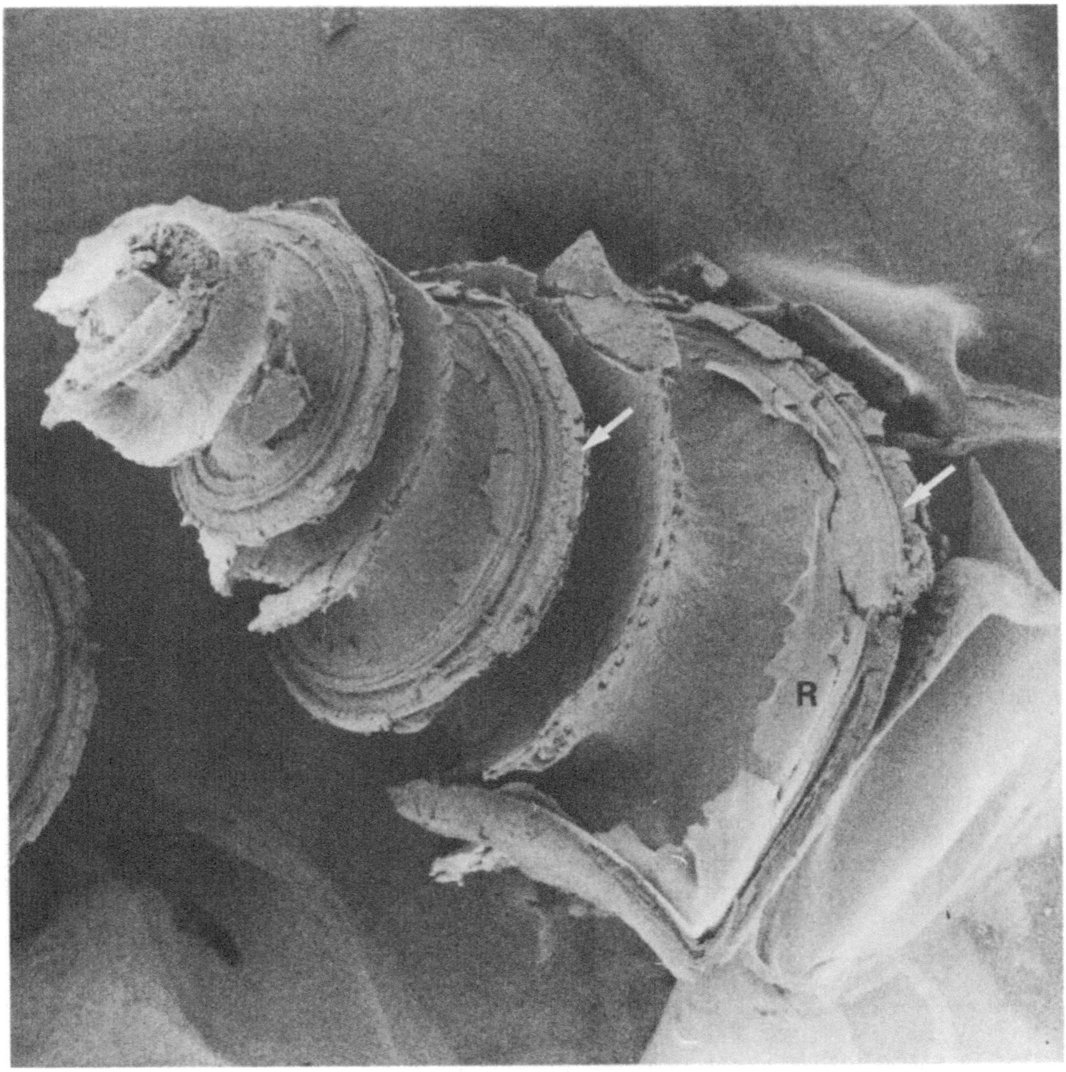

Figure 102 Cochlea (guinea pig). Four turns of the guinea pig's cochlea are exposed. R: Reissner's membrane; arrow: the location of the organ of Corti (× 45)

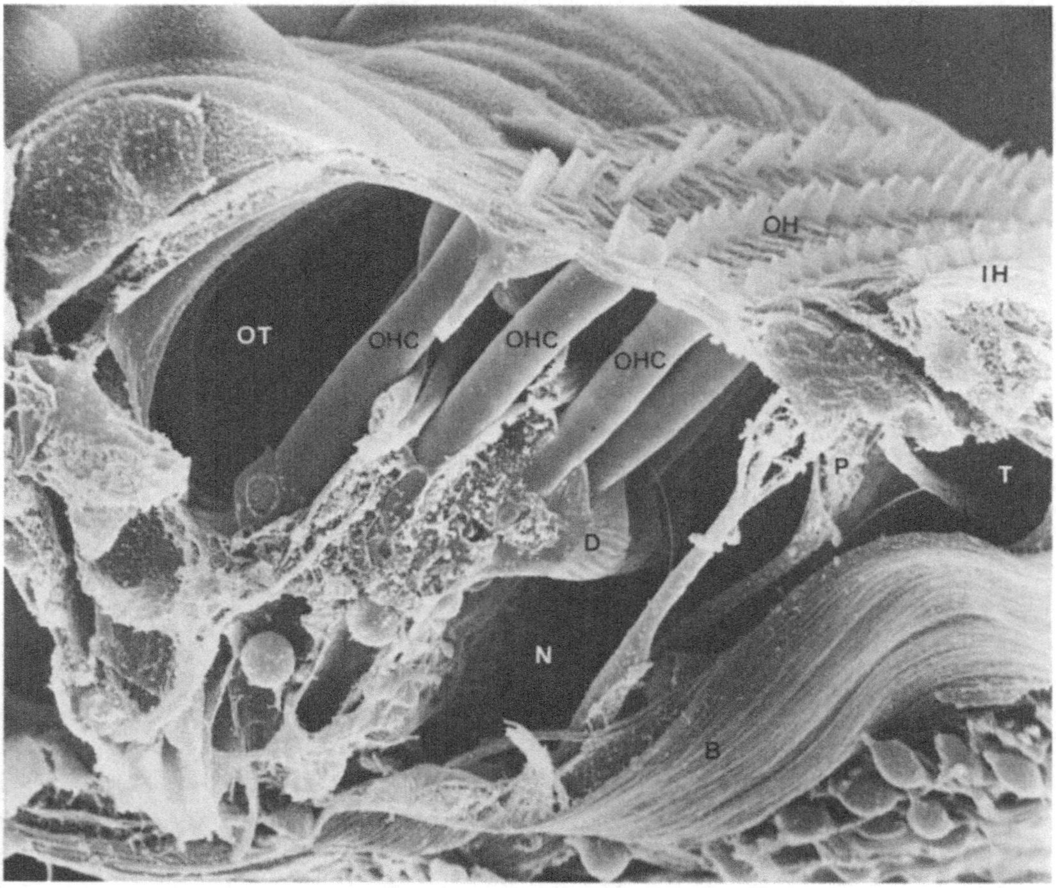

Figure 103 Cracked organ of Corti (guinea pig). IH: inner hair; OH: outer hair; N: Nuel's space; OT: outer tunnel; P: outer pillar cell; OHC: outer hair cell; D: Deiters' cell; T: tunnel of Corti; B: basilar membrane; (courtesy G. Bredberg) (× 1700)

a

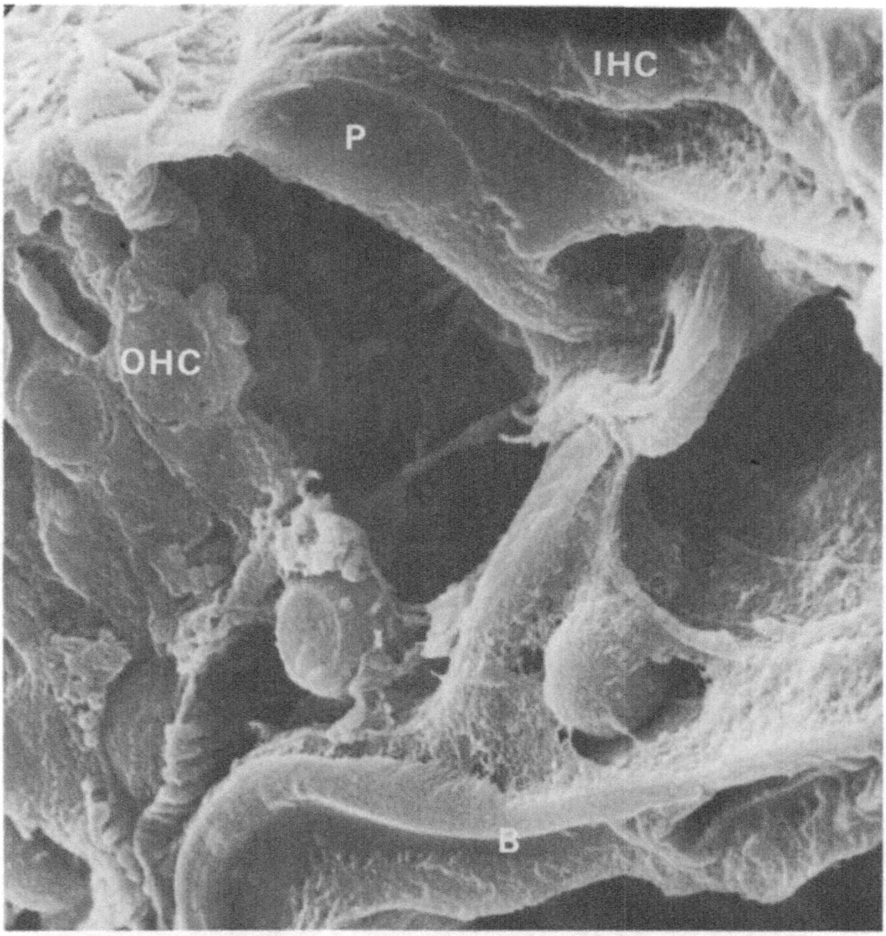

b

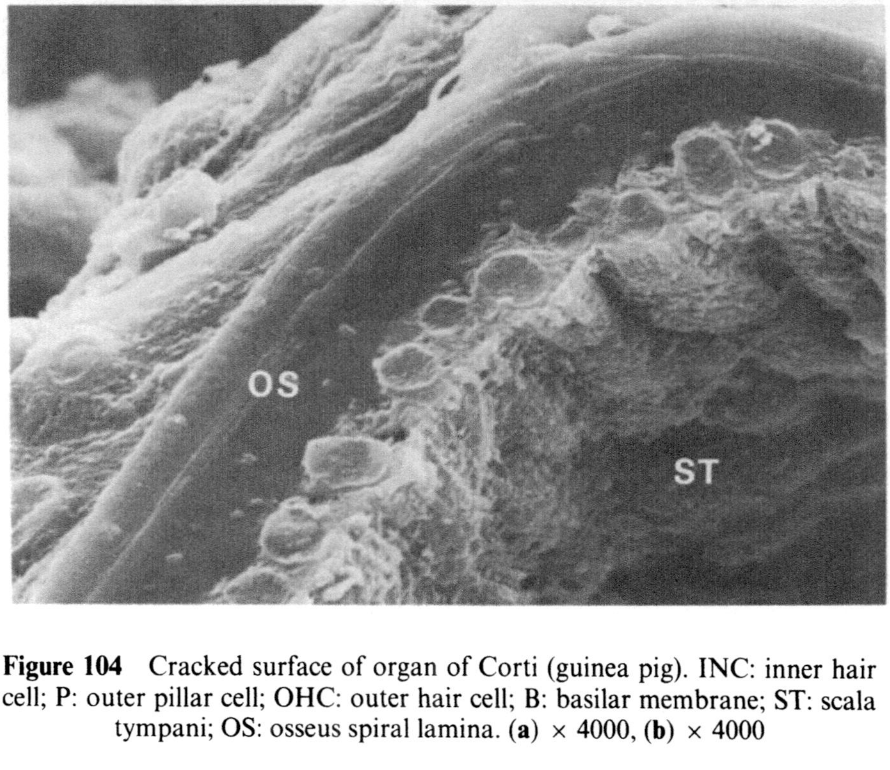

Figure 104 Cracked surface of organ of Corti (guinea pig). INC: inner hair cell; P: outer pillar cell; OHC: outer hair cell; B: basilar membrane; ST: scala tympani; OS: osseus spiral lamina. (**a**) × 4000, (**b**) × 4000

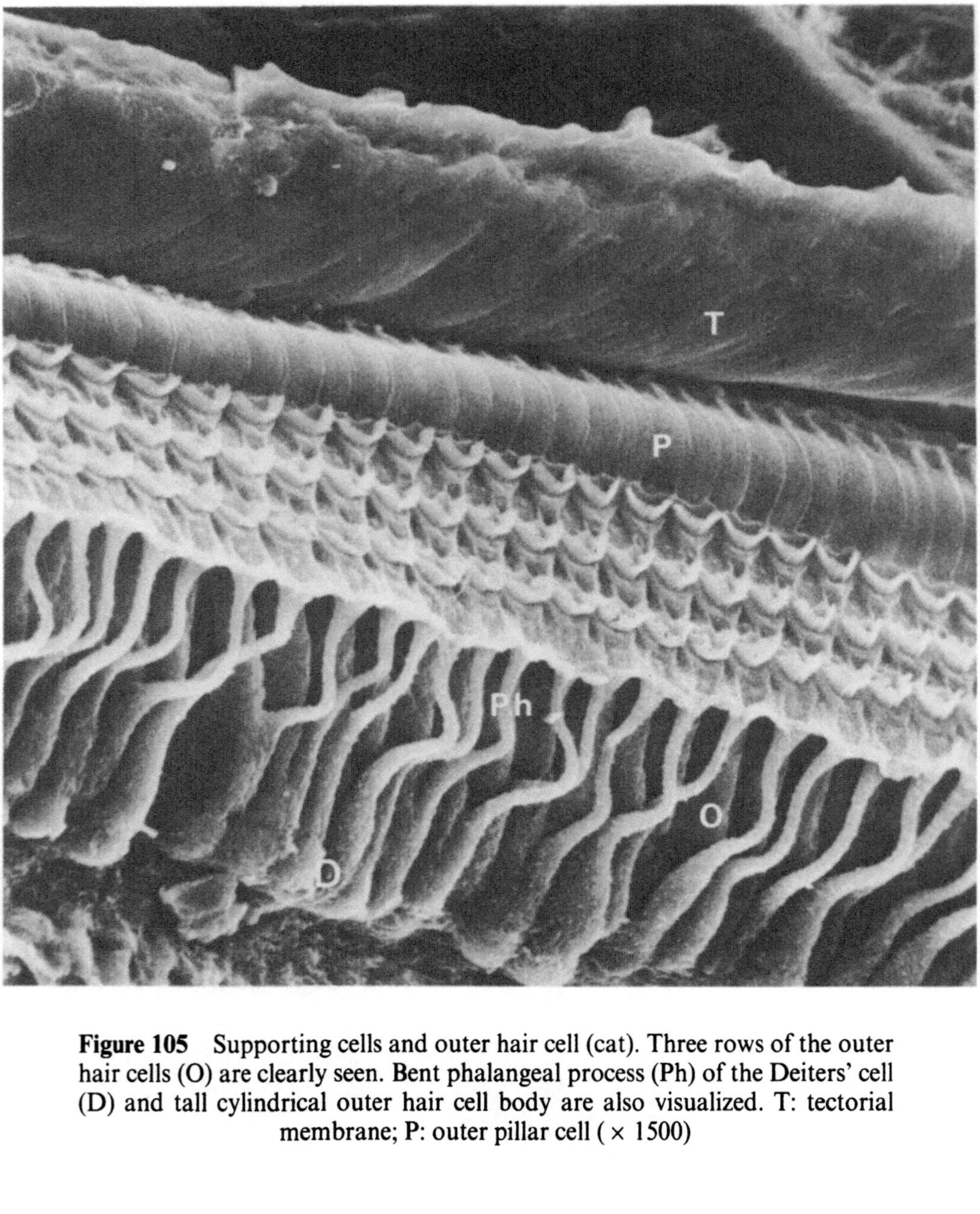

Figure 105 Supporting cells and outer hair cell (cat). Three rows of the outer hair cells (O) are clearly seen. Bent phalangeal process (Ph) of the Deiters' cell (D) and tall cylindrical outer hair cell body are also visualized. T: tectorial membrane; P: outer pillar cell (× 1500)

Figure 106 The outer hair cell and the supporting cell (cat). O: outer hair cell; D: Deiters' cell; Ph: phalangeal process of Deiters' cell. (**a**) × 4500, (**b**) × 4500

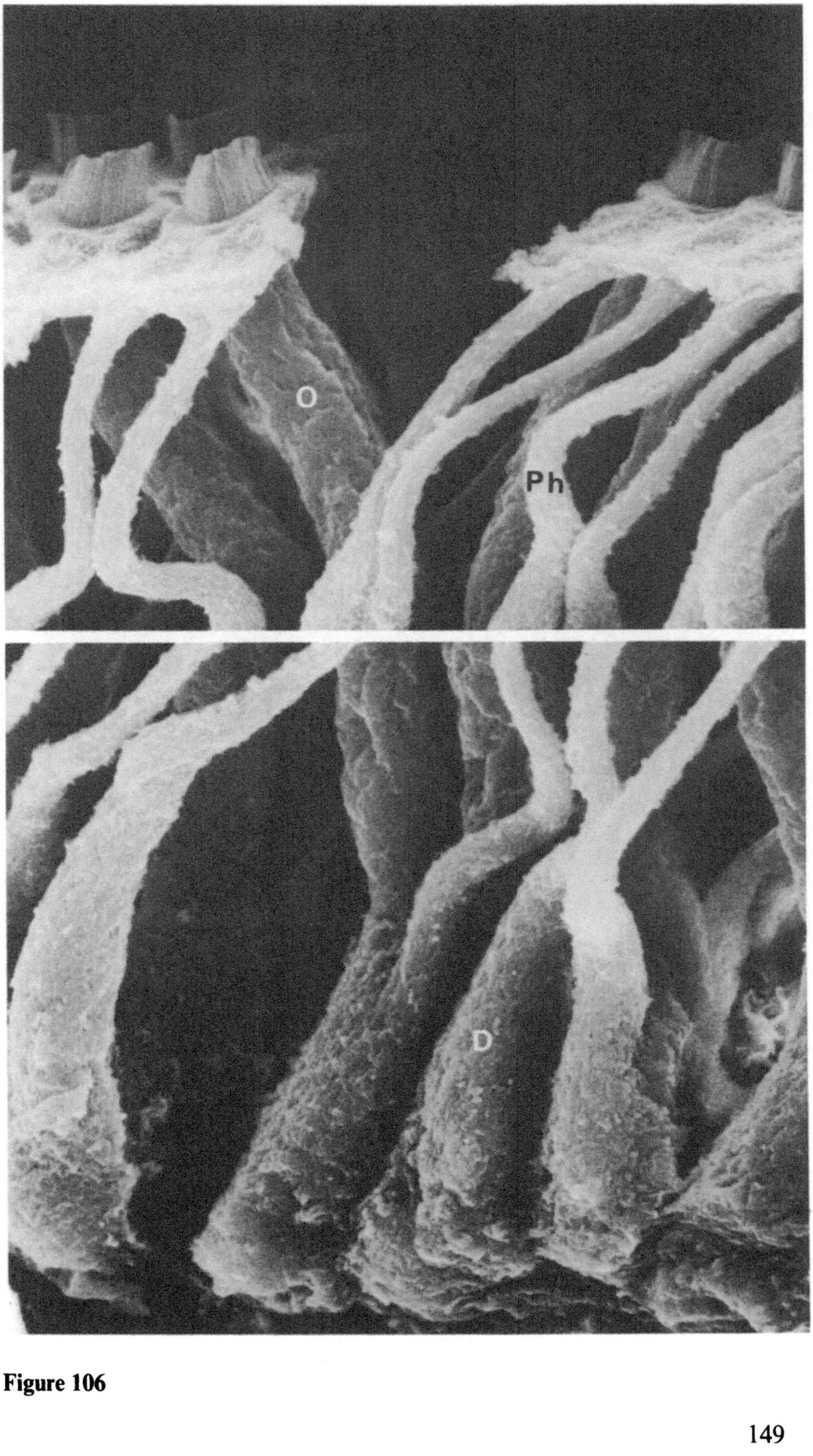

Figure 106

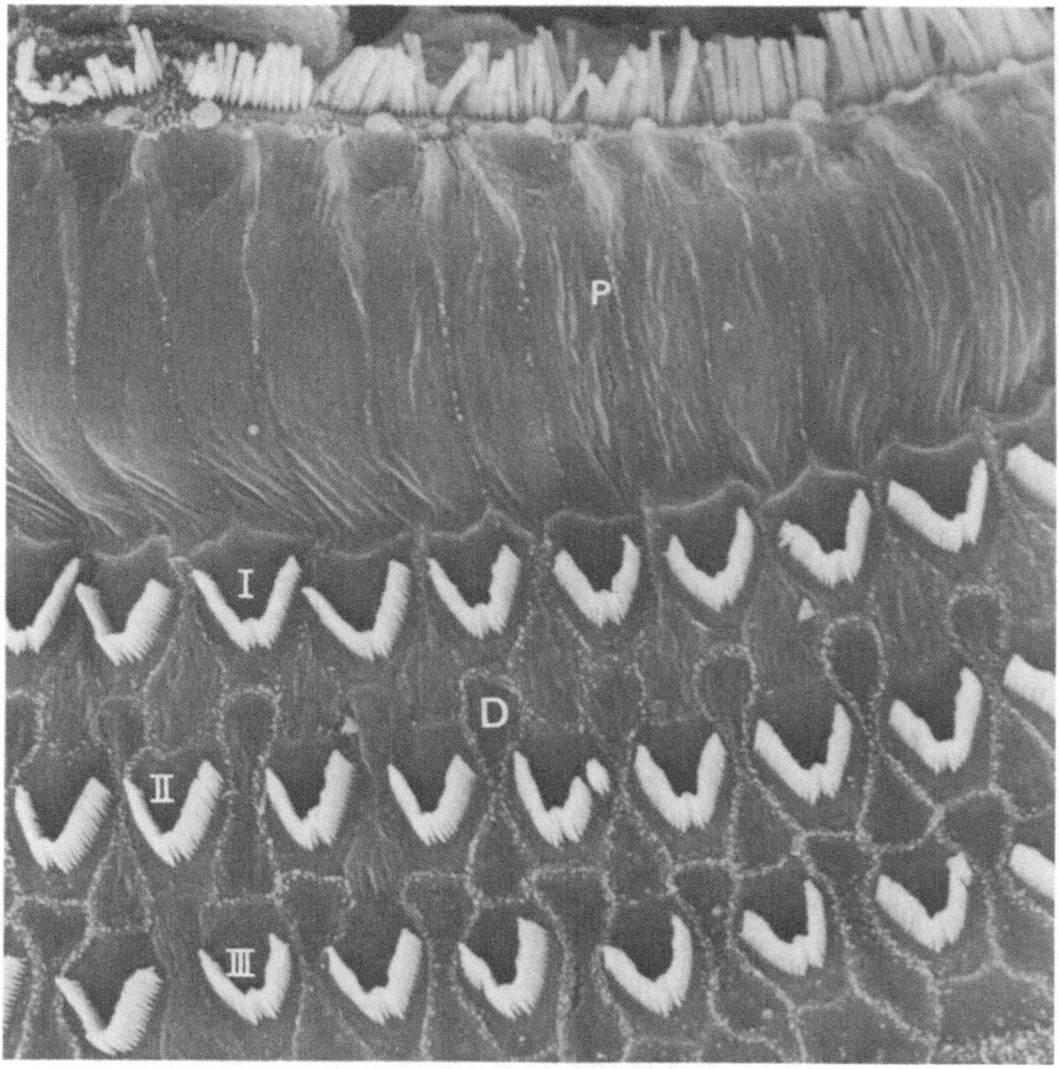

Figure 107 Inner and outer hair cell surface (rabbit). The single row of the inner hair cells and three rows (I, II, III) of the outer hair cells are arranged clearly. Outer hair cell cilia make W-shaped pattern. Top of phalangeal process (D) is dumb-bell-shaped. P: outer pillar cell (× 2200)

Figure 108 (**a**) The same specimen as Figure 107 (× 4500), (**b**) high magnification of the outer hair cell cilia. In rabbit each W-shaped arrangement of the outer hair cell cilia is composed of three rows of the cilia. D: top of phalangeal process (× 9000)

a

b

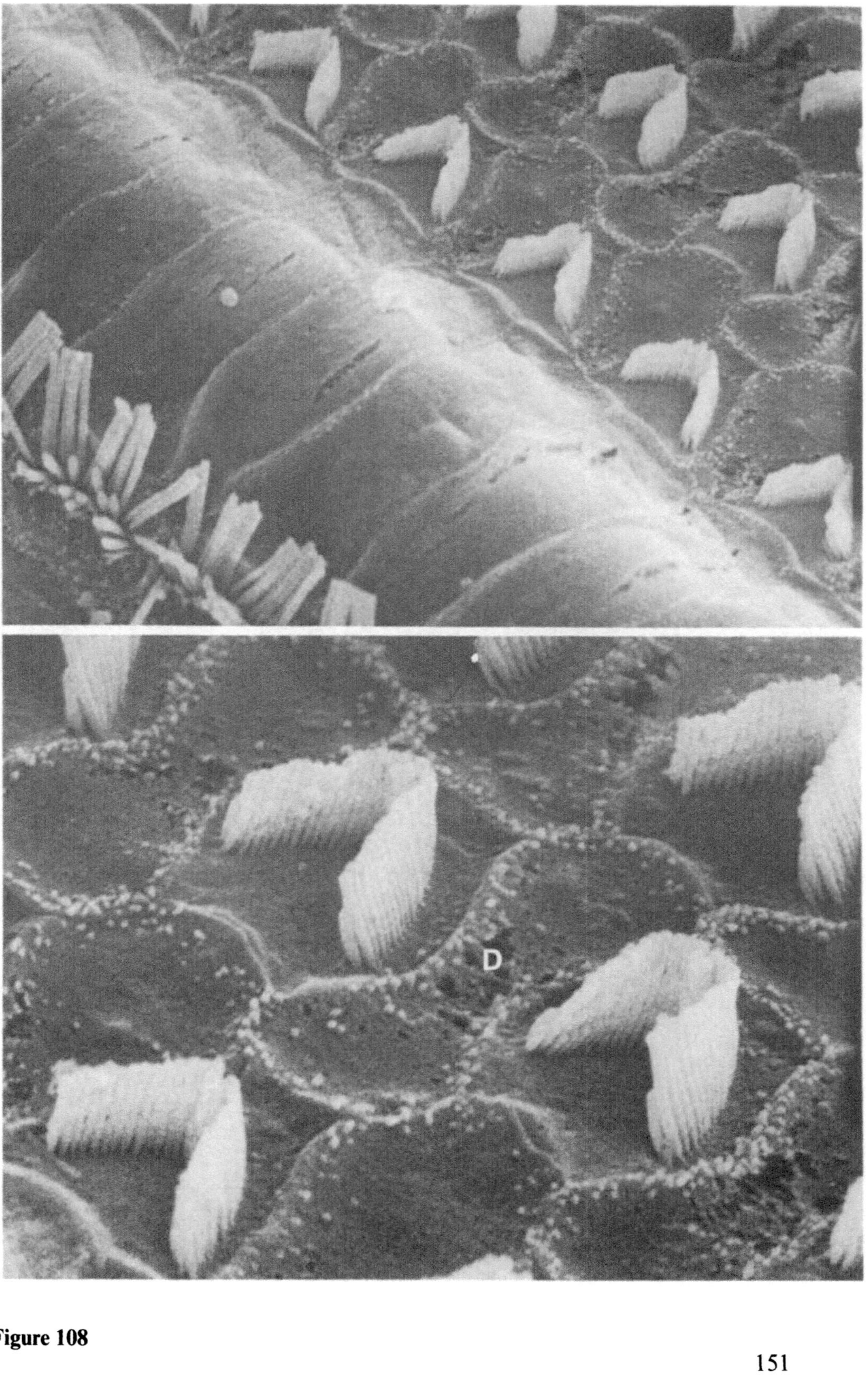

Figure 108

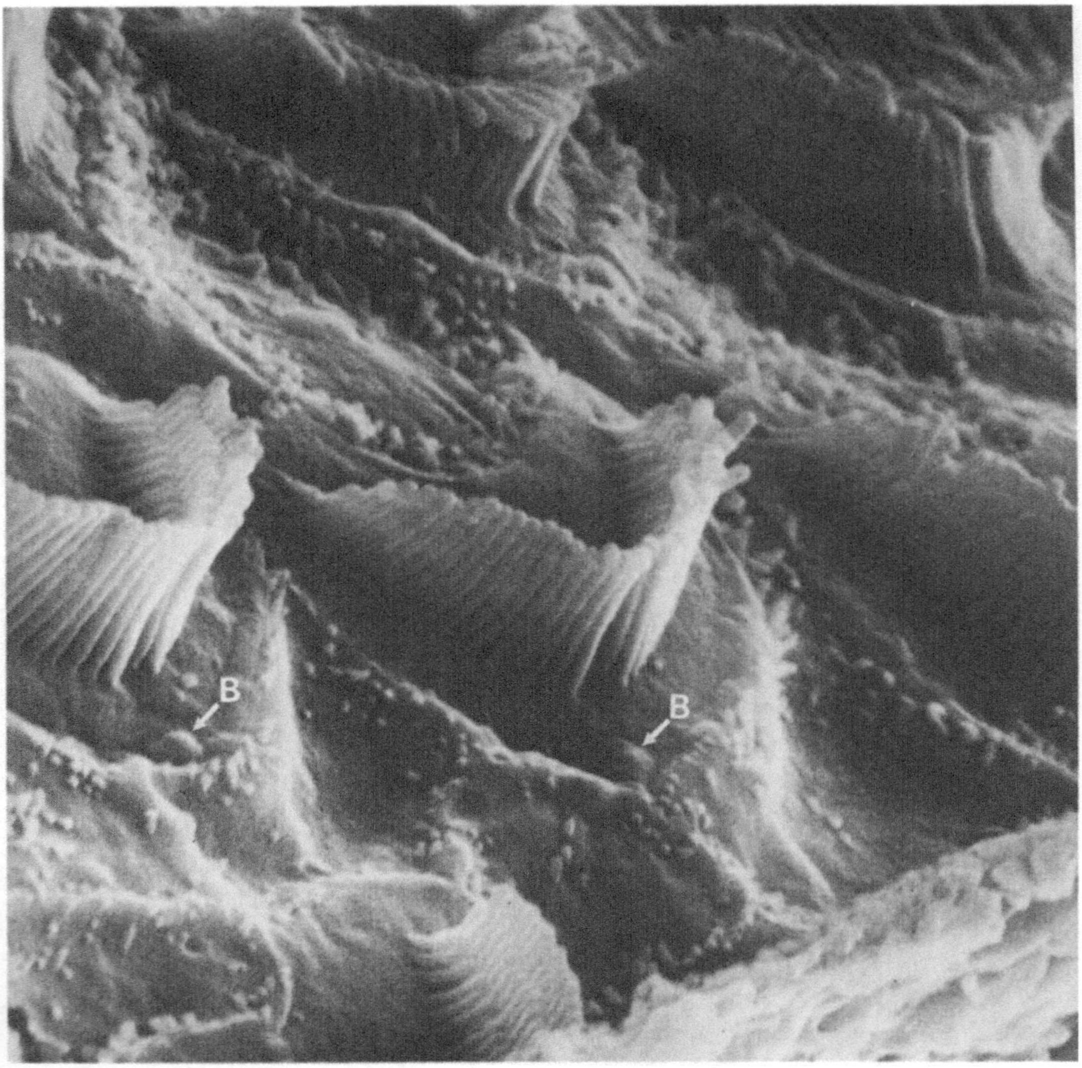

Figure 109 Surface of the outer hair cell (guinea pig). B: basal body (×15 000)

Figure 110 Cochlea (monkey). (**a**) The apical and second turns (× 100), (**b**) tall outer hair cell cilia of the apical turn. Tall cilia are arranged in three rows. Intracellular distance is short (× 1200)

a

b

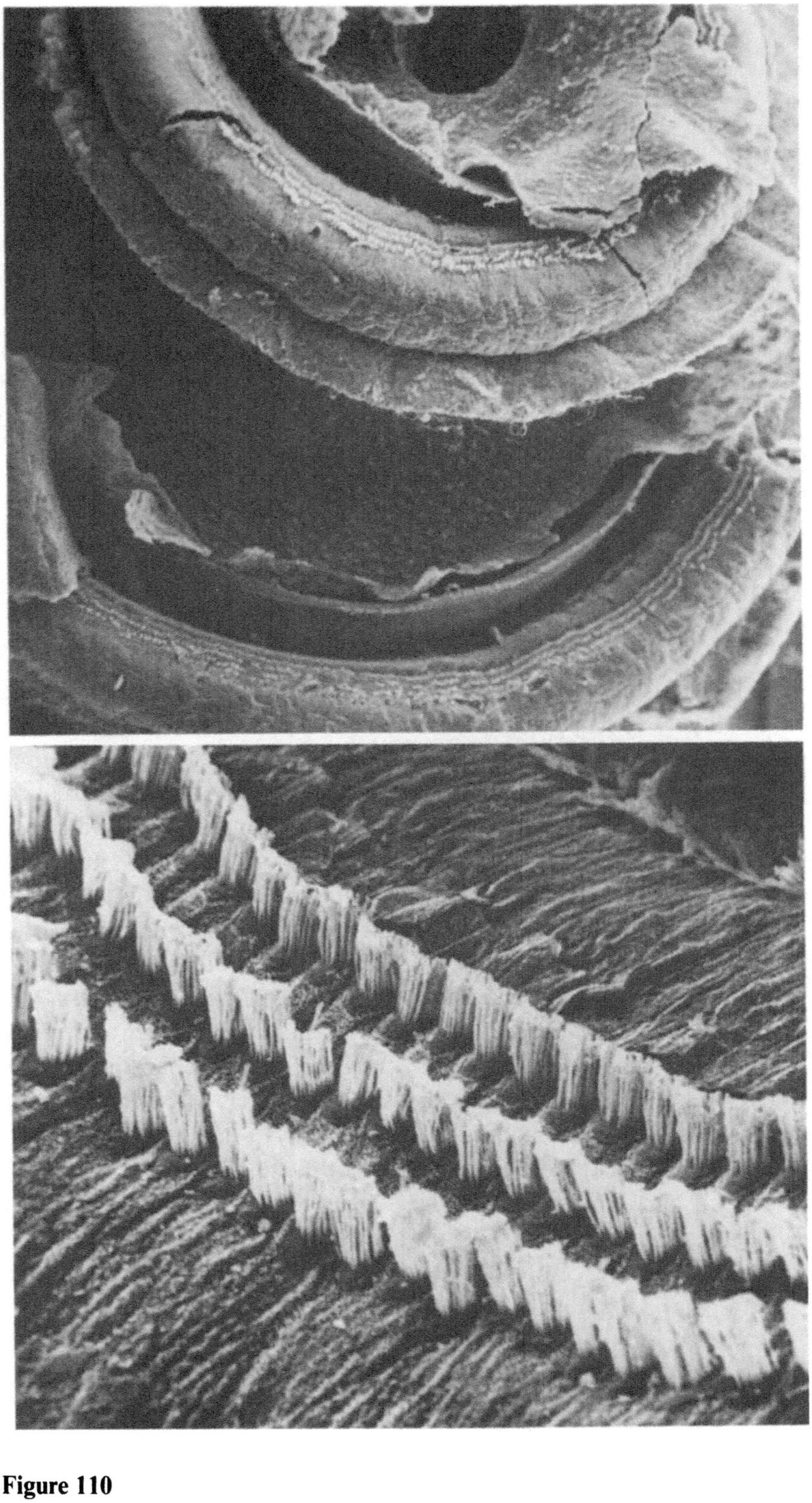

Figure 110

The outer and the inner hairs

Both outer and inner hairs are rod-shaped, tapering toward the root. They are arranged in steps from the shorter to the longer hairs. The number of steps of outer hairs is four or five in the human and monkey and three in the guinea pig, rabbit, dog and cat. The inner hairs are in two to four steps in most animals.

The outer hairs make a W-shaped arrangement in the basal turn but in the upper turn, they show a V pattern rather than a W. The inner hairs have only two steps in the lower basal turn, but four steps in the upper turn. Also they become longer in the upper turn.

The tectorial membrane

The tectorial membrane is divided into two layers, the upper and the lower layer. The upper layer is rich in fine radiating fibres and is thus also called the fibrous layer. Some of the fibres run longitudinally. Thicker fibres wind on the outer surface of the fibrous layer, creating a mesh pattern. The lower layer is called the granular layer and consists of a gelatin substance.

The tectorial membrane is divided into three zones, inner, middle and outer zones, at the plane vertical to the modiolus. The inner zone is above the spiral lamina and composed of sparse fibrous tissue and an uneven substance. The middle zone is located above the organ of Corti and is the widest. The outer zone includes the outer margin and is made of a dense substance. The outer margin appears separated from the Deiters' cell under the light microscope; however, electronmicroscopic study reveals that it touches the Deiters' cell. In the upper turn close to the helicotrema, the outer margin also touches the Hensen's cell. The marginal part which touches the Deiters' cell often forms a network, which is called the border plexus, or the marginal net.

The lower surface of the tectorial membrane has a layer of a dense substance at the border of the inner and the middle zone. This part is called the Hensen's stripe, and corresponds to the position of the inner hair cells. In the lower surface of the tectorial membrane, there are impressions where tops of the outer hairs reach. These outer hairs are the longest ones which form the outermost row of the W-shaped arrangement, thus making a W-shaped imprint on the tectorial membrane (Kimura, 1966; Iurato, 1976; Lindeman, 1971; Lim, 1972; Tanaka *et al.*, 1973). Granular substance accumulates in the area of the imprint and forms layers of high electron density. There is no imprint on the tectorial membrane above the inner hairs. Instead, the longest inner hairs touch the Hensen's stripe. Hoshino (1974, 1975) reported the insertion of the inner hairs into the tectorial membrane in a 10-day old kitten and the imprint of the inner hairs in the lower turn of an adult cat.

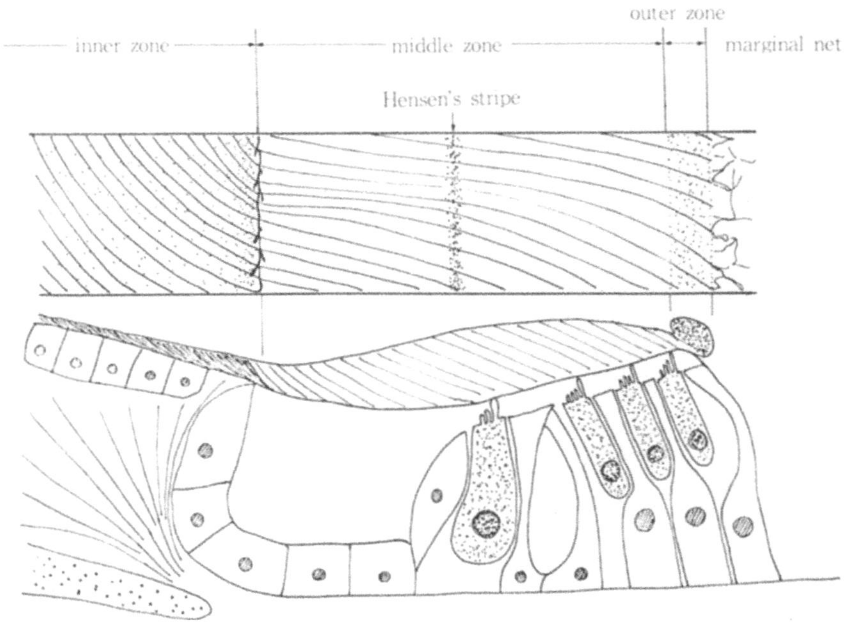

Figure 111 Schema of the tectorial membrane

References

1. Hoshino, T. (1974). Relationship of the tectorial membrane to the organ of Corti. A scanning electron microscopic study of cats and guinea pigs. *Arch. Histol. Japan.*, **37,** 25
2. Iurato, S. (1976). Organ of Corti. In *Submicroscopic structure of the inner ear*. p. 91. (Oxford: Pergamon)
3. Kimura, R. (1966). Hairs of the cochlear sensory cells and their attachment to the tectorial membrane. *Acta Otolaryngol.* (*Stockholm*), **61,** 55
4. Lim, D. (1972). Fine morphology of the tectorial membrane. Its relationship to the organ of Corti. *Arch. Otolaryngol.* **96,** 199
5. Lindeman, H. H., Ades, H. W., Bredberg, G. and Engström, H. (1971). The sensory hairs and the tectorial membrane in the development of the cat's organ of Corti. *Acta Otolaryngol.* (*Stockholm*), **72,** 229
6. Tanaka, T., Kosaka, N., Takiguchi, T. and Takahara, S. (1973). Observation on the cochlea with SEM. *Scanning Electron Microscopy*, **III,** 427

Figure 112 Outer and inner hair cell cilia (monkey). (**a**) Outer hair cell cilia of the basal turn. W-shaped sensory cilia are composed of four rows. There are approximately 130–140 cilia in a single W which shows a relatively wide tip angle (× 12 600). (**b**) Outer hair cell cilia of the second turn which shows a slightly narrower angle of W arrangement (× 12 600). (**c**) Outer hair cell cilia of the apical turn. The cilia arrangement is narrow V-shaped rather than W with tall outermost cilia (× 12 600). (**d**) Inner hair cell cilia of the basal turn. The cilia form two linear rows (× 8400). (**e**) Inner sensory cilia of the second turn. Cilia increase in number. There are more cilia in this turn than the basal, thus forming four rows (× 12 600). (**f**) Inner sensory cilia of the apical turn. The cilia are arranged in a wide V, showing tall outermost cilia (× 12 600)

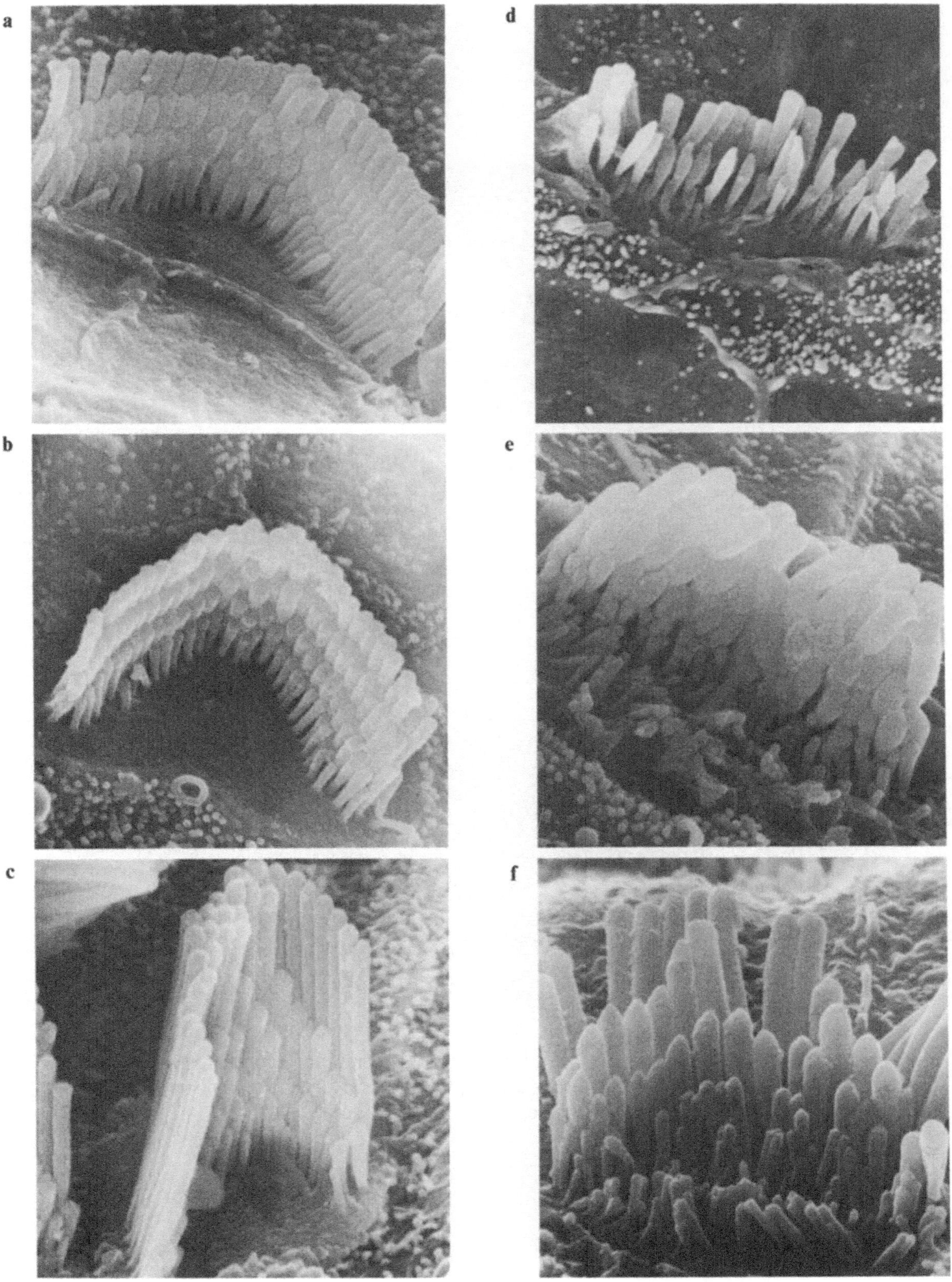

Figure 112

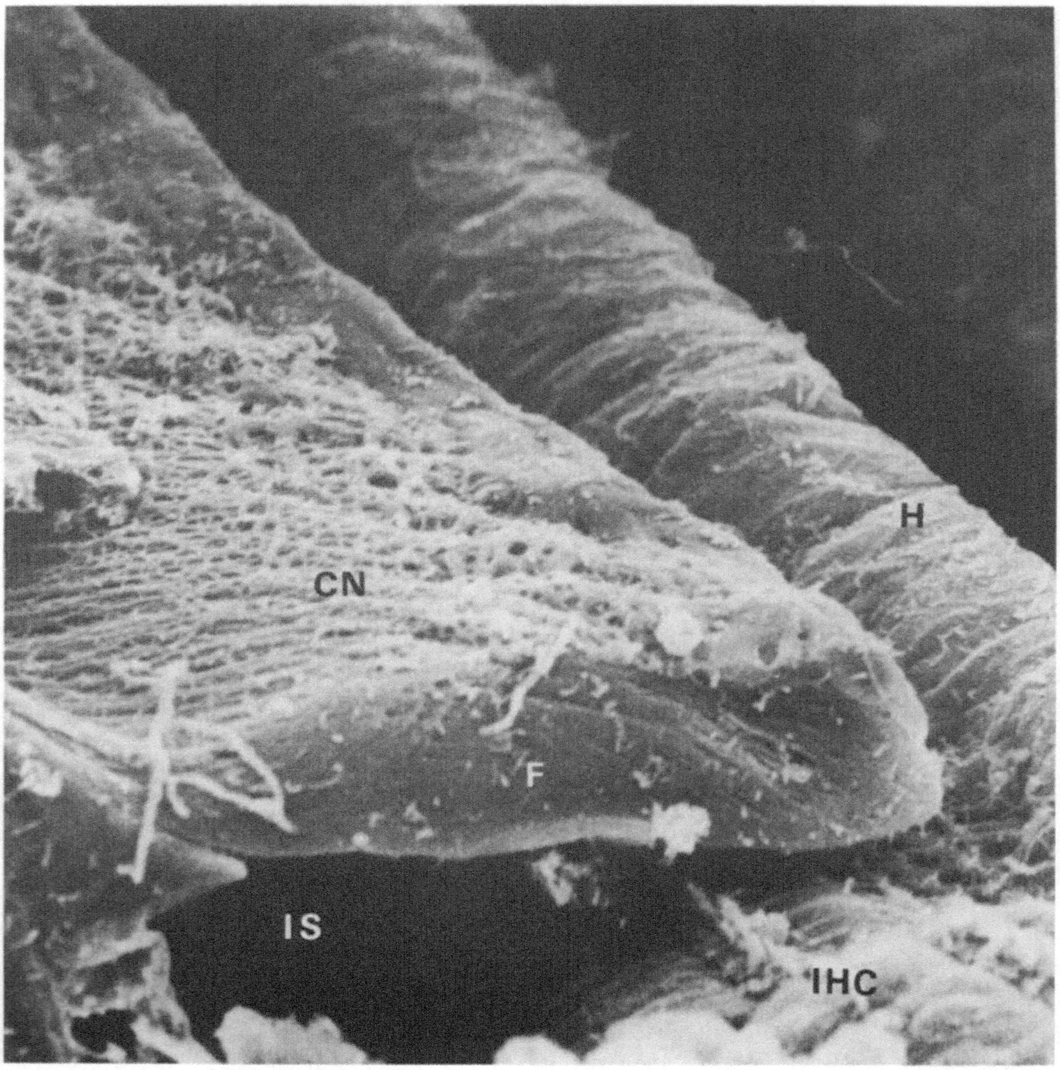

Figure 113 Cracked surface of the tectorial membrane (guinea pig). CN: cover net (surface of the fibrous layers); F: fibrous layer; H: Hensen's cell; IS: internal spiral sulcus; IHC: inner hair cell (× 900)

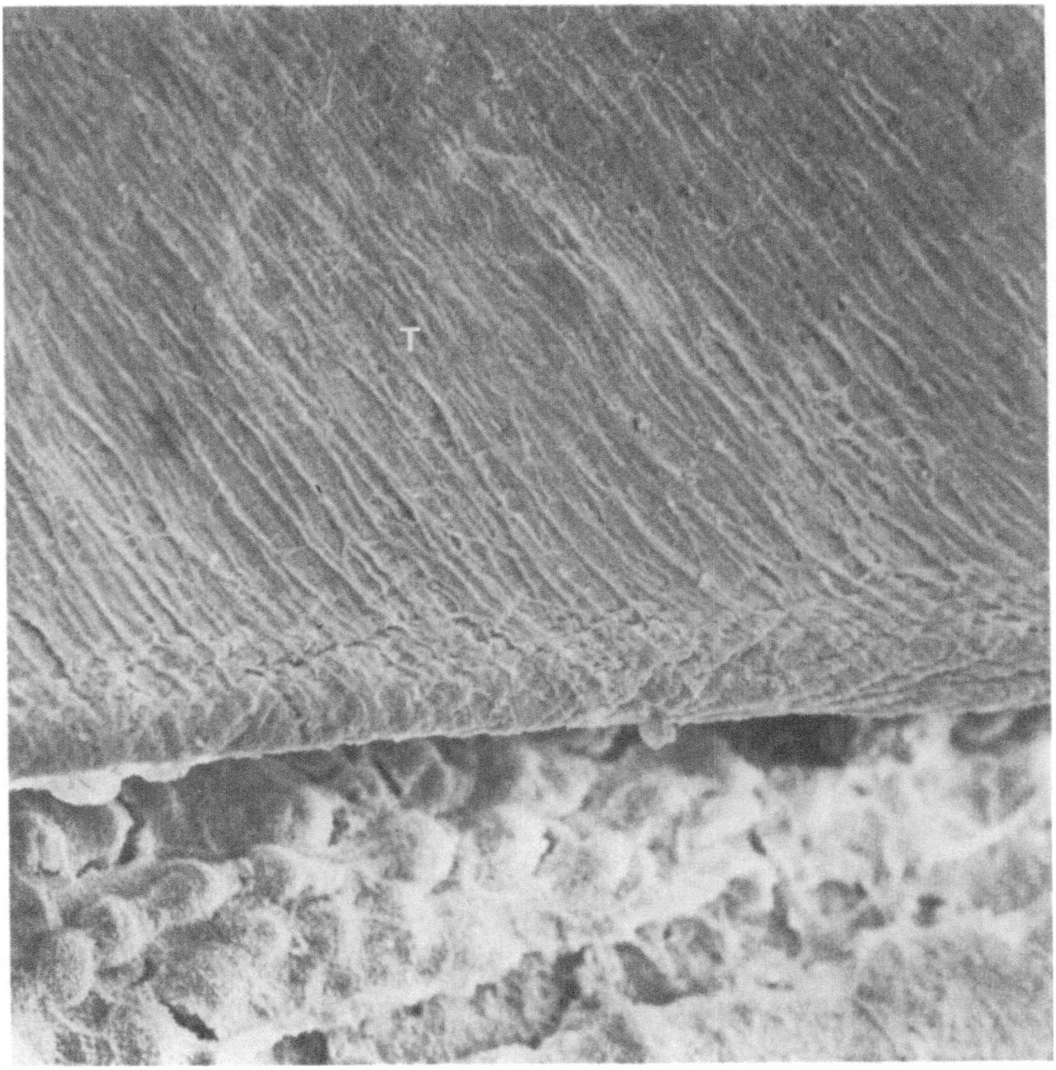

Figure 114 Surface of the tectorial membrane (T) (monkey) (× 1500)

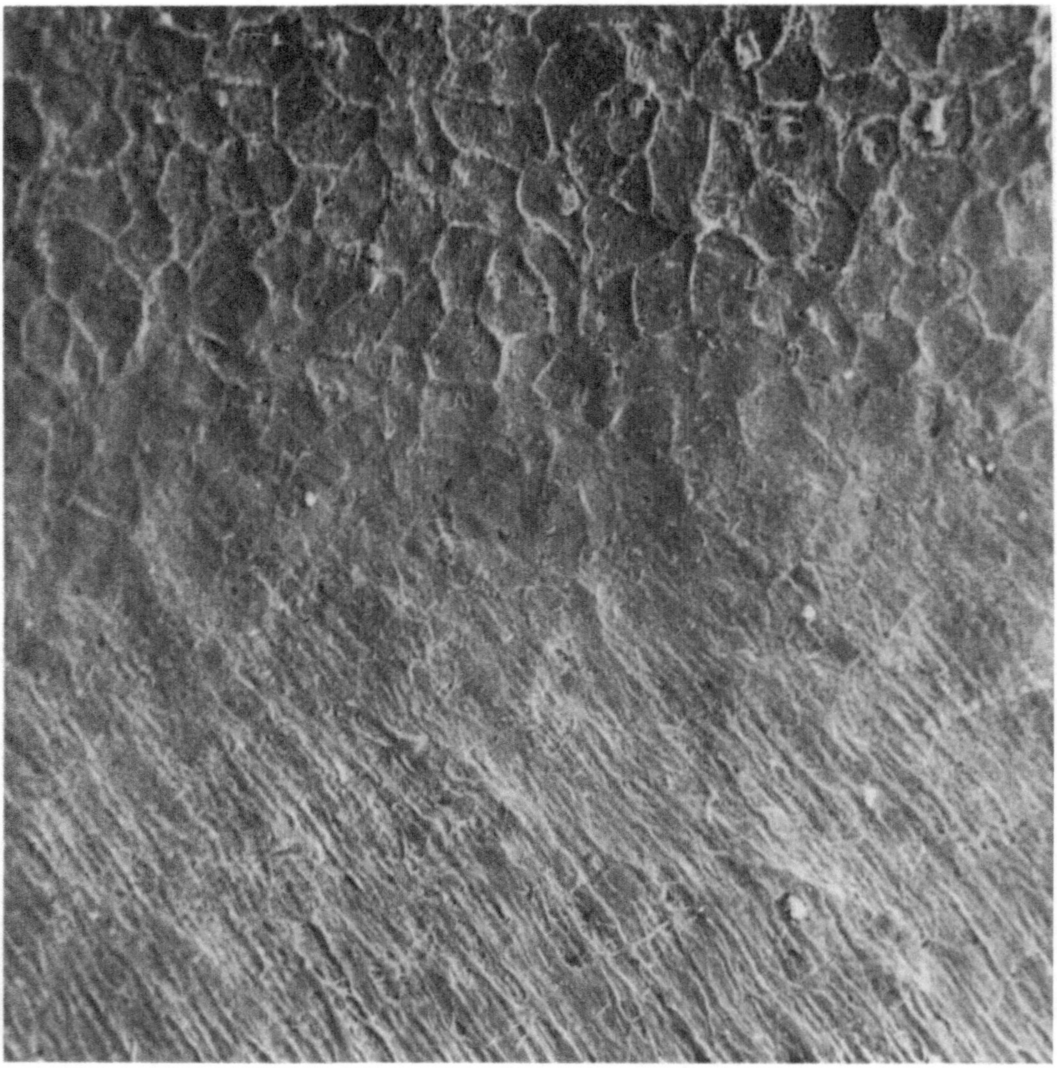

Figure 115 Surface of the tectorial membrane facing the organ of Corti (monkey). Flat polygonal cells are observed (× 1500)

Figure 116 Surface of the tectorial membrane (monkey). (**a**) Fibres are well visualized (× 4000), (**b**) high magnification of (a). Fine fibres form a network, connecting neighbouring thick fibres (× 13 000)

a

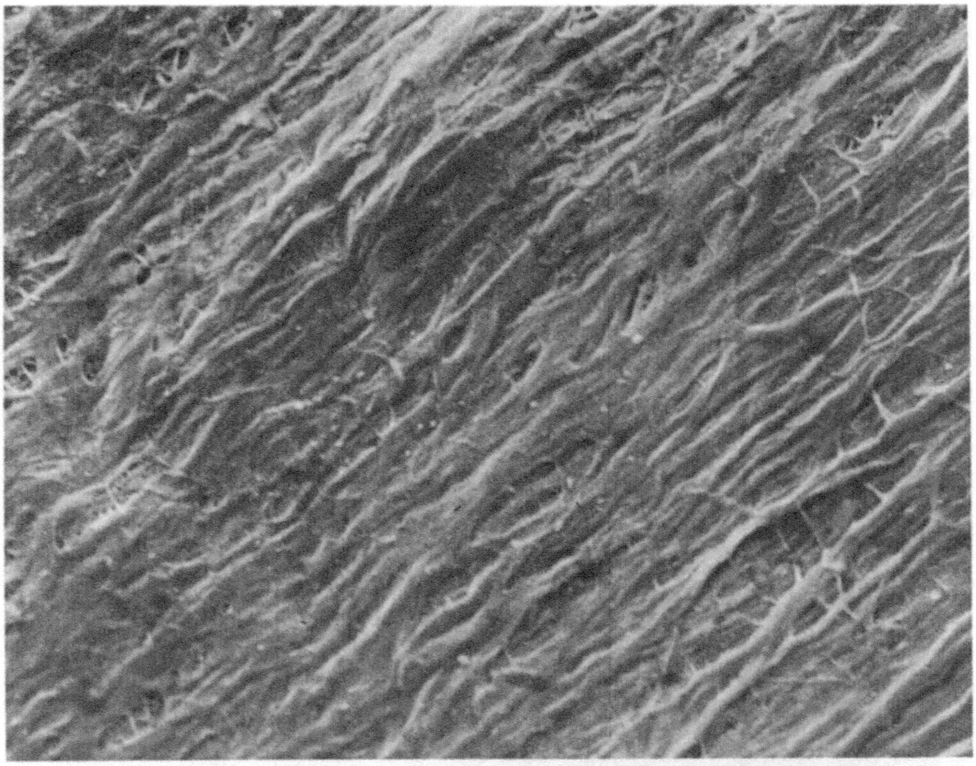

b

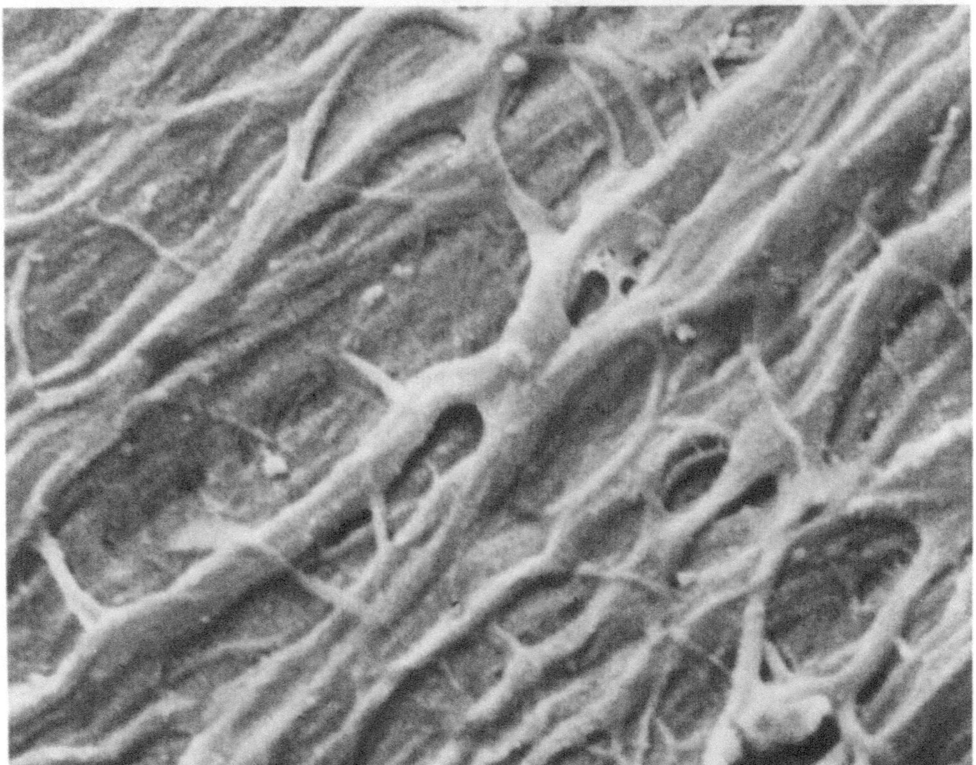

Figure 116

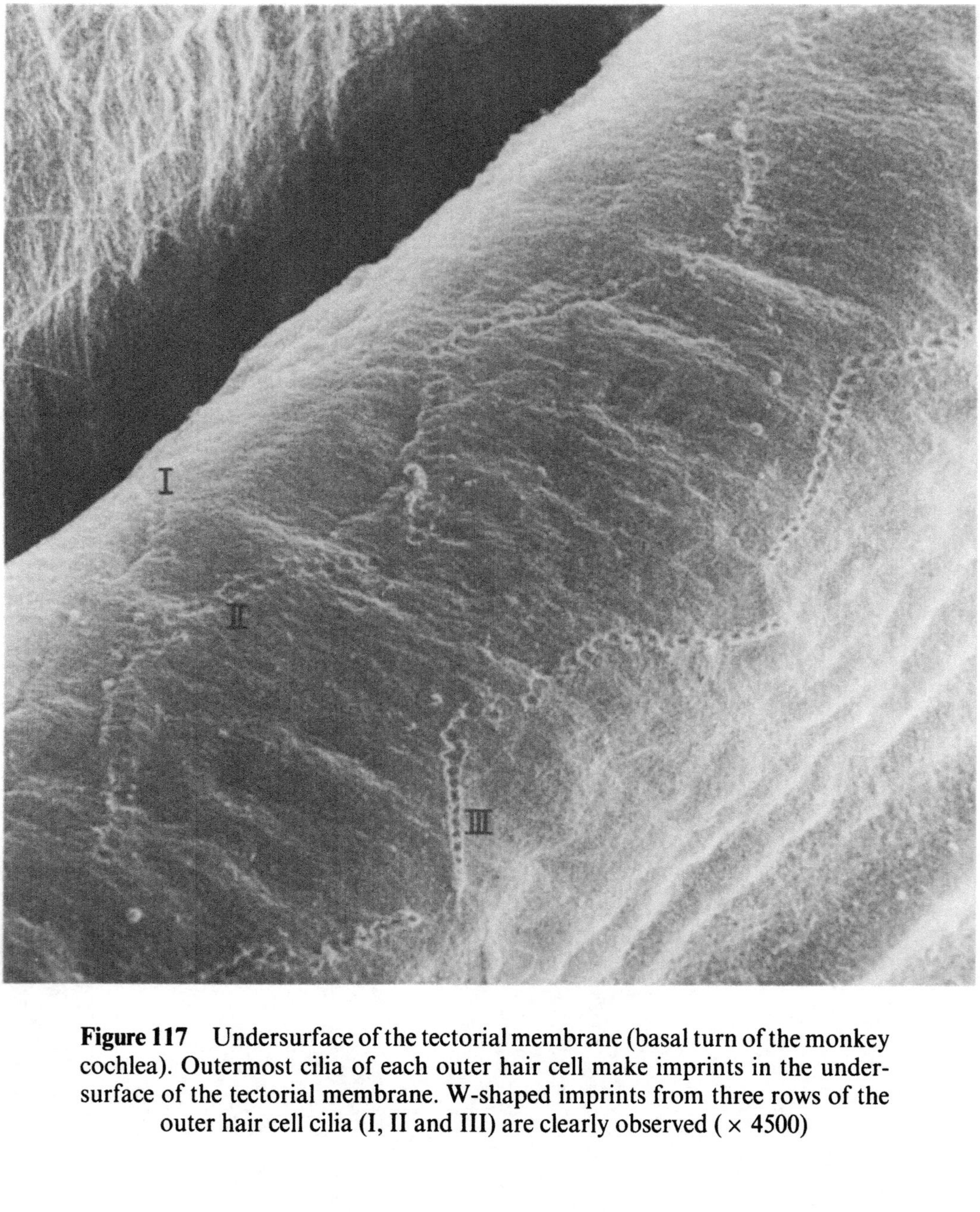

Figure 117 Undersurface of the tectorial membrane (basal turn of the monkey cochlea). Outermost cilia of each outer hair cell make imprints in the under-surface of the tectorial membrane. W-shaped imprints from three rows of the outer hair cell cilia (I, II and III) are clearly observed (× 4500)

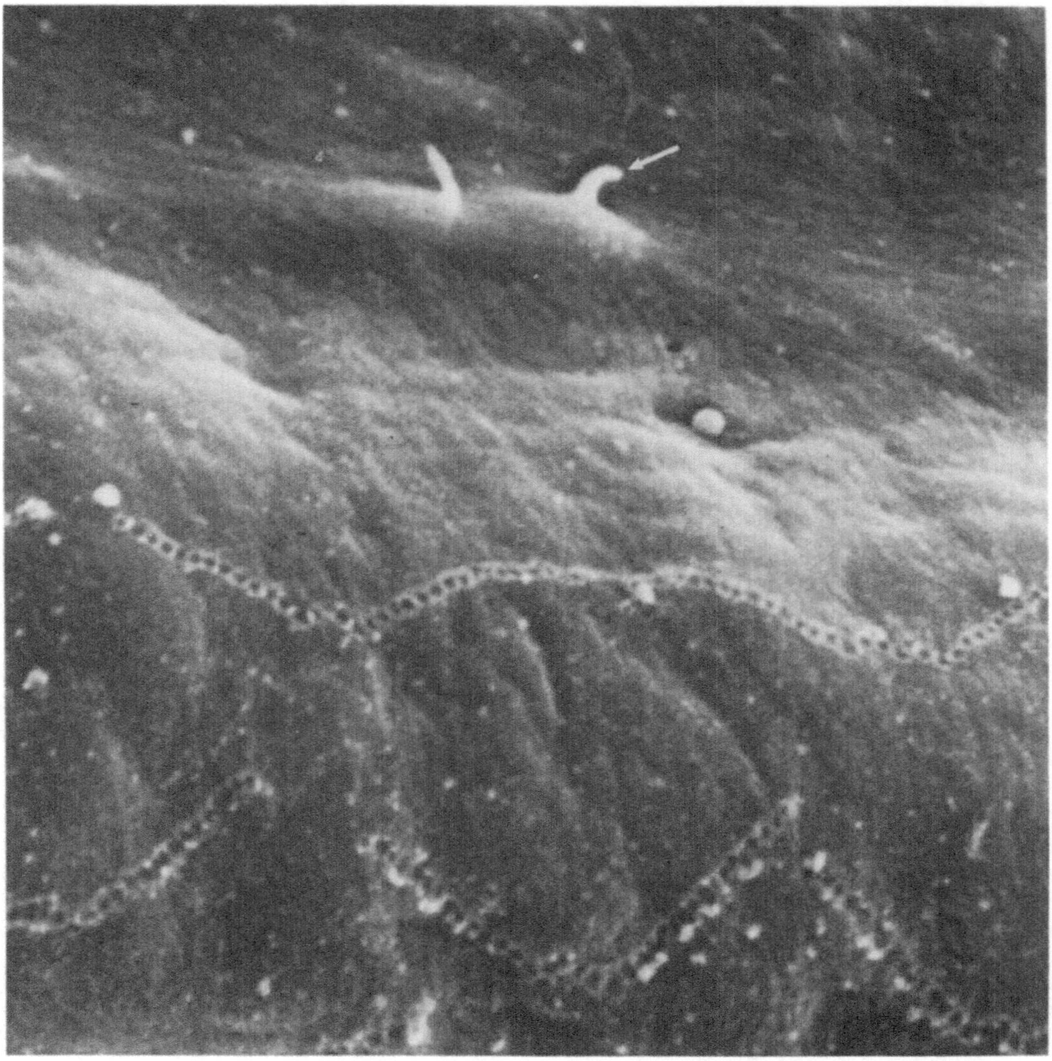

Figure 118 Undersurface of the tectorial membrane (basal turn monkey). W-shaped imprints made from outer hair cell cilia are well visualized. The arrow shows trabeculae of the Hensen's stripe which attaches to the inner hair cell cilia (× 9000)

a

b

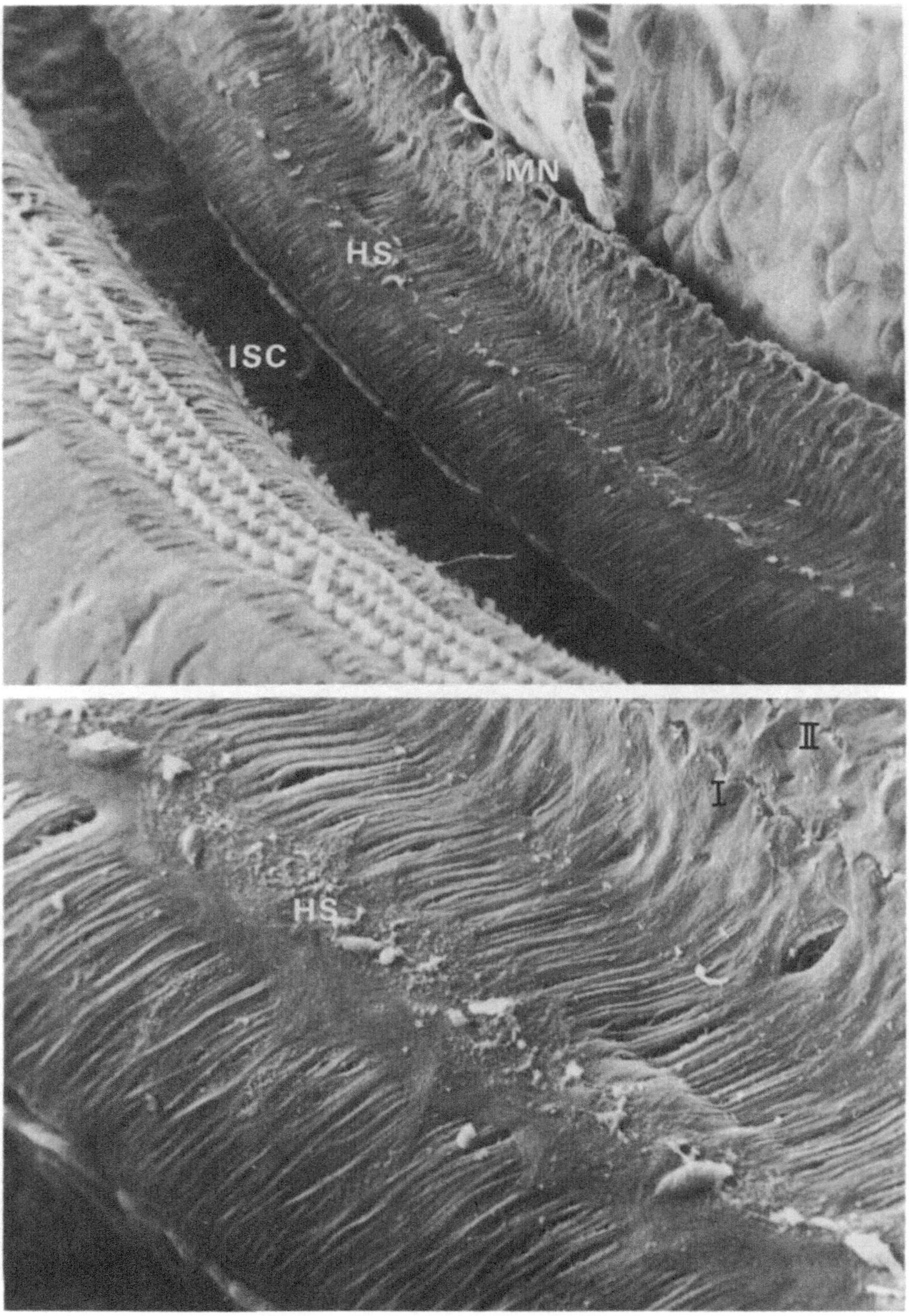

Figure 119 Undersurface of the tectorial membrane (apical turn, monkey). (**a**) The part facing the inner hair cell cilia is called Hensen's stripe (HS). Outer margin of the tectorial membrane is marginal net (MN), which attaches to the Deiters' and Hensen's cells (× 1000) ISC: inner sulcus cell. (**b**) High magnification of the Hensen's stripe (HS) and the imprints of the first and the second row outer hair cell cilia (× 3000)

Reissner's membrane

Reissner's membrane is a very thin membrane first reported by Reissner in 1851. In the embryonic stage it is structured by the inner ectodermal layer and several outer mesodermal layers. During the individual's growth the outer layers decrease in number, ending up in two cell layers, inner and outer.

The cochlear canal is divided by Reissner's membrane and the basilar membrane into three spaces, the scala vestibuli, the scala media (cochlear duct) and the scala tympani. The scalae vestibuli and tympani contain perilymphatic fluid and the scala media contains the endolymphatic fluid.

Reissner's membrane is approximately 2-3 μm thick and separates the scala vestibuli and the cochlear duct, extending from the osseous spiral lamina to the lateral wall. Histologically it consists of two cellular layers as mentioned before, a single layer of polygonal epithelial cells on the endolymphatic side (cochlear duct side) and flat cells on the perilymphatic side (scala vestibuli side). The polygonal cells of the endolymphatic side have large oval nuclei and vacuoles, mitochondria, rough endoplasmic reticulum, Golgi apparati and free lysosomes in their cytoplasm. Many microvilli are found on this side, the greatest number being seen in the part closer to the osseous spiral lamina.

The cells on the perilymphatic side have very little cytoplasm with large oval nuclei and fewer vacuoles, mitochondria, and less rough endoplasmic reticulum and lysosomes than the cells on the endolymphatic side.

Between the inner and outer cells there is a basement membrane 0.25 μm or less thick. The inner side of this membrane continues to the basement membrane of the superficial cells of the limbus. The outer side disappears near the stria vascularis.

The function of Reissner's membrane is not yet clear, but it is speculated that fluid transportation takes place between the endolymphatic and the perilymphatic spaces, because of its permeability. This function is possibly due to the microvilli, pinocytotic vacuoles and the cells of the endolymphatic side with high ATPase activity.

References

1. Chou, J. T. Y. (1963). Respiration of Reissner's membrane of the guinea pig. *J. Laryngol.*, **77**, 374
2. Duvall, A. J. and Rhodes, V. T. (1967). Reissner's membrane. *Arch. Otolaryngol.* **86**, 143
3. Iurato, S. (1967). *Submicroscopic structure of the inner ear*, p. 76. (Oxford: Pergamon)
4. Kikuchi, K. and Hilding, D. A. (1965). The development of the organ of Corti in the mouse. *Acta Otolaryngol.* (*Stockholm*).), **60**, 207
5. Lawrence, M., Walsk, D., and Litton, W. B. (1961). Circulation of the inner ear fluids. *Ann. Otolaryngol.*, **70**, 753
6. Rauch, S., Köstlin, A., Schnieder, E. A. and Schindler, D. (1963). Arguments for the permeability of Reissner's membrane. *Laryngoscope*, **73**, 135
7. Watanuki, K. (1968). Some morphological observation of Reissner's membrane. *Acta Otolaryngol.* (*Stockholm*), **66**, 40

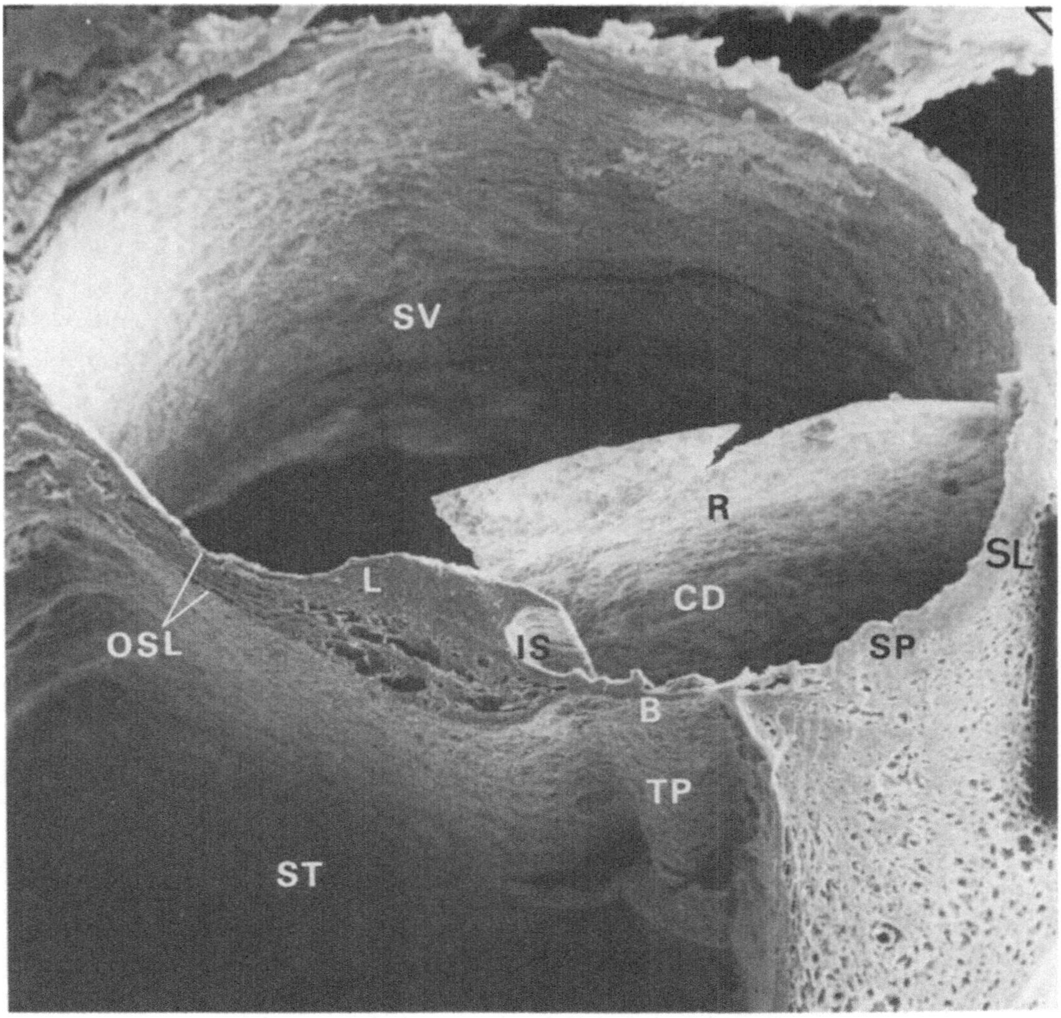

Figure 120 Cracked surface of the cochlea (guinea pig). SV: scala vestibuli; ST: scala tympani; R: Reissner's membrane; SL: spiral ligament; SP: spiral prominence; IS: internal spiral sulcus; CD: cochlear duct; L: limbus; B: basilar membrane; TP: tympanic pannicle; OSL: osseous spiral lamina (× 50)

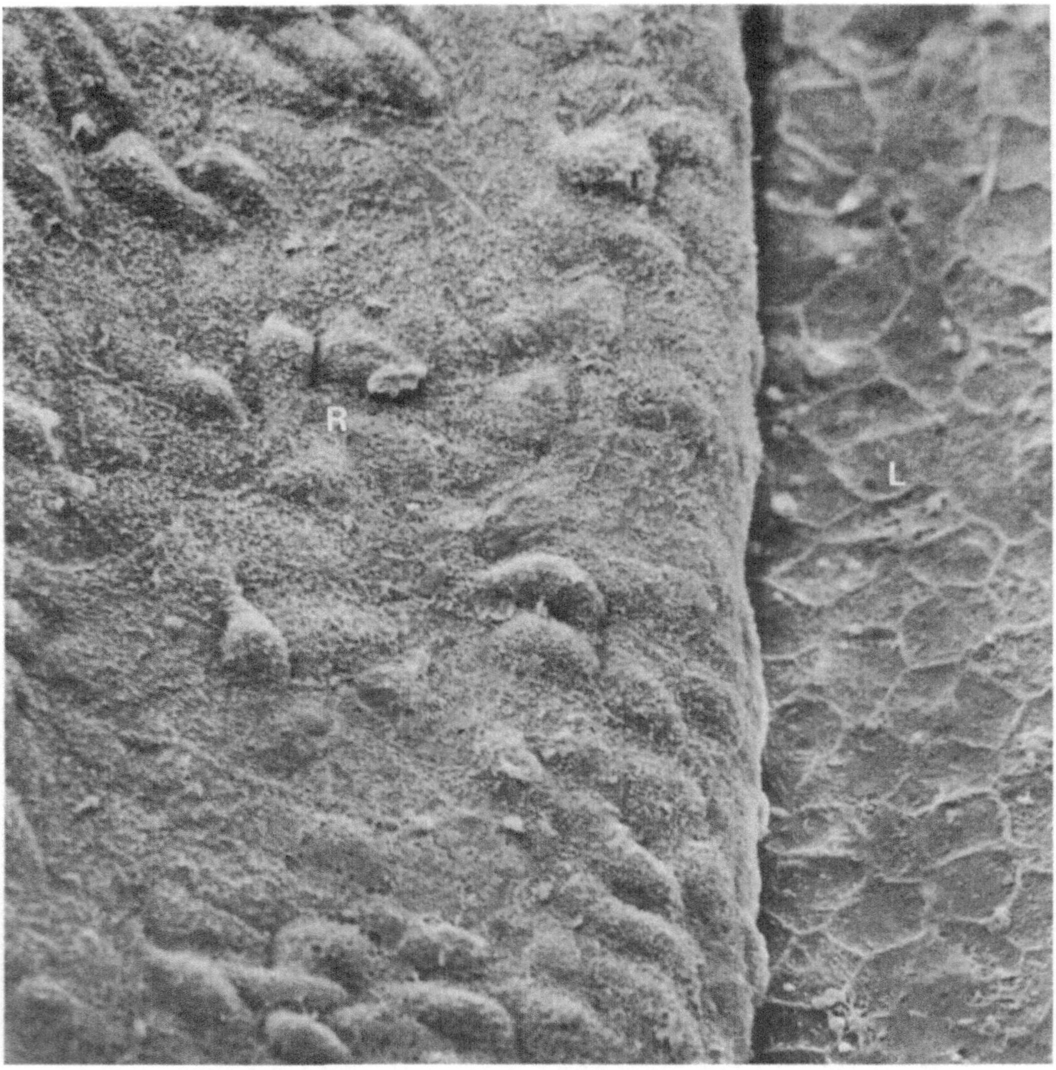

Figure 121 Perilymphatic side of Reissner's membrane (R). Reissner's membrane extends from the osseous spiral lamina (L) to the lateral wall. Protrusions observed on the polygonal cells appear to be nuclei (× 1500)

Figure 122 Endolymphatic side of the Reissner's membrane (monkey). (**a**) This portion is covered with dome-like cells (× 5200), (**b**) both long and short microvilli are seen on the cell surface (× 13 000)

a

b

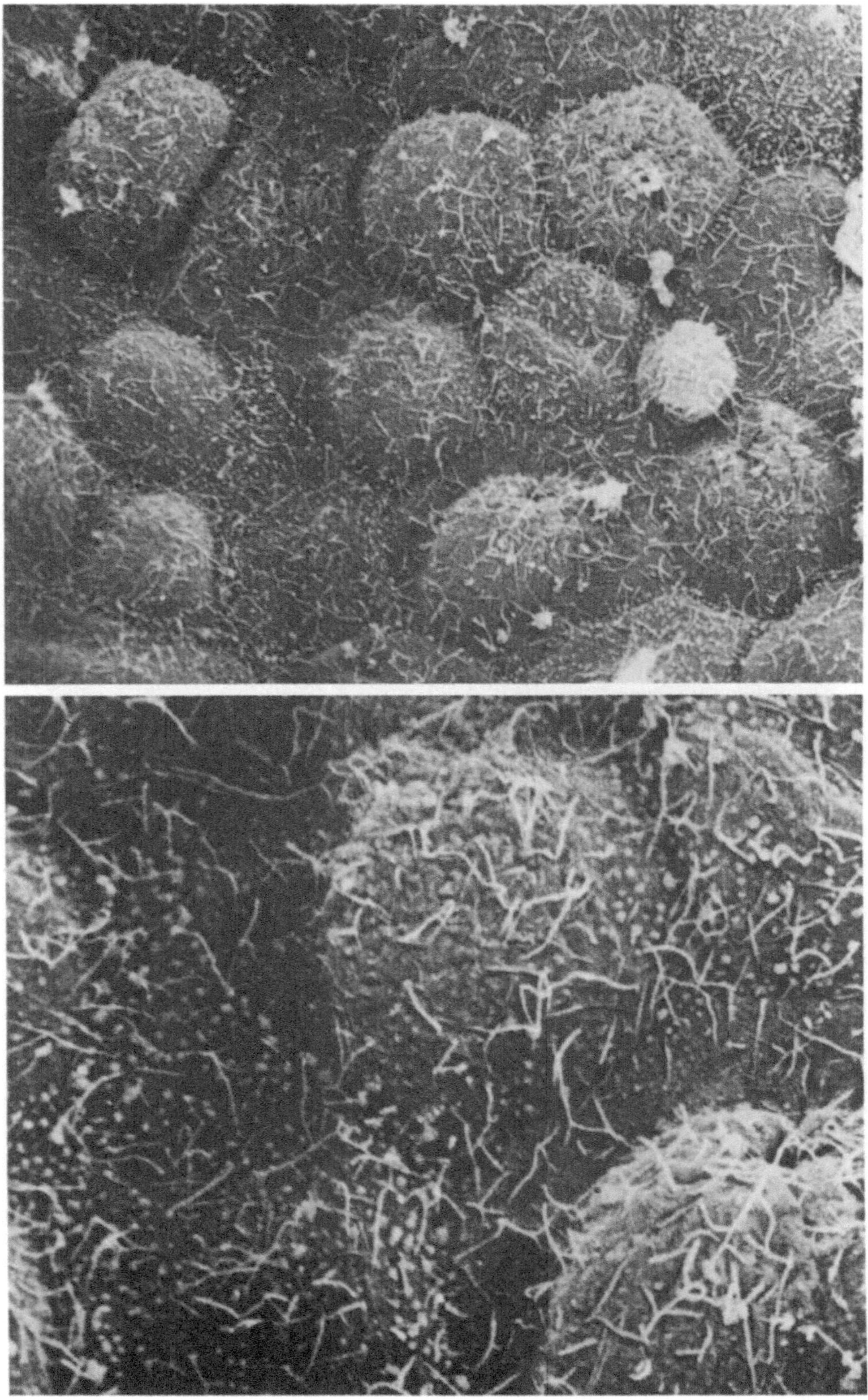

Figure 122

The stria vascularis

This is an important portion which forms the outer wall of the cochlear duct. Its morphological structures are three cell layers, the spiral ligament and the network of the arterioles. The three kinds of cells are, the marginal cells on the endolymphatic space, the basal cells on the spiral ligament and the intermediate cells.

The marginal cell is a big cell which is well stained by osmium. In the lower part of the cell body, there are many extensions with a large number of mitochondria, which permeate into the deeper cells. This structure has to do with the electrophysiological mechanism of the cell discharge. (Hinojosa and Rodriguez-Echandia, 1966).

The intermediate cell is located below the marginal cell. This is a slightly smaller cell with brownish pigment, and is chromophobic.

The basal cell layer is located deeper than the other two and faces the spiral ligament. This cell is flat with a long extension to the intermediate or marginal cells. Detailed study on these three cells was done using specimens taken from patients with Ménière's disease by Kimura and Schuknecht (1970).

The function of the stria vascularis is secretion and absorption of the endolymphatic fluid. The marginal cell probably controls electrolyte concentration. Innumerable vessels are distributed in the epithelia of the stria vascularis. Axelsson (1968) demonstrated in his detailed study that the structural components are a relatively small number of arterioles and collecting venules.

References

1. Hinojosa, R. and Rodriguez-Echandia, E. L. (1966). The fine structure of the stria vascularis of the cat inner ear. *Am. J. Anat.*, **118**, 631
2. Kimura, R. and Schuknecht, H. (1970). The ultrastructure of the human stria vascularis. Part I. *Acta Otolaryngol.* (*Stockholm*), **69**, 415

Figure 123 Stria vascularis (guinea pig). (**a**) Luminal surface of the stria vascularis (ST). Surface structure of the stria vascularis appears somewhat different between two portions, upper (U) and lower (L) portions, above and below the spiral prominence (SP). R: Reissner's membrane; SL: spiral ligament (× 100). (**b**) Surface structure of the portion (U) above the spiral prominence (S). Pentagonal or hexagonal smooth cells are arranged like a pavement with few microvilli (× 3000)

a

b

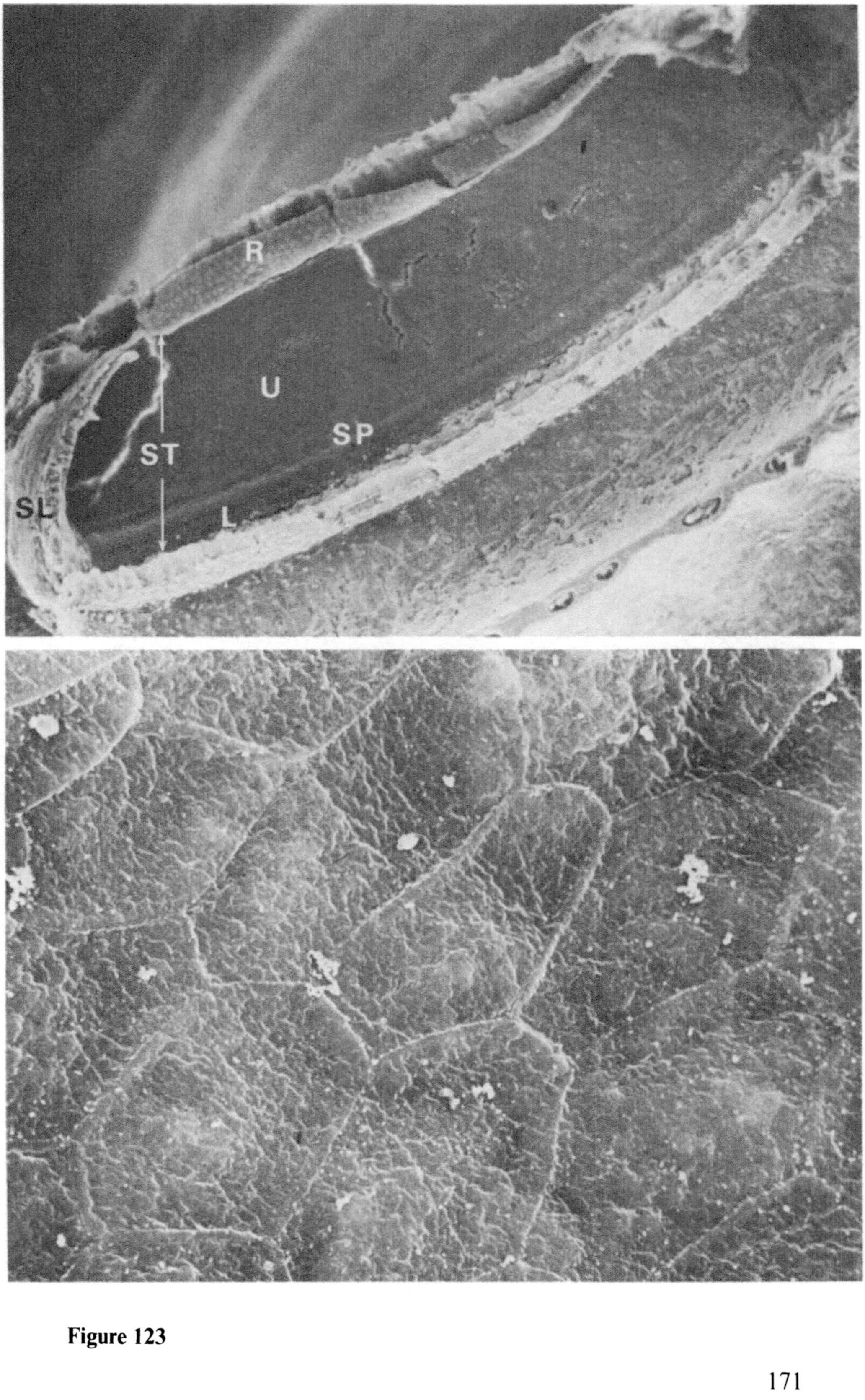

Figure 123

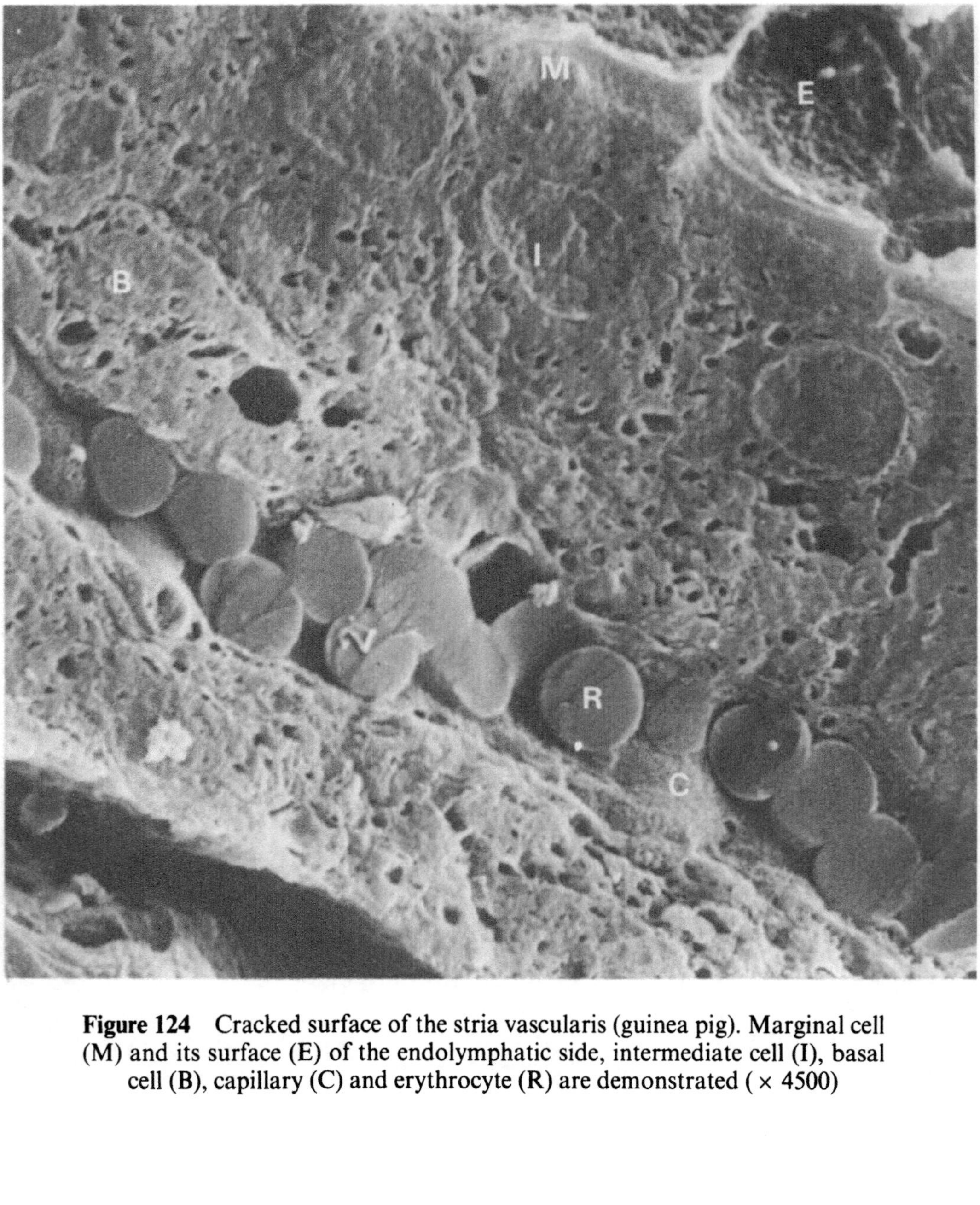

Figure 124 Cracked surface of the stria vascularis (guinea pig). Marginal cell (M) and its surface (E) of the endolymphatic side, intermediate cell (I), basal cell (B), capillary (C) and erythrocyte (R) are demonstrated (× 4500)

Figure 125 Stria vascularis (guinea pig). (**a**) Cells from the area of spiral prominence. This portion is characterized by its long cells (× 3000). (**b**) Cells in the area below the spiral prominence. Cells are shorter than those of the upper portion shown in Figure 123 (b), but with larger numbers of microvilli (× 3000)

a

b

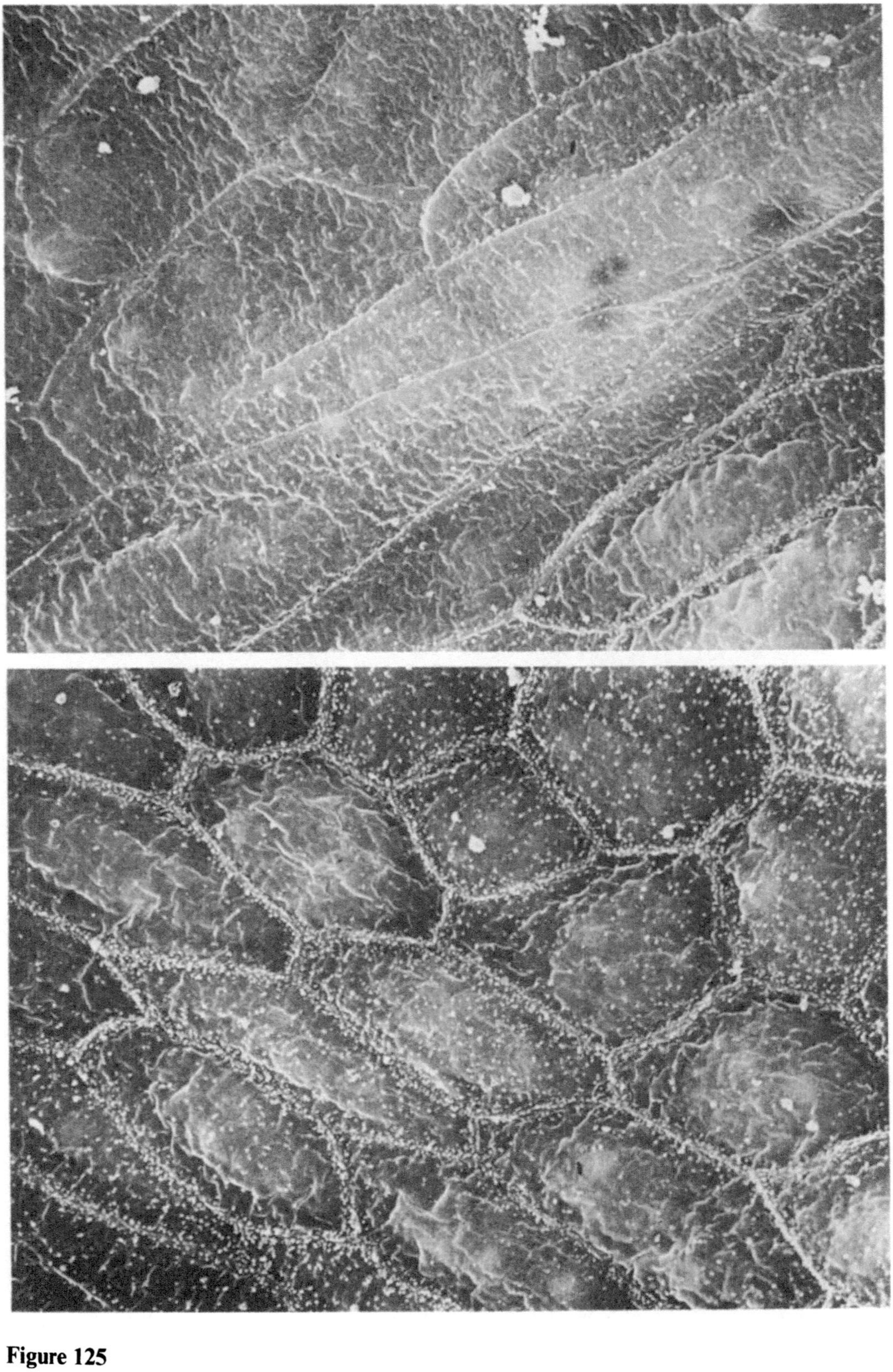

Figure 125

The mesothelial cell

The mesothelial cell, which is mesodermal in origin, covers the basal lamina of the side of the scala tympani. During the embryonic period, it fills the perilymphatic space. As the individual grows it gradually disappears from the perilymphatic space due to migration to the basal lamina of the side of the scala tympani. Morphological structure is different between the apical and basal turns. In the basal turn, the cell layers are thick and densely arranged like other cochlear wall cells (Watanuki, 1969; Hoshino, 1975). This probably serves for protection. In the apical turn, the cells are spindle-shaped and are sparsely distributed. These cells have fine processes on both ends. The mesothelial cell was found to be phagocytotic (Angelborg, 1974). It is also called the tympanic border cell, basilar membrane cell, tympanic covering layer, or tympanic pannicle.

References

1. Angelborg, C. *et al.* (1974). The tympanic covering layer. An electron microscopic study in guinea pig. *Acta Otolaryngol* (*Stockholm*) *Suppl.*, **319**, 43
2. Hoshino, T. (1975). The structure of the cochlea. *Otolaryngology* (*Tokyo*), **47**, 951
3. Watanuki, K. *et al.* (1969). Fundamental structures of the basilar membrane of the cochlea. *Audiology*, **12**, 478

a

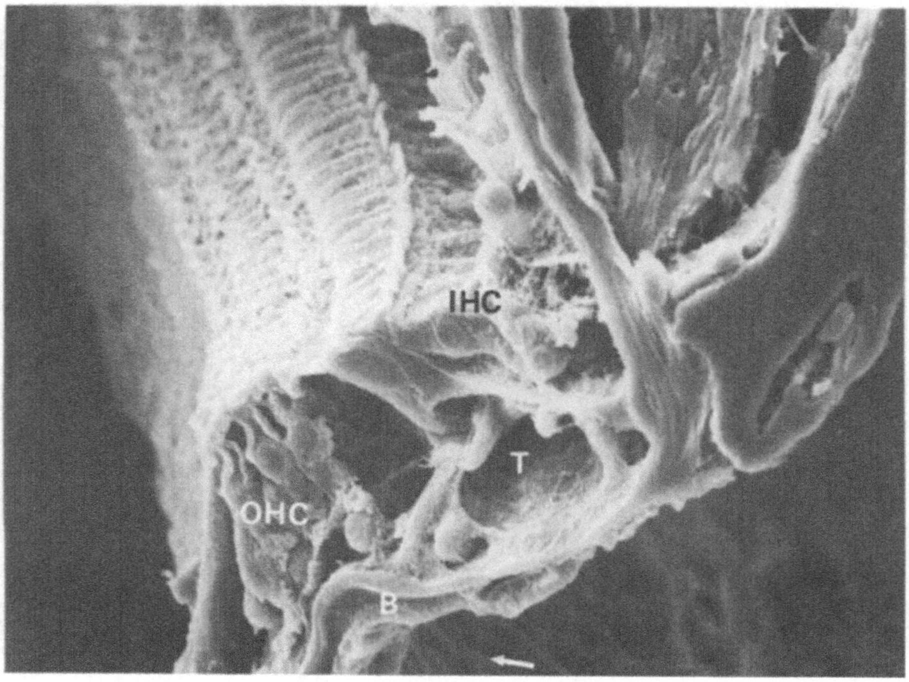

Figure 126

b

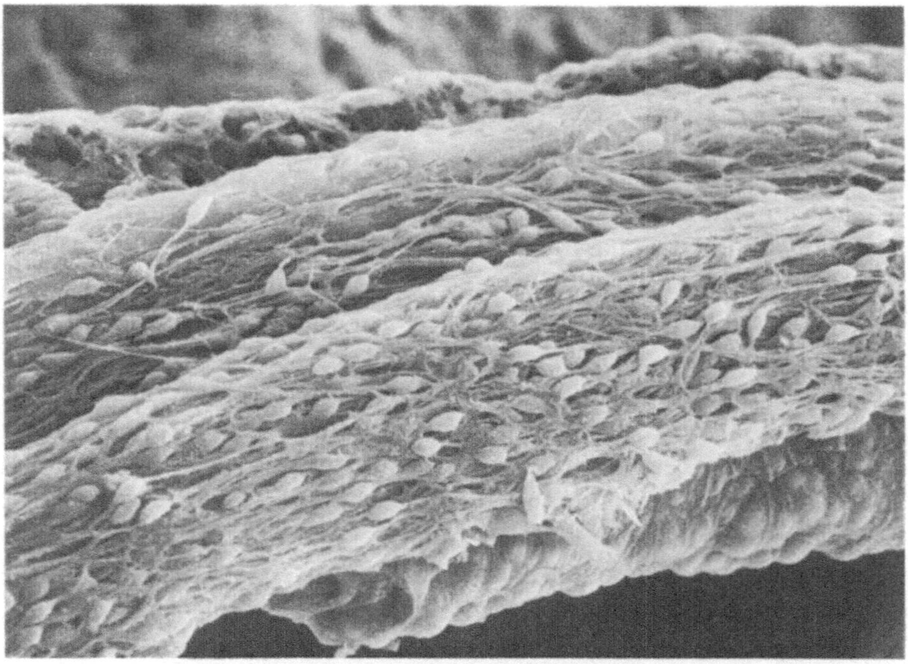

c

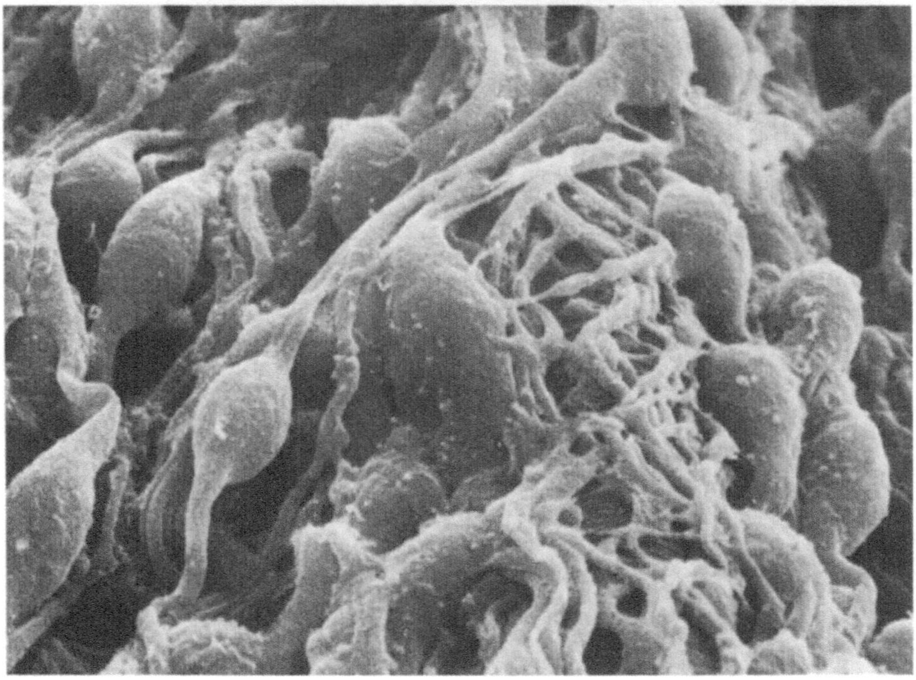

Figure 126 Cells of the basement lamina (guinea pig). (**a**) Organ of Corti and its cracked surface. IHC: inner hair cell; OHC: outer hair cell; B: basal cell; T: tunnel of Corti; arrow: cell of the basement lamina (× 1300), (**b**) cells of the basement lamina in the second turn. Fine processes extend from both ends of the spindle-shaped cells (× 600), (**c**) high magnification of the basement lamina in the third turn (× 4000)

The spiral ganglion

The spiral ganglion, the ganglion of the cochlear nerve, is located in the osseous spiral lamina. In humans, the number of ganglion cells is 23 000–28 000 (Guild, 1932). There are more ganglion cells in the upper basal to the lower middle turns and less in the lower basal and apical turns.

The ganglion cell is a bipolar cell with axons from both the ends. The nerve fibre reaches the hair cells of the organ of Corti after running through the habenula perforata. The afferent fibres run into the internal acoustic meatus, forming the trunk of the cochlear nerve. In the spiral ganglion cells of warm blooded animals, both myelinated and unmyelinated cells are found and the former comprise more than 90% of the whole. Both cells are surrounded by the rough endoplasmic reticulum.

The ganglion cells are classified into light cells and dark cells. Electronmicroscopically, the former are poor in rough endoplasmic reticulum but the latter are rich in Nissl bodies and organelles (Suzuki *et al.*, 1963). Myelinated cells are mostly dark cells, while unmyelinated ones are light cells. It is known that this relationship is reversed in some animals.

References

1. Ballantyne, J. and Engström, H. (1969). Morphology of the vestibular ganglion cells. *J. Laryngol. Otol.*, **93**, 19
2. Guild, S. R. (1952). Correlations of histologic observations and the acuity of hearing. *Acta Otolaryngol* (*Stockholm*), **17**, 207.

Figure 127 Cracked surface of the spiral ganglion cells (guinea pig). (**a**) Spiral ganglion cell (G) is a bipolar cell with elliptical cracked surface (× 400), (**b**) high magnification of (a). Large nuclei (N) slightly shifted to one side of the cytoplasm are seen (× 4000)

a

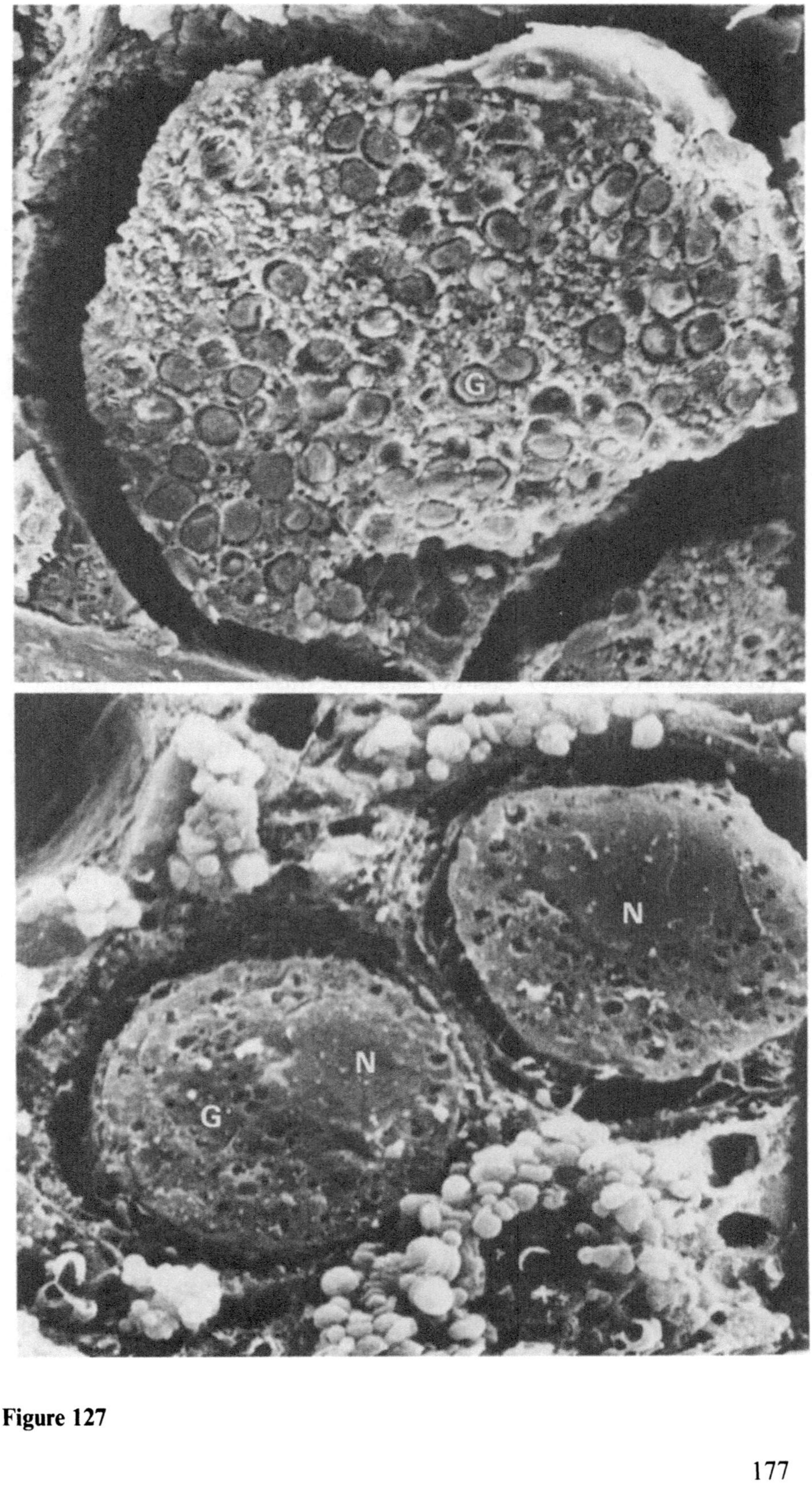

b

Figure 127

The innervation of the organ of Corti

(1) *The afferent nerve fibres*

The primary auditory neuron is the bipolar spiral ganglion cell. The axon reaches the medulla through the habenula perforata and the internal auditory meatus. The dendritic process makes contact with the hair cells through the habenula perforata.

The number of cochlear nerve fibres in humans is 31 000 on average, of which 90% innervate the inner hair cells. A single nerve fibre innervates one or two inner hair cells and a single inner hair cell receives several nerve fibres. The remaining cochlear nerve fibres, i.e. 5–10%, innervate the outer hair cells (Spoendlin, 1966, 1971; Morrison, 1975).

(2) *The efferent nerve fibres*

These fibres are termed the olivocochlear bundle by Rasmussen. Three quarters originate from the contralateral superior olivary nucleus (crossed olivocochlear bundle) and one quarter from the ipsilateral superior olivary nucleus (uncrossed olivocochlear bundle). They run with the vestibular nerve and join the cochlear nerve in the internal auditory meatus after forming Oort's anastomosis. The crossed olivocochlear bundle comprises the tunnel radial fibres in the cochlea which synapse at the base of the outer hair cells. The uncrossed olivocochlear bundle is the inner spiral bundle which synapses underneath the inner hair cells.

The nerve endings

Abundant cochlear nerve endings are distributed on the bottom of the hair cells. The afferent nerve ending is 0.5–1.0 μm in diameter and is termed a nongranulated or type I ending by Engström (1958).

The efferent nerve ending is large and goblet-shaped and has many synaptic vesicles and mitochondria. This ending is termed granulated or type II ending and is also differentiated from the afferent ending by a double layer structure and subsynaptic cisterna at the hair cell side.

References

1. Engström, H. (1958). On the double innervation of the sensory epithelia of the inner ear. *Acta Otolaryngol. (Stockholm)*, **49**, 109
2. Morrison, D., Schindler, R. A. and Wersäll, J. (1975). A quantitative analysis of the afferent innervation of the organs of Corti in the guinea pig. *Acta Otolaryngol. (Stockholm)*, **79**, 11
3. Spoendlin, H. (1966). The organization of the cochlear receptor. *Arch. Otolaryngol.* **13**, 1
4. Spoendlin, H. (1971). Degeneration behaviour of the cochlear nerve. *Arch. Klin. Exp. Ohren Nasen Kehlkopfheilkd.*, **200**, 275

a b

c

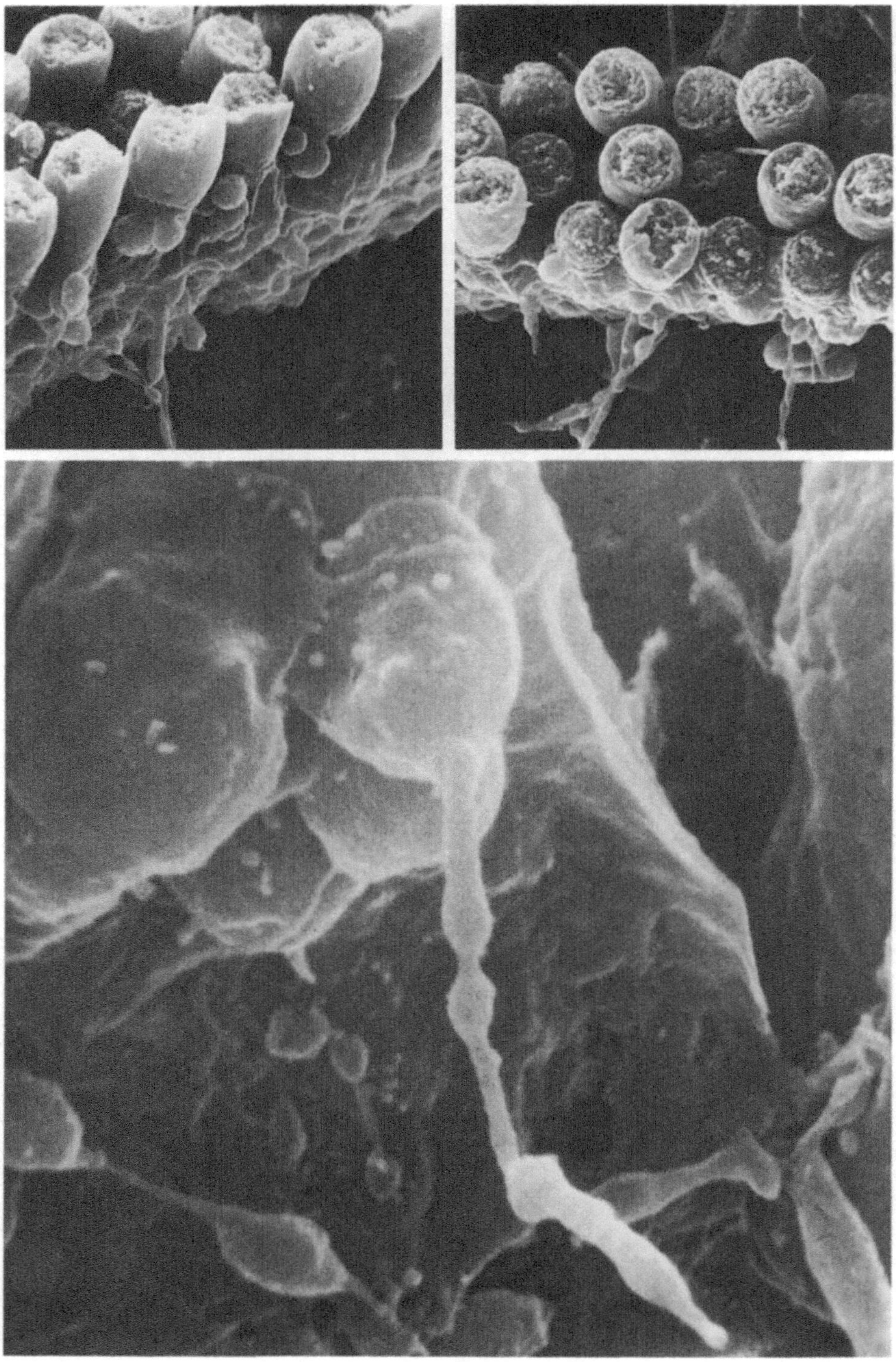

Figure 128 Nerve endings of the outer hair cells (guinea pig). (**a**) × 2100, (**b**) × 2100, (**c**) × 15000

a

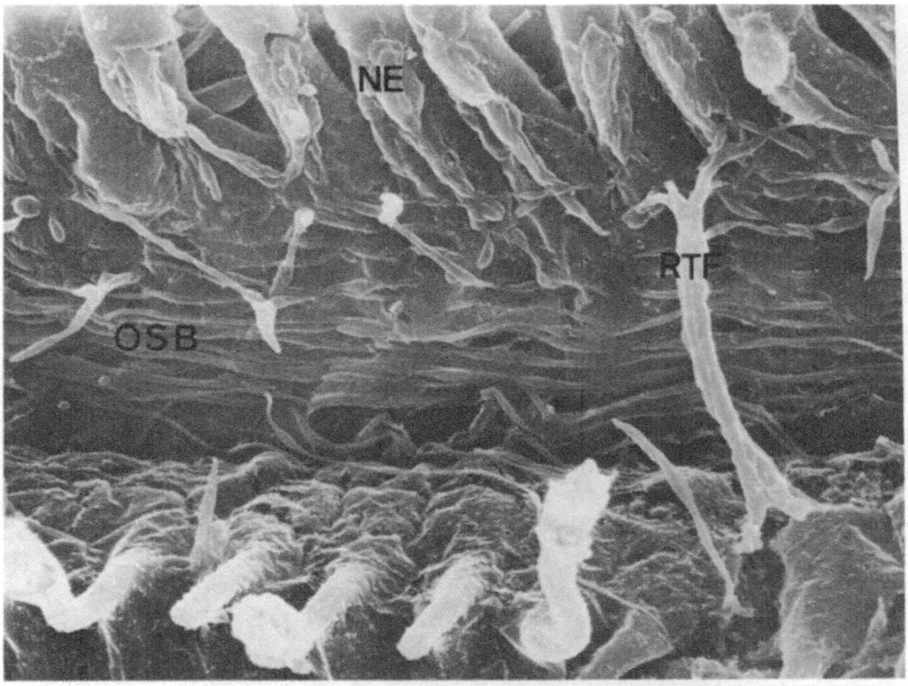

b

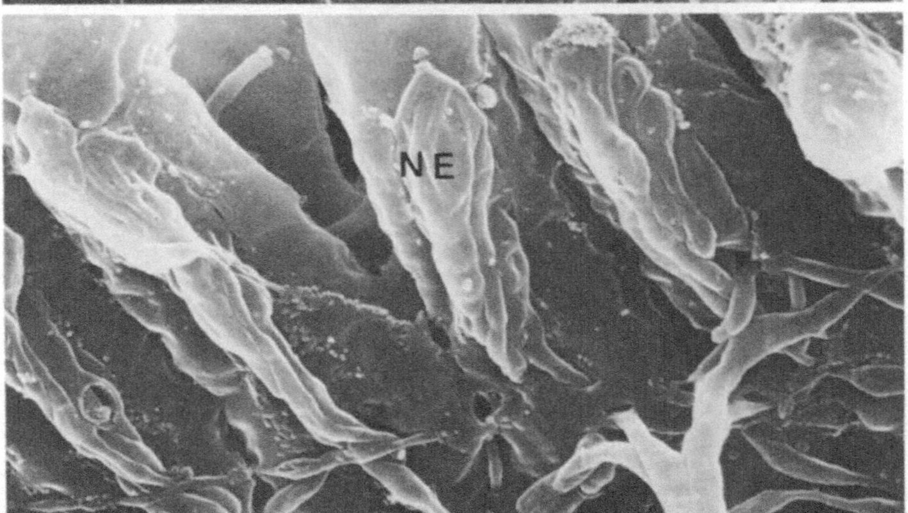

Figure 129 Lower portion of the basal turn (guinea pig's cochlea). (**a**) Medial and lateral walls of the space of Nuel seen from above. Nerve endings (NE) are entirely exposed into the Nuel's space, and are arranged in clusters on the lower pole of the outer hair cells. Nerve fibres of the outer spiral bundle (OSB) and radiating tunnel fibre (RTF) are demonstrated (× 2200). (**b**) High magnification of (a) shows the complexity of the relation of the NE with the RTF and OSB (× 5500)

a

b

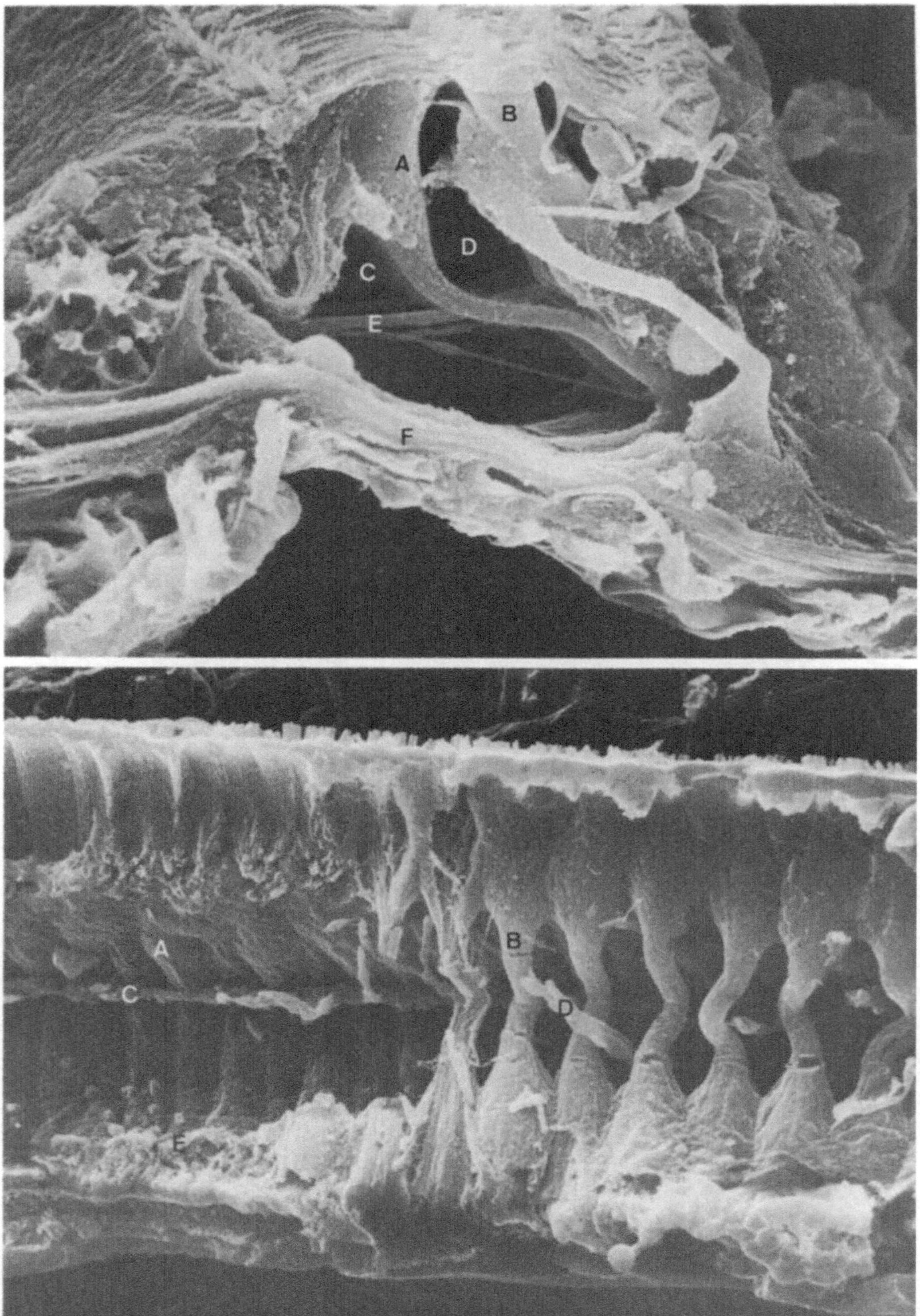

Figure 130 (**a**) Cracked specimen of the organ of Corti (guinea pig). A: outer pillar cell; B: outer hair cell, first row; C: tunnel of Corti; D: space of Nuel; E: radiating tunnel fibre; F: basilar membrane (× 2000). (**b**) A: inner pillar cell; B: outer pillar cell; C: tunnel spiral bundle; D: radiating tunnel fibre; E: basilar membrane (× 1300)

a

b

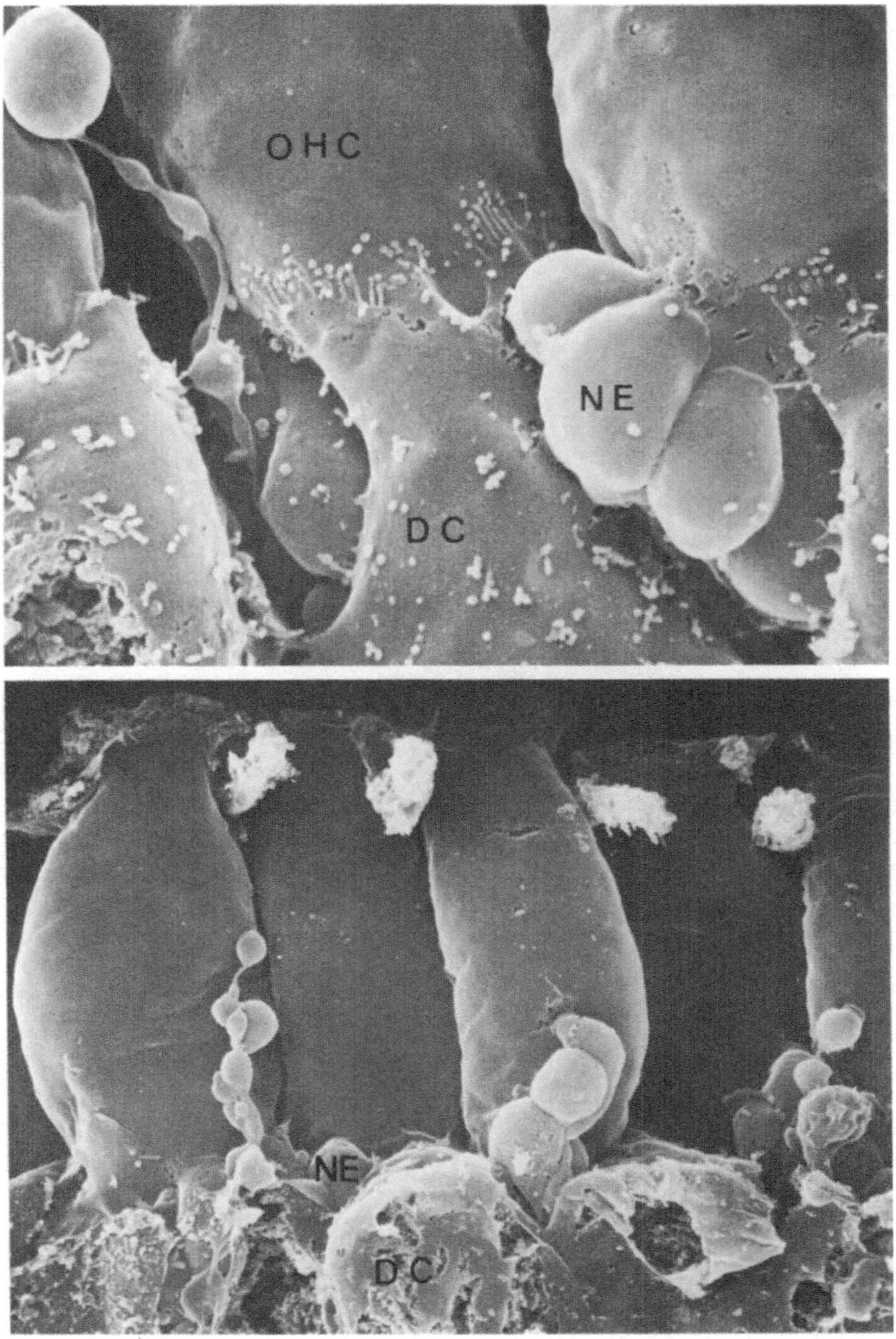

Figure 131 Lower portion of the second turn of guinea pig's cochlea. **(a)** Few nerve endings are seen on the lower end of outer hair cells owing to the Deiters' cells becoming bigger and covering the lower pole of outer hair cells and some nerve endings. On the left, a high nerve ending is seen in contact with the left outer hair cell while its fibre is running in close contact with the middle outer hair cell. DC: Deiters' cell; OHC: outer hair cell; NE: nerve ending (× 8250). **(b)** Several outer hair cells with some high nerve endings. Deiters' cells are bulged and cover the nerve endings in the lower portion. NE: nerve ending; DC: Deiters' cell (× 4000)

a

b

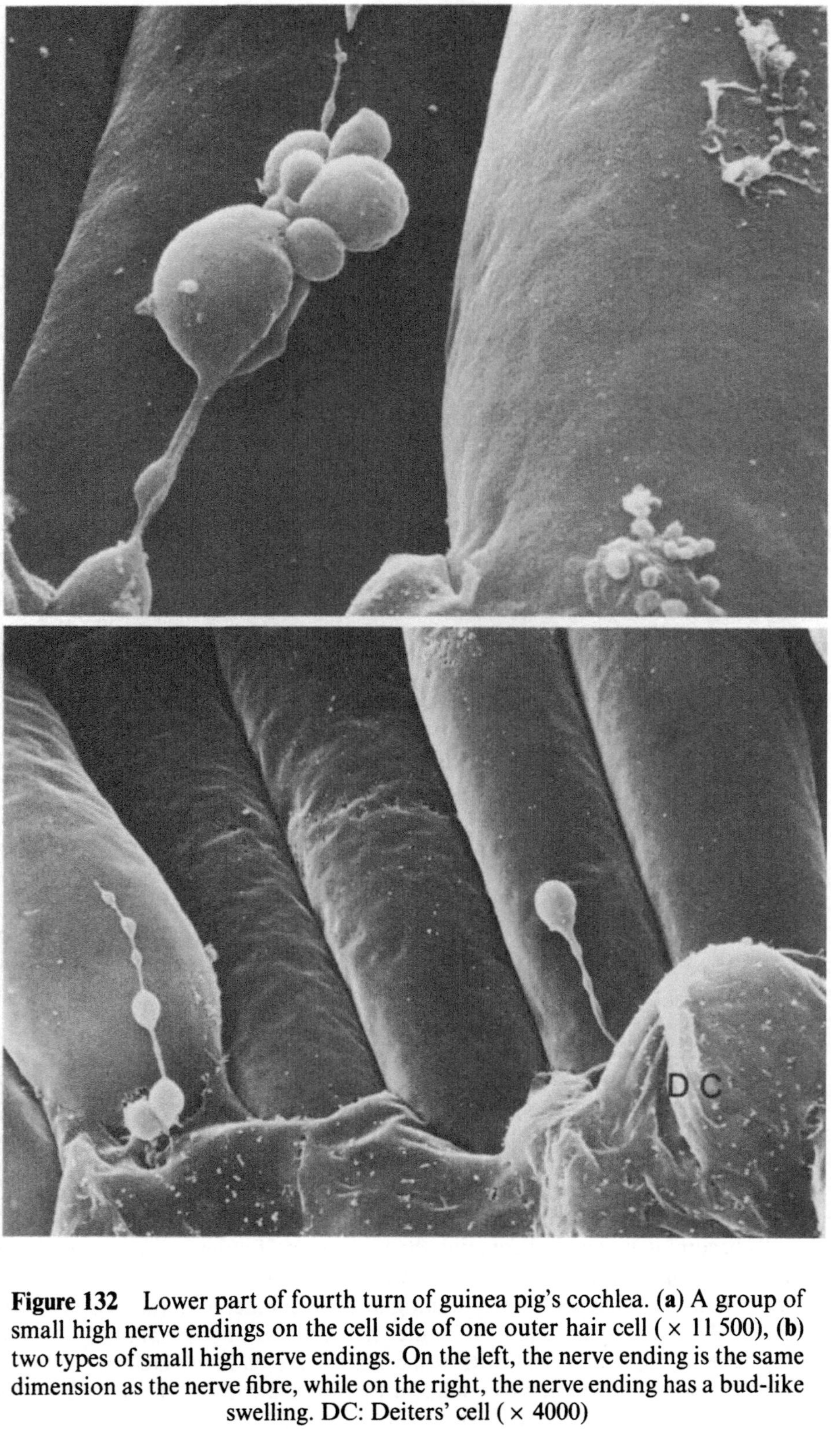

Figure 132 Lower part of fourth turn of guinea pig's cochlea. (**a**) A group of small high nerve endings on the cell side of one outer hair cell (× 11 500), (**b**) two types of small high nerve endings. On the left, the nerve ending is the same dimension as the nerve fibre, while on the right, the nerve ending has a bud-like swelling. DC: Deiters' cell (× 4000)

a

b

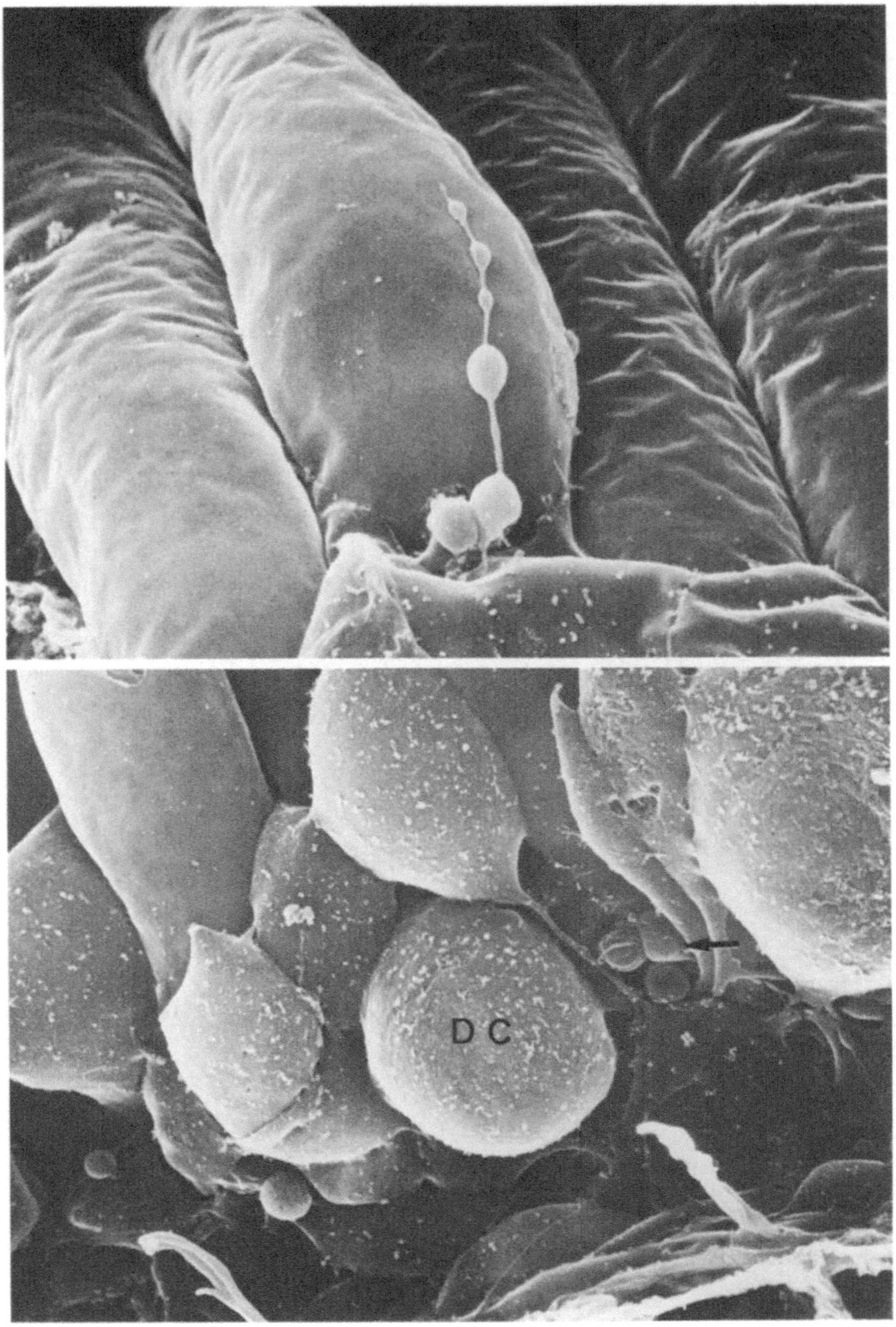

Figure 133 (**a**) Lower part of the fourth turn of guinea pigs' cochlea. High magnification of the picture in Figure 132(b). The nerve fibre has four swellings before terminating in the same dimension as the nerve fibre (× 5500). (**b**) Deiters' cells (DC) are bulged and cover the lower end of outer hair cells. Occasionally, Deiters' cells are smaller, hence the small nerve endings that can be seen (arrow) (× 4000)

The vascular system of the inner ear

The internal auditory artery forms the labyrinthine artery after branching from the anterior inferior cerebellar artery. The anterior inferior cerebellar artery is one of the branches of the basilar artery. The labyrinthine artery runs through the internal auditory meatus with the cochlear nerve and the facial nerve and is finally divided into the common cochlear artery and the anterior vestibular artery. The common cochlear artery further branches into two arteries, the main cochlear and the vestibulo-cochlear artery. The latter has two branches, the cochlear ramus and the posterior vestibular artery.

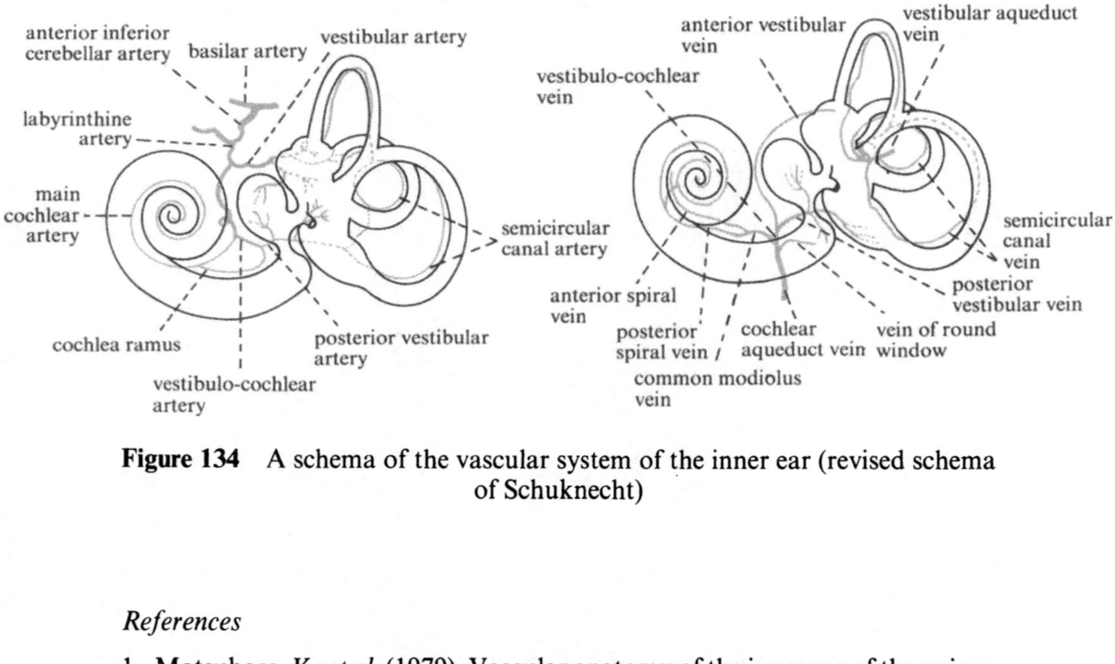

Figure 134 A schema of the vascular system of the inner ear (revised schema of Schuknecht)

References

1. Matsubara, K. *et al.* (1979). Vascular anatomy of the inner ear of the guinea pig. *Auris. Nasus. Larynx.*, **6**, 1
2. Schuknecht, H. F. (1974). *Pathology of the Ear.* (Harvard University Press)

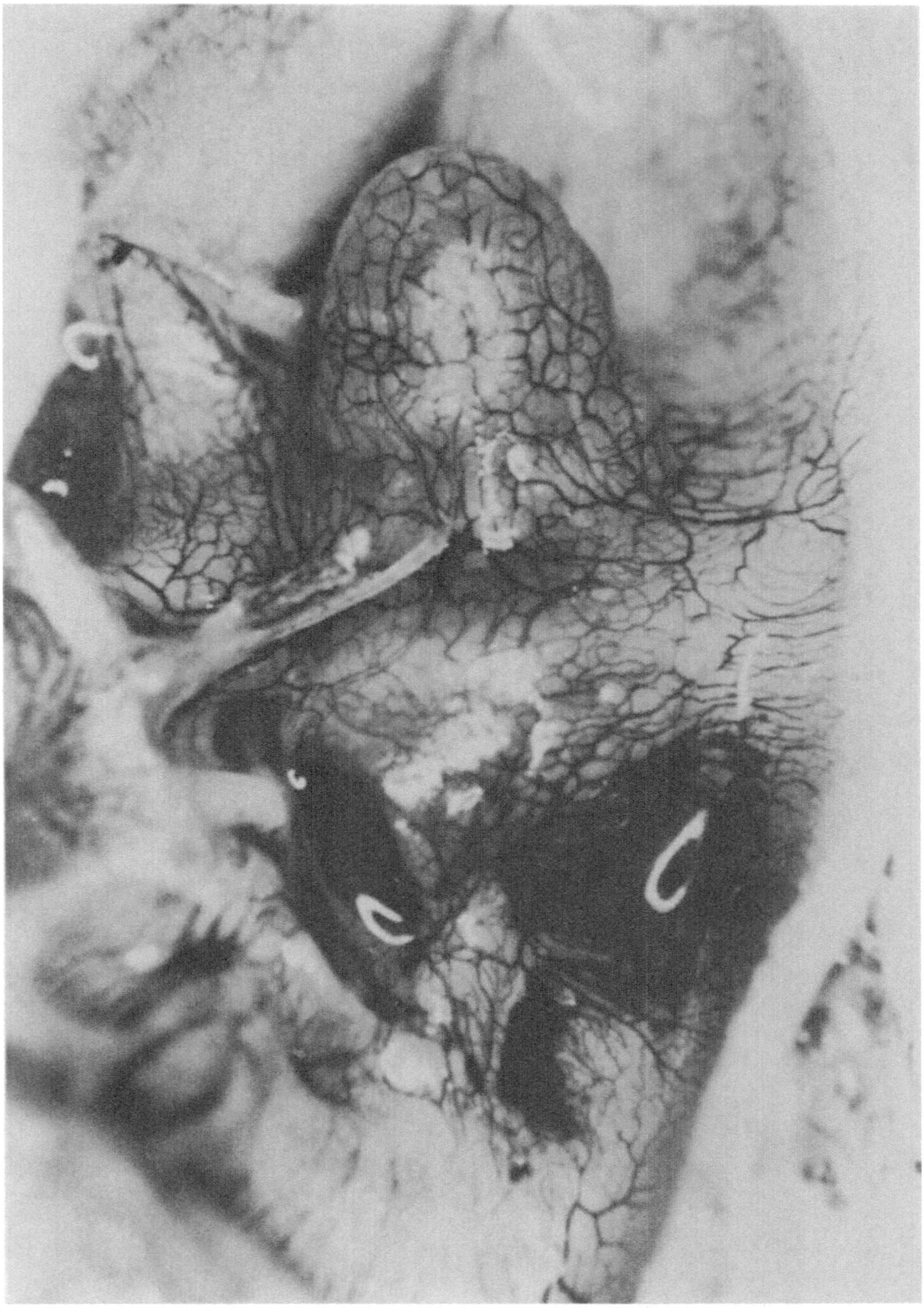

Figure 135 Vascularization of bony cochlea (guinea pig). (Indian ink method) (courtesy K. Sato)

a

b

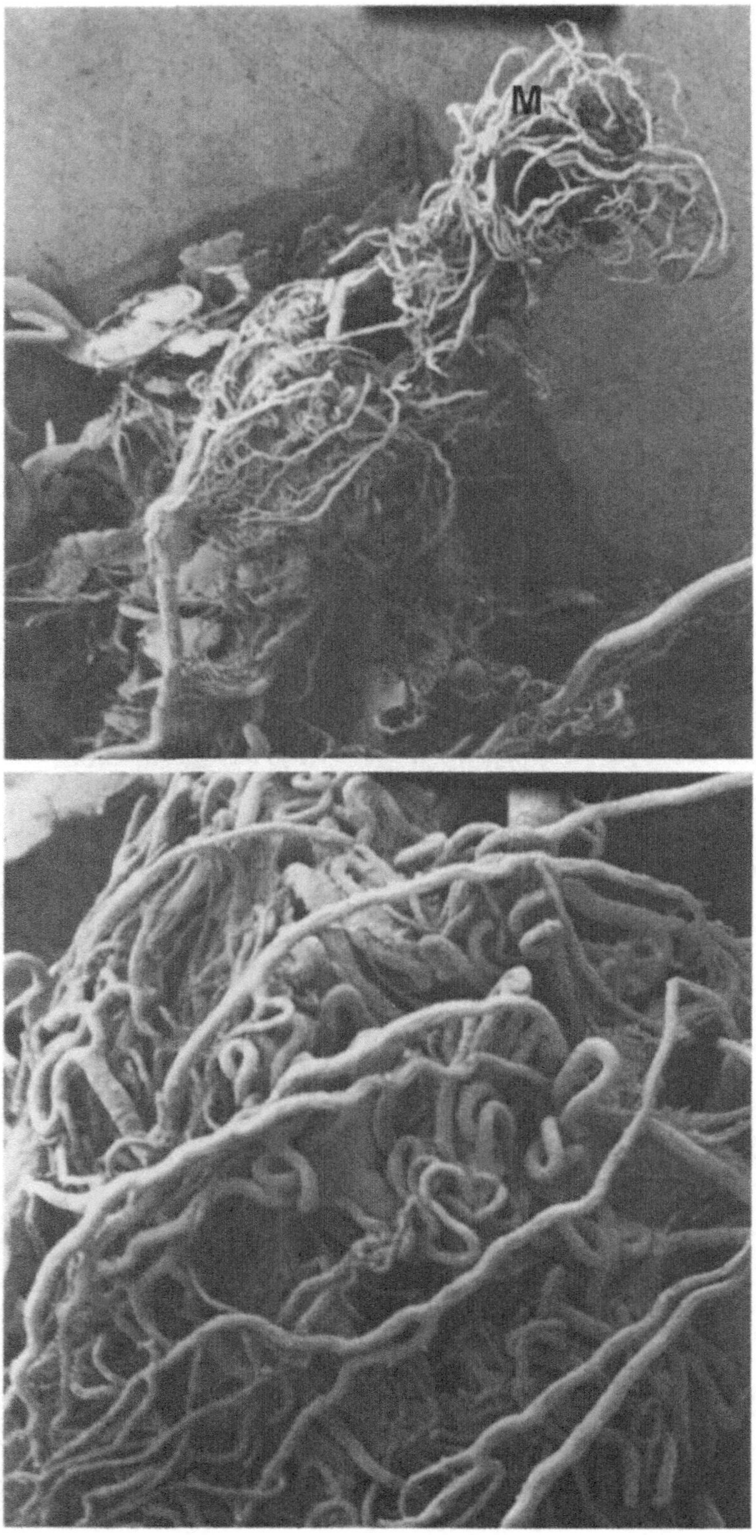

Figure 136 Vascular system of the guinea pig's cochlea. Vascular cast of the guinea pig was made by injection of methacrylate resin. This method was reported by Matsubara, *et al.* in detail (1979). (**a**) Vascular cast of the guinea pig cochlea. M: modiolus (× 20), (**b**) vascular network of basal turn (× 100)

Morphological Changes of the Middle and Inner Ear

Morphological changes of the vestibular organ by aminoglycosides

It is well known that dihydrostreptomycin selectively affects the auditory system, while streptomycin sulphate affects the vestibular organ. A great number of studies on the effect of other aminoglycoside agents have been done. In this chapter, changes of the vestibular organ due to intratympanic injection of gentamycin and intraperitoneal injection of streptomycin sulphate are described.

Guinea pigs with a mean weight of 300 g were used in this study. A small silicone tube was inserted into the middle ear bulla for intratympanic application of gentamycin. Gentamycin (4 mg) was administered daily during a period of 10 days and the cochlea was removed and inspected either 1 or 60 days after the treatment was completed. Streptomycin sulphate (250 mg/kg) was injected intraperitoneally every other day and the cochlea was inspected 2, 4 and 6 weeks after the treatment.

It has been long considered that only hair cells are disrupted by the ototoxic drugs; however, our study revealed that the otolithic organs are also affected prior to the hair cells.

References

1. Harada, Y. (1967). The ototoxicity of streptomycin and dihydrostreptomycin. *J. Hiroshima Med. Ass.*, **20**, 893
2. Harada, Y. (1973). Comparison between the lateral semicircular canal lesion in Ménière's disease and vestibular lesions with ototoxic agents. *Equilibrium Res.*, **3**, 2
3. Harada, Y. *et al.* (1976). The effect of ototoxic drugs on metabolic disorder of statoconia. *Ear Res.*, **7**, 60
4. Harada, Y. (1977). The injury of vestibular neurosensory epithelium caused by ototoxic drugs. *Otologia (Fukuoka)*, **23**, 604
5. Harada, Y. (1978). Comparative anatomy of otolithic organ and otolith. *Ear Res.*, **9**, 55

Figure 137 Damage of the crista (guinea pig). (**a**) Lateral semicircular canal crista of the guinea pig treated with intratympanic injection of gentamycin 4 mg for 10 days. Sensory cells are lost in the middle part of the crista (× 260).
(**b**) High magnification of (a). Sensory cilia are fused or lost (× 3000)

a

b

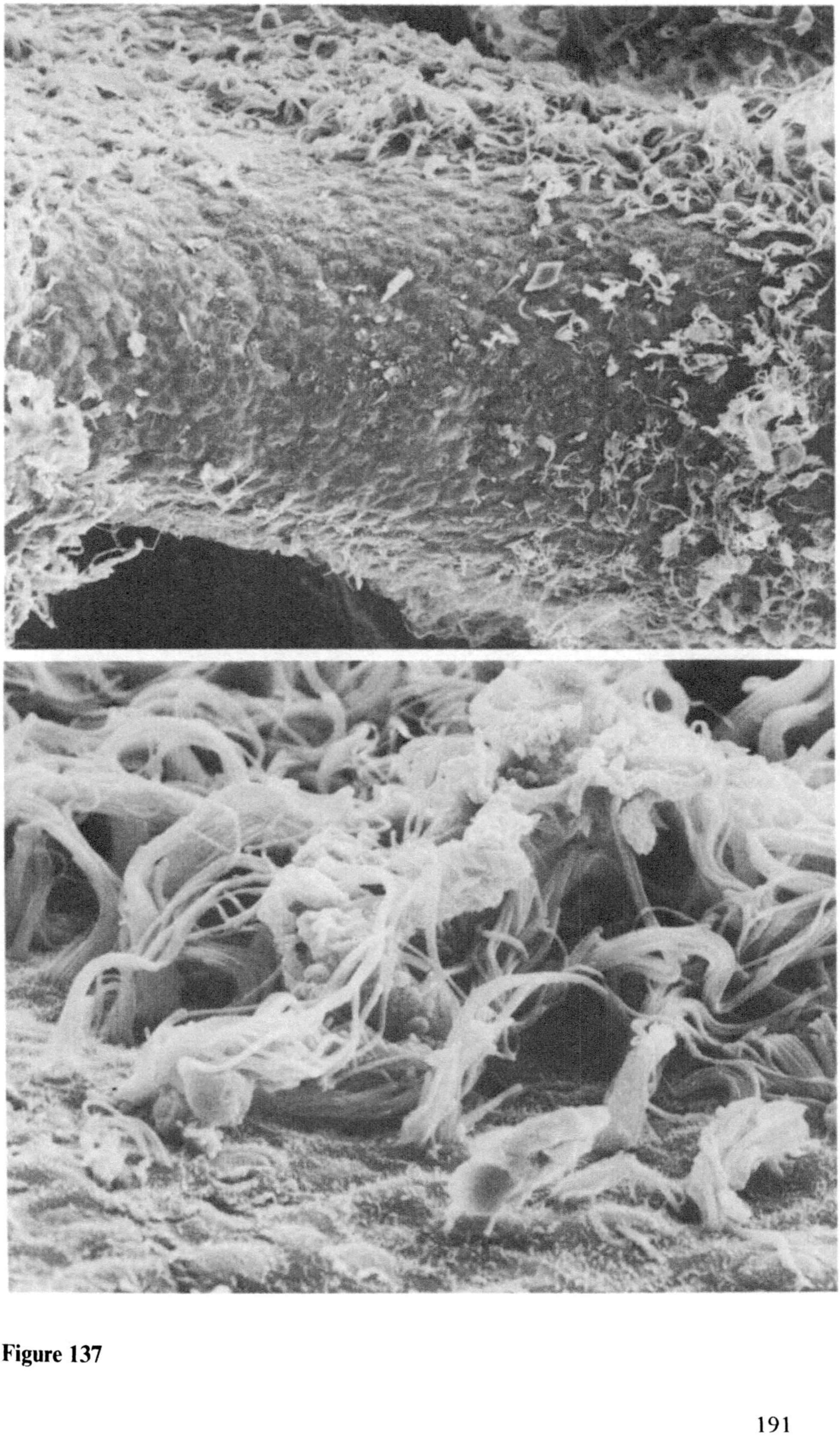

Figure 137

a

b

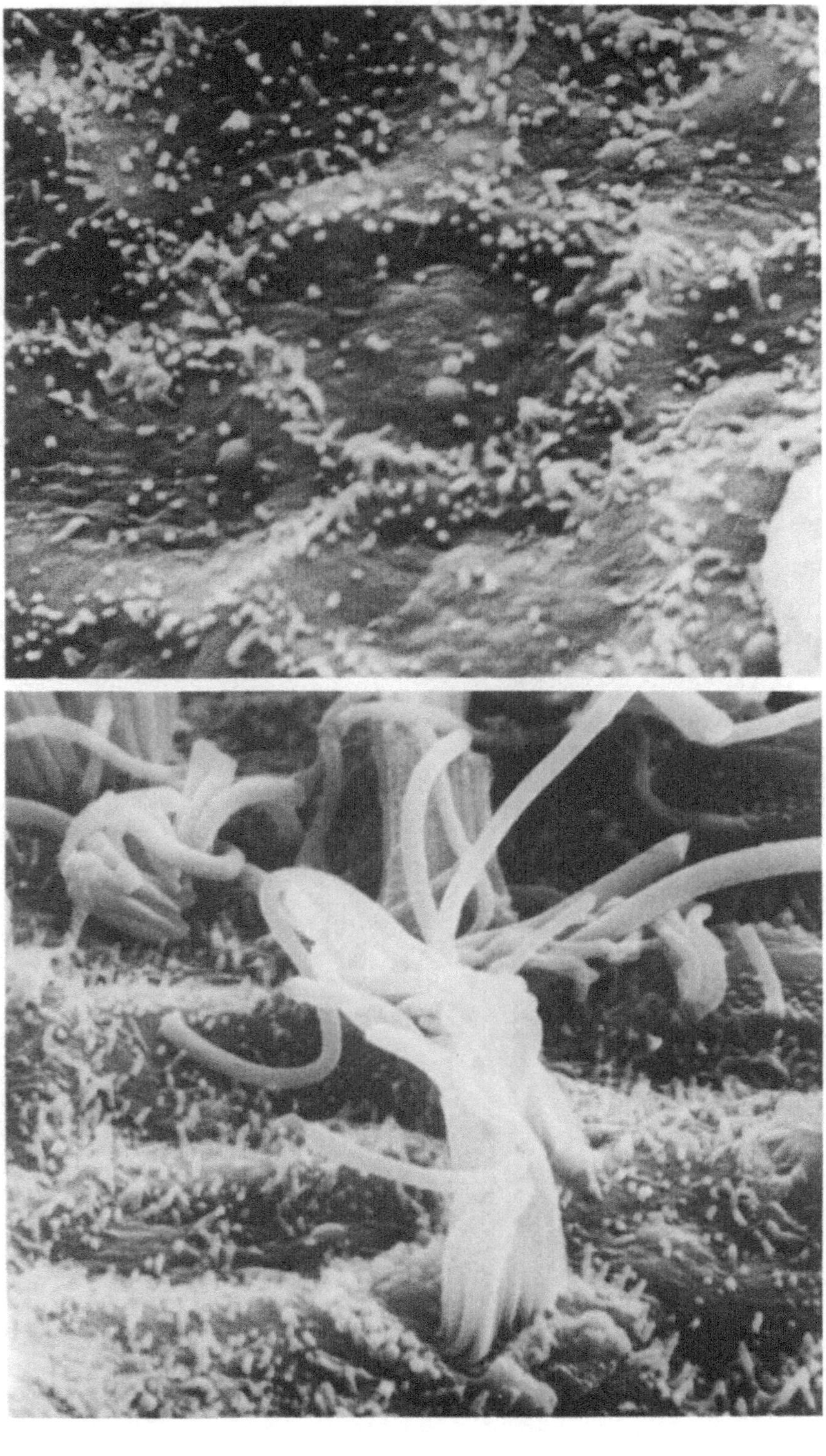

Figure 138 **(a)** The middle part of the crista. This part is well cleared of degenerated cells and replaced by the supporting cells (× 13 000). **(b)** Change of the sensory cilia. Cilia appear floppy with disturbed arrangement (× 13 000)

a

b

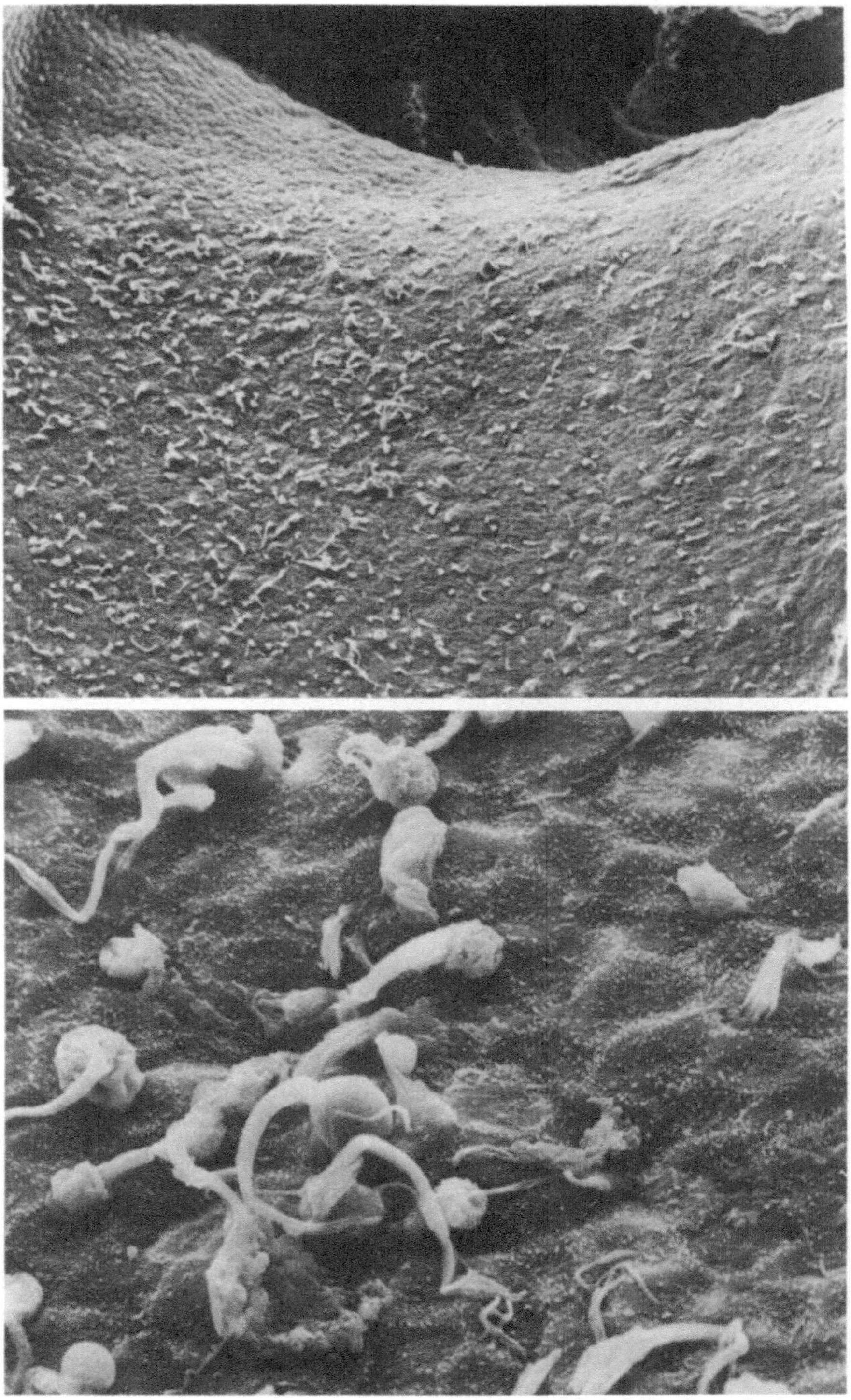

Figure 139 (**a**) Change of the utricular macula sensory cilia due to intratympanic injection of gentamycin (× 400). (**b**) High magnification of (a) (× 4000)

(I) *Changes of the vestibular organ due to intratympanic injection of gentamycin (guinea pig).*

Acute Experiment Severe degenerative changes were seen in the sensory epithelia. In the cristae of the semicircular canals, intensive changes were found, especially in the central portion. In all animal loss of the sensory cilia was observed and this extended to the whole area of the sensory epithelia in a few animals. Similar changes were found in the utricular macula. Degenerative change of the sensory cilia proceeded from fusion to disappearance of the cilia and this progression was common in all animals.

Chronic Experiment Further changes of the vestibular sensory epithelia were observed 2 months after intratympanic injection of gentamycin. Almost the whole population of sensory cilia of the cristae disappeared and the cristae appeared shrunken. Vesicular changes were observed on the surface of the sensory cilia which remained only in the peripheral part of the cristae. Changes of the cilia ranged from slight degeration to disappearance. Similar findings were observed in the utricular macula. According to these results, it is postulated that sensory cilia never regenerate like the tracheal cilia do.

Figure 140 (**a**) Crista showing loss of a great number of cilia 2 months after intratympanic injection of gentamycin (× 400), (**b**) crista without a healthy sensory cell. Fused cilia are situated in the corner of the cells (× 4000)

a

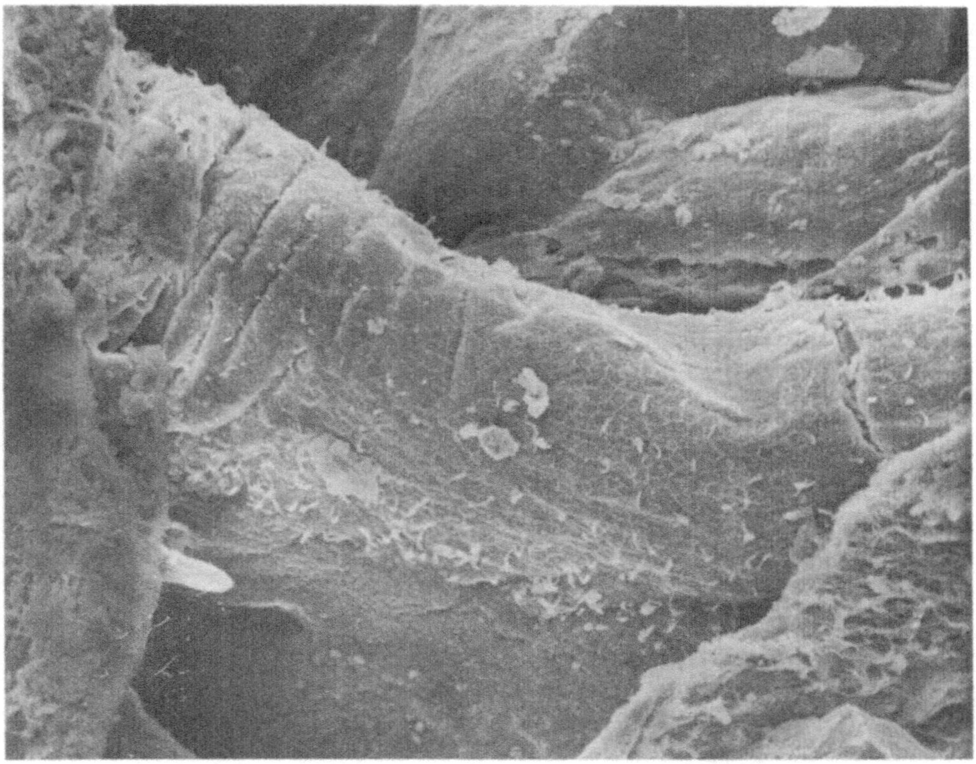

b

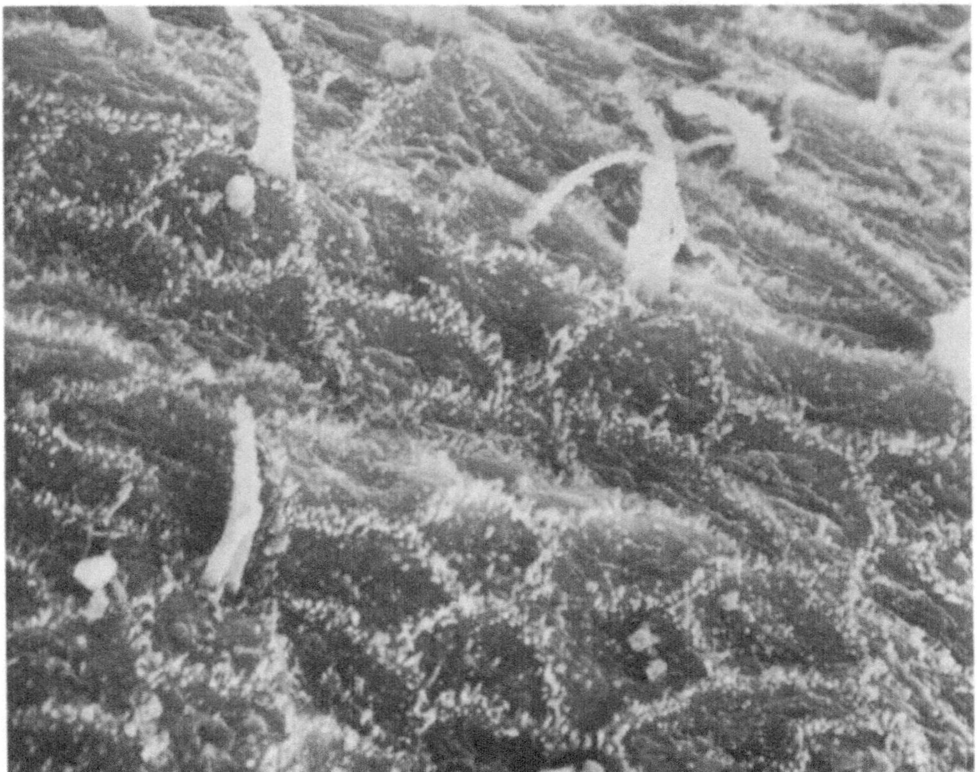

Figure 140

(2) *Changes of the vestibular organ due to intraperitoneal injection of streptomycin sulphate*

Guinea pigs were given an intraperitoneal injection of streptomycin sulphate (250 mg/kg) every other day for 2, 4, 6 and 8 weeks. Changes of the sensory epithelia did not develop as fast as with intratympanic injection. Only slight changes of the cilia were observed in the 2 week injection group. However, in the 4 week injection group, various changes were found in the central part of the crista, such as fusion, ballooning and slanting of the cilia. These changes were less severe than with intratympanic injection. The cilia also decreased in numbers. The periphery of the crista did not show any remarkable change in the 4 week injection group. However, in the 8 week injection group, the peripheral changes became recognizable.

Figure 141 Damage of the crista due to intraperitoneal injection of streptomycin (guinea pig). (**a**) Decreased cilia in the middle part of the crista (× 300), (**b**) disturbed pattern and ballooning of the cilia (arrow) (× 3000)

a

b

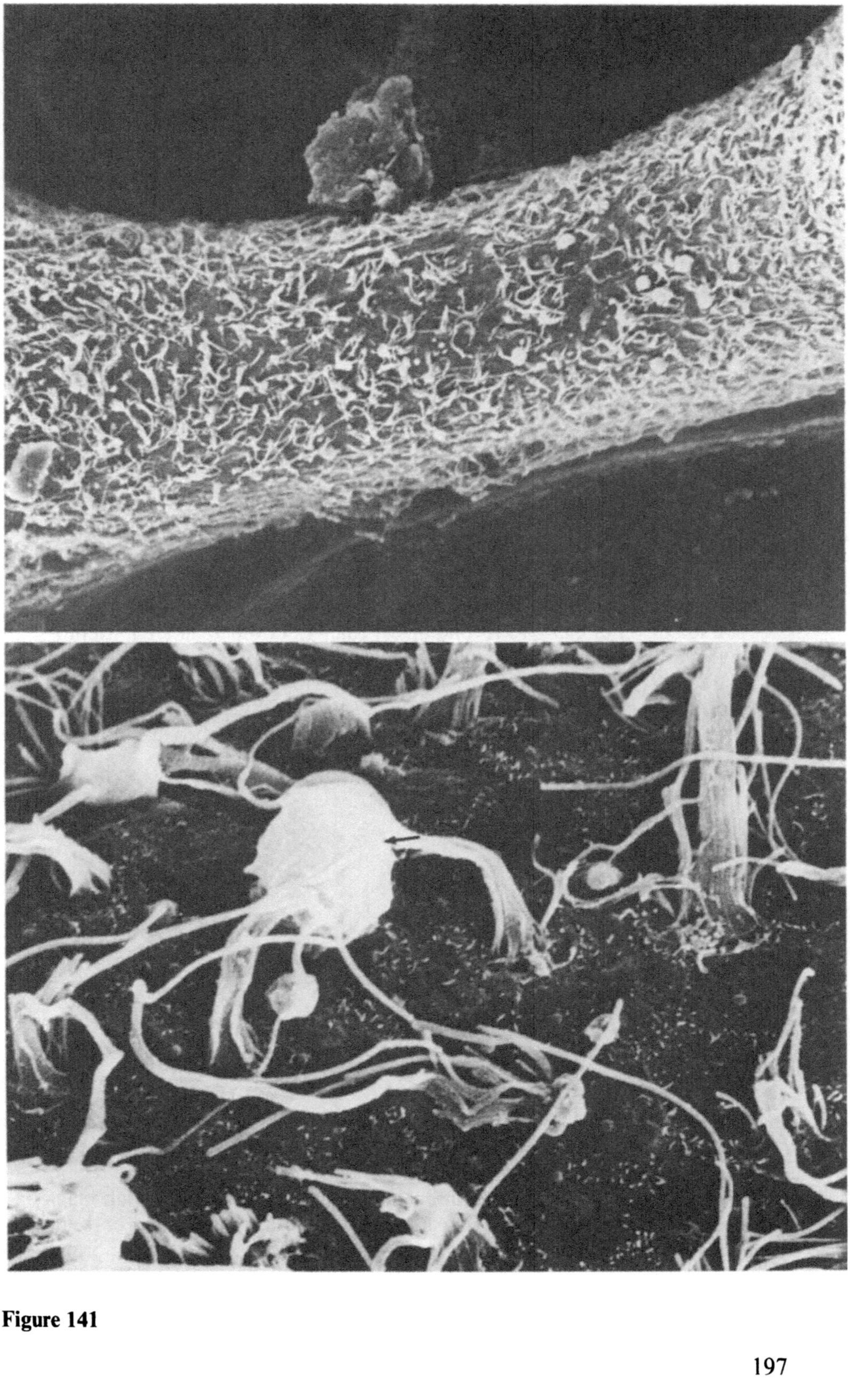

Figure 141

(3) *Changes of the otoconia*

Very few studies on the changes of the otoconia due to streptomycin sulphate injection have been performed. Only one study was done (Watanuki, 1971) on the changes of the otolithic layer. Initial changes in the otolithic layer developed after seven injections during a period of 2 weeks. The otoconia started falling from the portion of the striola. The longer the period of injection, the more severe the changes and the otolithic layer becomes thinner.

In the 2 week injection group, the otoconia in the otolithic layer were reduced in number and tended to be replaced by large otoconia. The otoconia showed some changes in the shape. They had jagged surfaces, were split in the central part, and had formation of layers in the end of the crystal.

It was also observed that changes in the otoconia precede those in the sensory cilia (Harada, 1973, 1978). The otoconia, which fall off the otolithic membrane, are transferred to the dark cell area where the otoconia are decalcified and finally absorbed.

References

1. Harada, Y. (1978). Morphological changes in the vestibular sensory organs after streptomycin intoxication. *Scanning Electron Microscopy*, **II**, 1977.
2. Harada, Y. *et al.* (1977) Morphological changes of otoconia after streptomycin intoxication. *Practica Otologica* (*Tokyo*), **70**, 1973
3. Harada, Y., Graham, M. D., Pulec, J. L. and House, W. F. (1978). Human otoconia in surgical specimens. *Arch. Otolaryngol*, **104**, 371
4. Harada, Y. and Sugimoto, Y. (1977). Metabolic disorder after streptomycin intoxication. *Acta Otolaryngol.* (*Stockholm*), **84**, 65

Figure 142 Otolithic layer of the utricle: the guinea pig treated with intraperitoneal injection of streptomycin for 2 weeks. Specimen was taken 2 weeks after cessation of injection. (**a**) Otoconia markedly reduced in the striola region (arrow). Large otoconia are predominantly observed (× 130). (**b**) High magnification of the striola region. The large otoconium is multilayered on both ends and looks cracked in the centre (arrow). Small otoconia appear normal (× 2500)

a

b

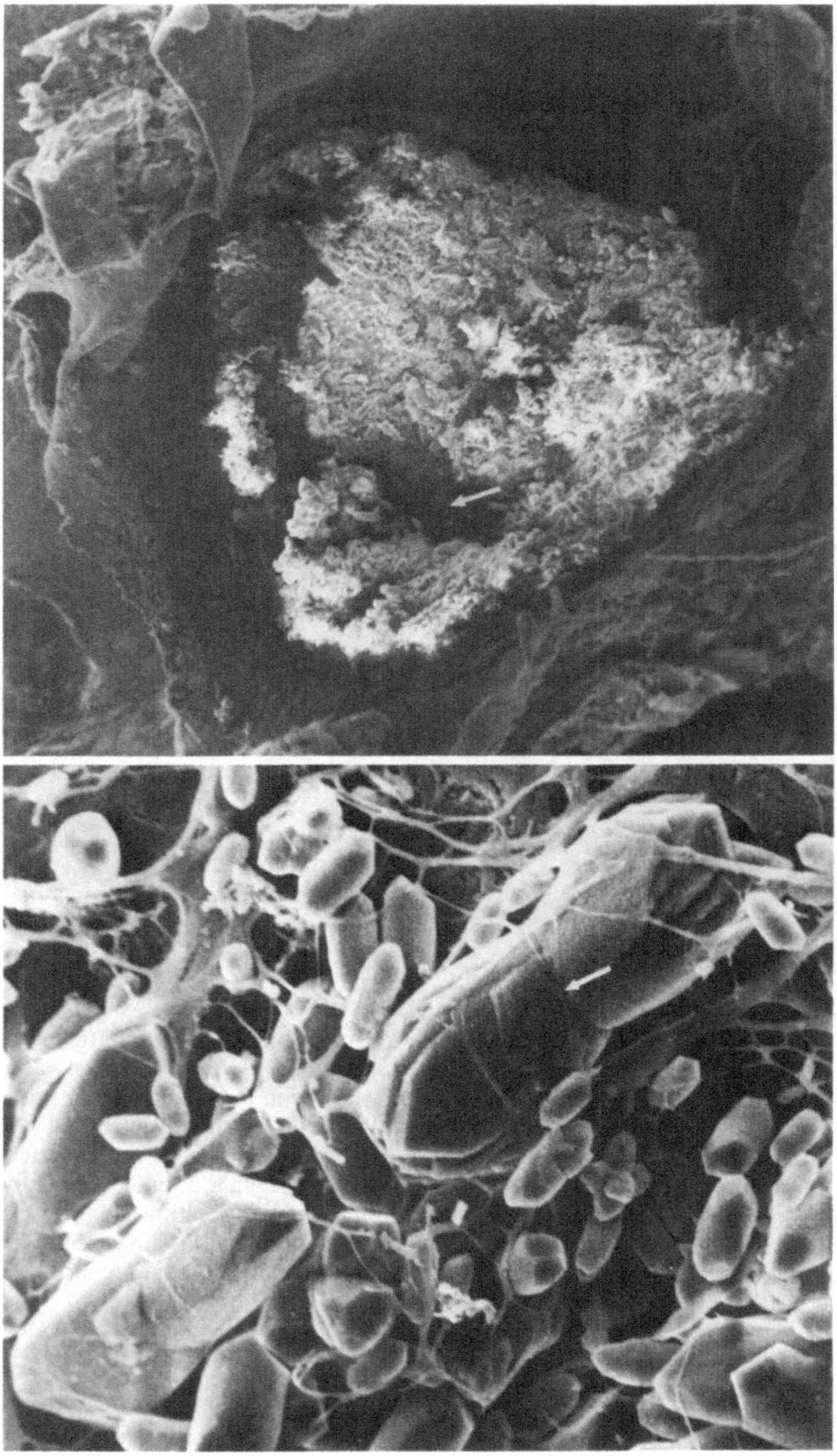

Figure 142

a b

c d

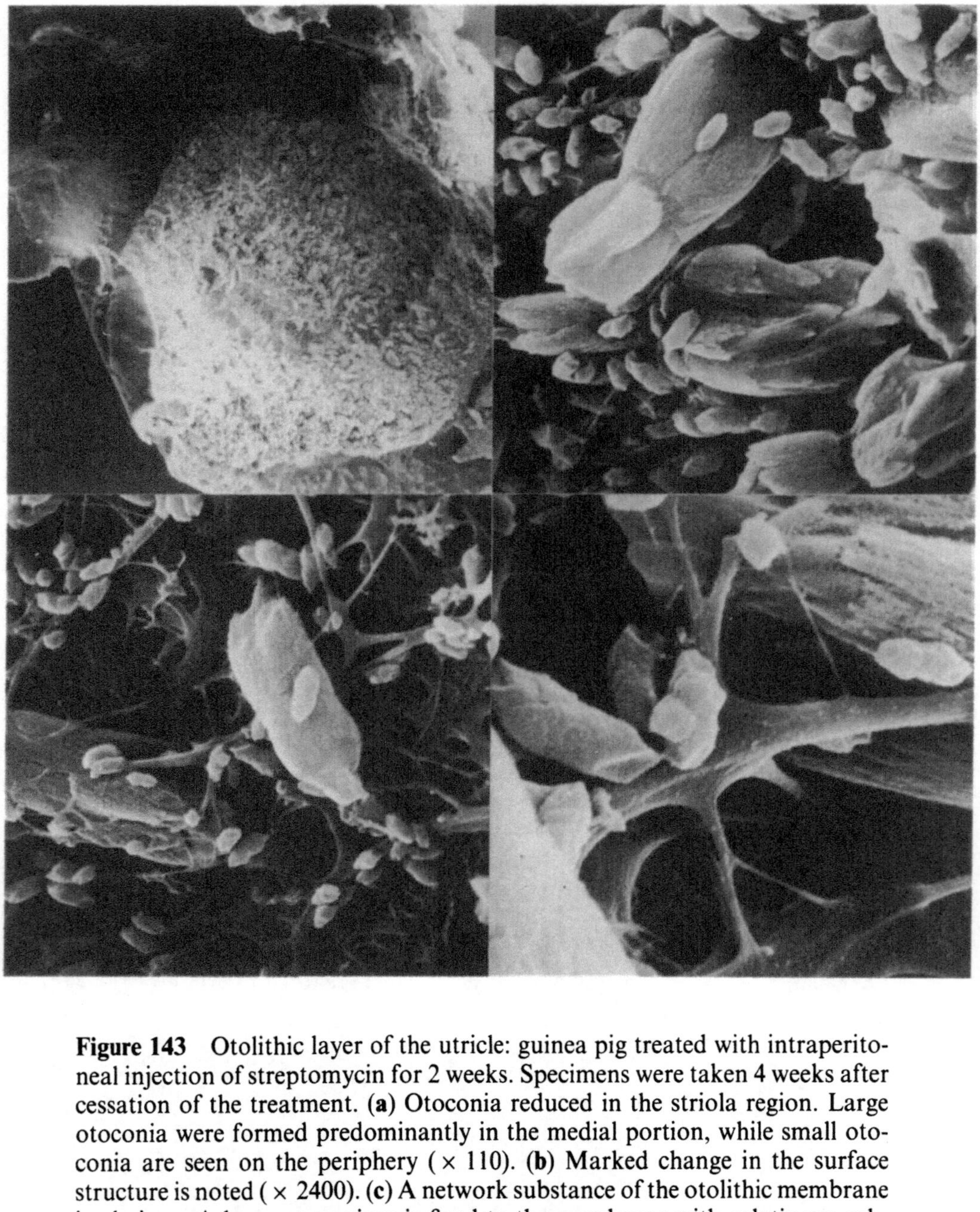

Figure 143 Otolithic layer of the utricle: guinea pig treated with intraperitoneal injection of streptomycin for 2 weeks. Specimens were taken 4 weeks after cessation of the treatment. (**a**) Otoconia reduced in the striola region. Large otoconia were formed predominantly in the medial portion, while small otoconia are seen on the periphery (× 110). (**b**) Marked change in the surface structure is noted (× 2400). (**c**) A network substance of the otolithic membrane is obvious. A large otoconium is fixed to the membrane with gelatinous substance (× 2400). (**d**) Gelatinous substance extends from the otolithic membrane and attaches to the otoconia. A few deformed small otoconia are also seen (× 8000)

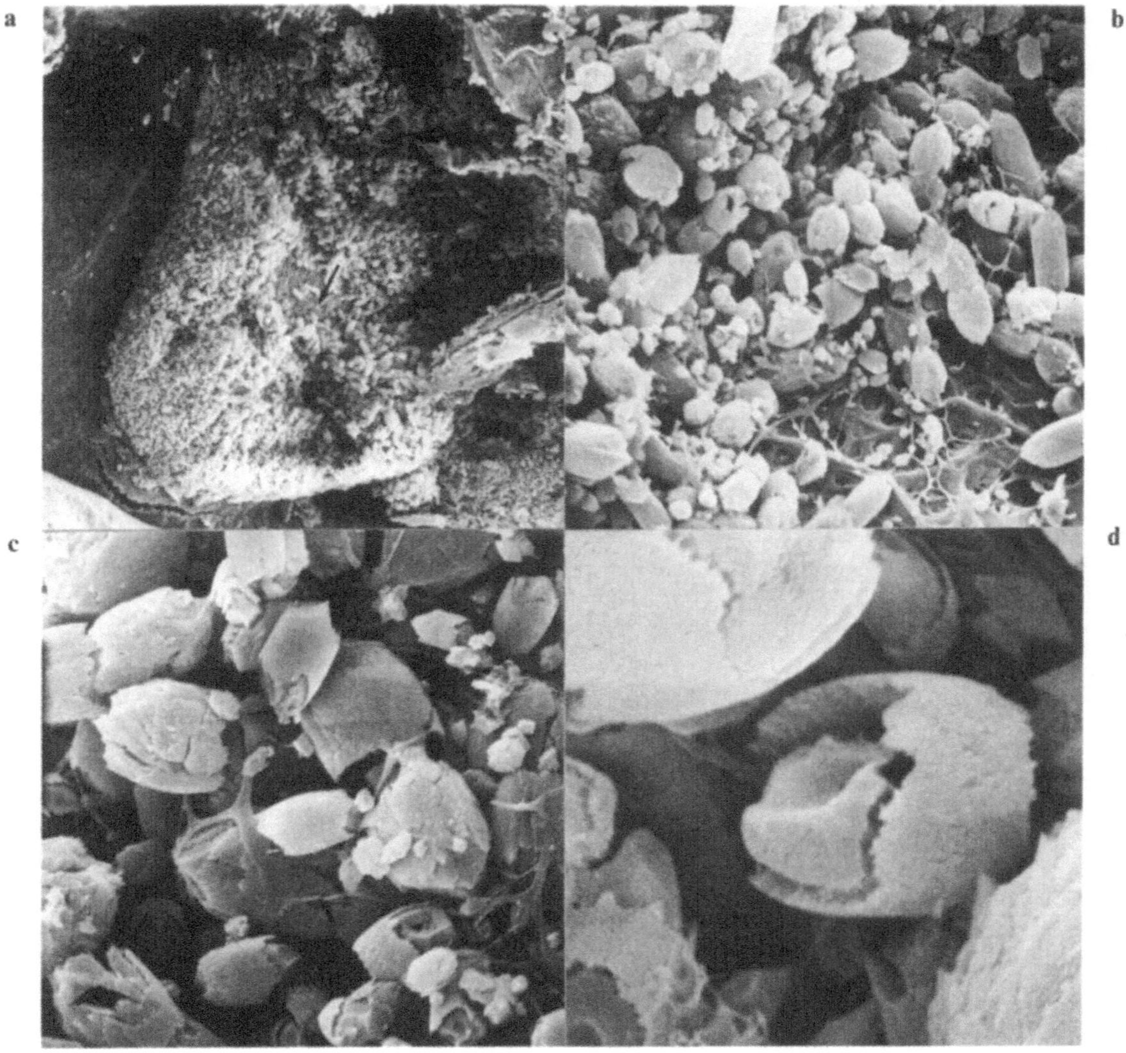

Figure 144 Otolithic layer of the utricle: guinea pig treated with streptomycin for 6 weeks. Specimen taken 4 weeks after cessation of the treatment. (**a**) Otolithic layer in the striola region appears remarkably thin with fairly wide area which misses otoconia (arrow) (× 100). (**b**) Number of small otoconia are deformed and cracks are seen in the equatorial portion of some otoconia (× 800). (**c**) Marked deformity of the otoconia. Both large and small otoconia are cracked in the centre (× 2400). (**d**) Crack in a small otoconium. Typical crystalline shape is already lost (× 8000)

(4) *Collapse of the otoconia*

Harada (1977) first reported collapse and degeneration of the otoconia due to streptomycin sulphate. As mentioned before, a split of the otoconia and multiple layer formation in the end of the crystal were observed in the course of collapse. The otolithic layer became thin from the striola, as small otoconia moved toward the dark cell area.

Streptomycin sulphate affects not only the vestibular sensory cells, but also the supporting cells of the sensory epithelia by inhibiting secretion of calcium. This possibly implicates metabolic disturbance and finally leads to collapse of the otoconia.

Figure 145 **(a)** Degenerated otoconia, the striola region (× 4000). **(b)** Degenerated otoconia; a portion apart from the striola (× 4000)

a

b

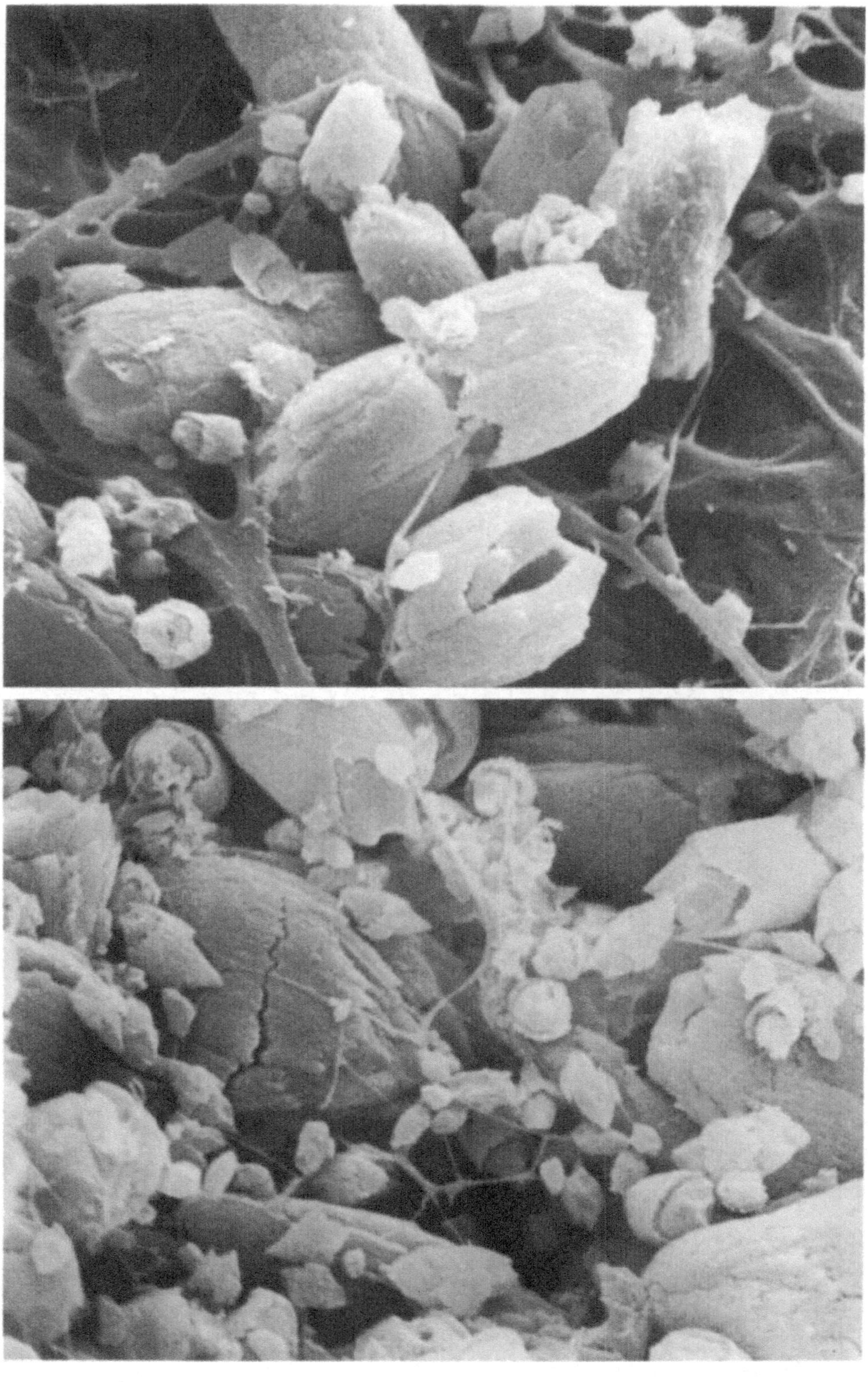

Figure 145

a

b

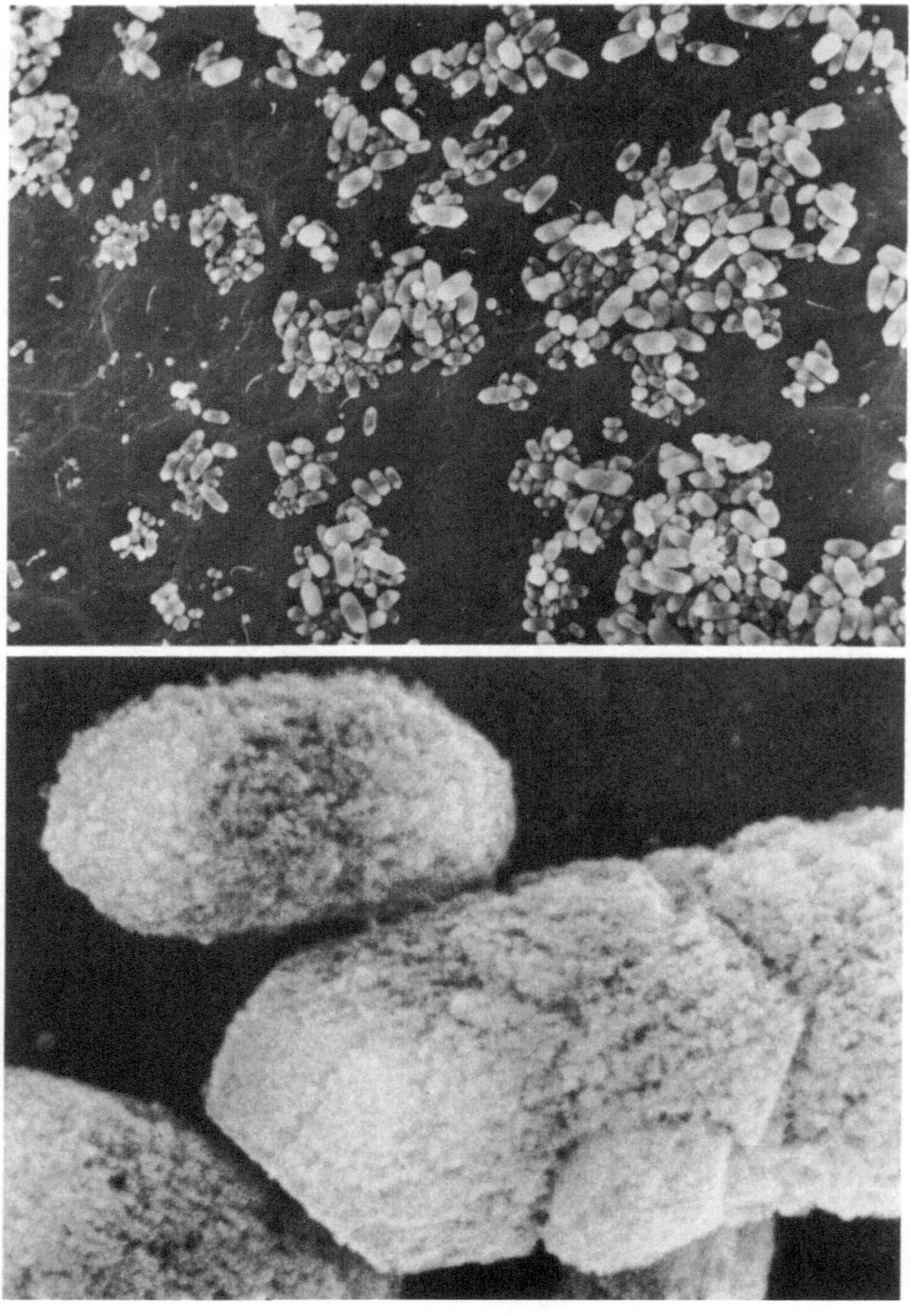

Figure 146 (**a**) Streptomycin-injected guinea pig: otoconia are disposed on the utricular dark cells after detaching from the otolithic membrane (× 1100). (**b**) High magnification of (a) (× 22 000)

(5) *Regeneration of the otoconia*

Harada (1977) first demonstrated turnover of the otoconia. In his studies, it was shown that the supporting cells of the macula produce otoconia, while the vestibular dark cells absorb them (Harada, 1977, 1978).

The author occasionally found changes of the otolithic layer and decrease in the otoconia, while carrying out experiments on inner ear damage due to streptomycin sulphate. After injecting streptomycin every other day for 4 to 8 weeks, changes in the otoconia and the otolithic layer, as mentioned in the previous section, developed. However, the otoconia accumulated again in the otolithic layer after ceasing the treatment. Two months after the cessation of the streptomycin sulphate injection, the otoconia started regenerating and accumulating in the otolithic layer. At this point the otoconia were not crystal-shaped. They slowly regained the original shape later on.

a

b

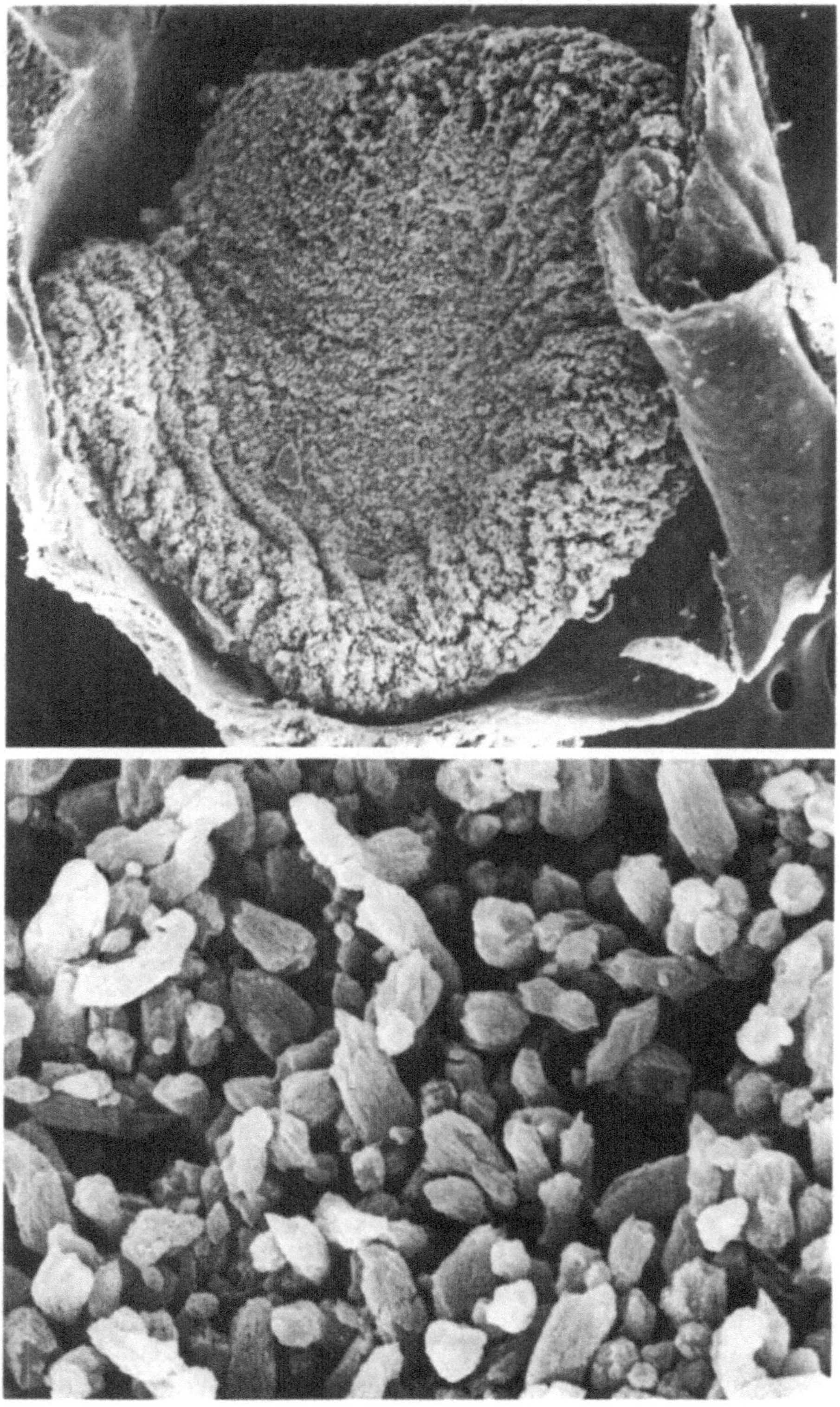

Figure 147 (**a**) Regeneration of the otoconia. About 8 weeks after cessation of streptomycin injection. The otolithic layer becomes thicker with a number of small otoconia visible (× 140). (**b**) Regenerated otoconia. Each otoconium is not typically crystalline yet (× 4000)

Morphological changes of the middle ear mucosa in sensory otitis media

In the middle ear mucosa, five cell types have been described: basal cell, intermediate cell, ciliated cell, non-ciliated cell with granules, and non-ciliated cell without granules (Hentzer, 1970; Shimada and Lim, 1972). Secretory cells have only little secretory capacity.

The mucosa in secretory otitis media consists mainly of secretory cells, and the number of ciliated cells is decreased. Intercellular spaces are widened, and the epithelium is thicker than the normal mucosa.

Aetiological factors of secretory ototis media are tubal dysfunction, infection, inflammation and allergy. The morphological changes of middle ear in secretory otitis media were examined under scanning electron microscope.

References

1. Hentzer, E. (1970). Ultrastructure of middle ear mucosa in secretory otitis media. *Acta Otolaryngol.* (*Stockholm*), **73**, 394
2. Lim, D. J. (1976). Recent advances in middle ear effusion. *Ann. Otol.*, **85**, Suppl., 25
3. Moller, P. and Dalen, H. (1981). Ultrastructure of the middle ear mucosa in secretory otitis media. *Acta Otolaryngol.*, **91**, 95
4. Shimada, T. and Lim, D. J. (1972). Distribution of ciliated cells in the human middle ear. *Ann. Otol.*, **81**, 203
5. Tom, M. (1980). Middle ear epithelia in chronic secretory otitis. *Arch. Otolaryngol.*, **106**, 593

a

b

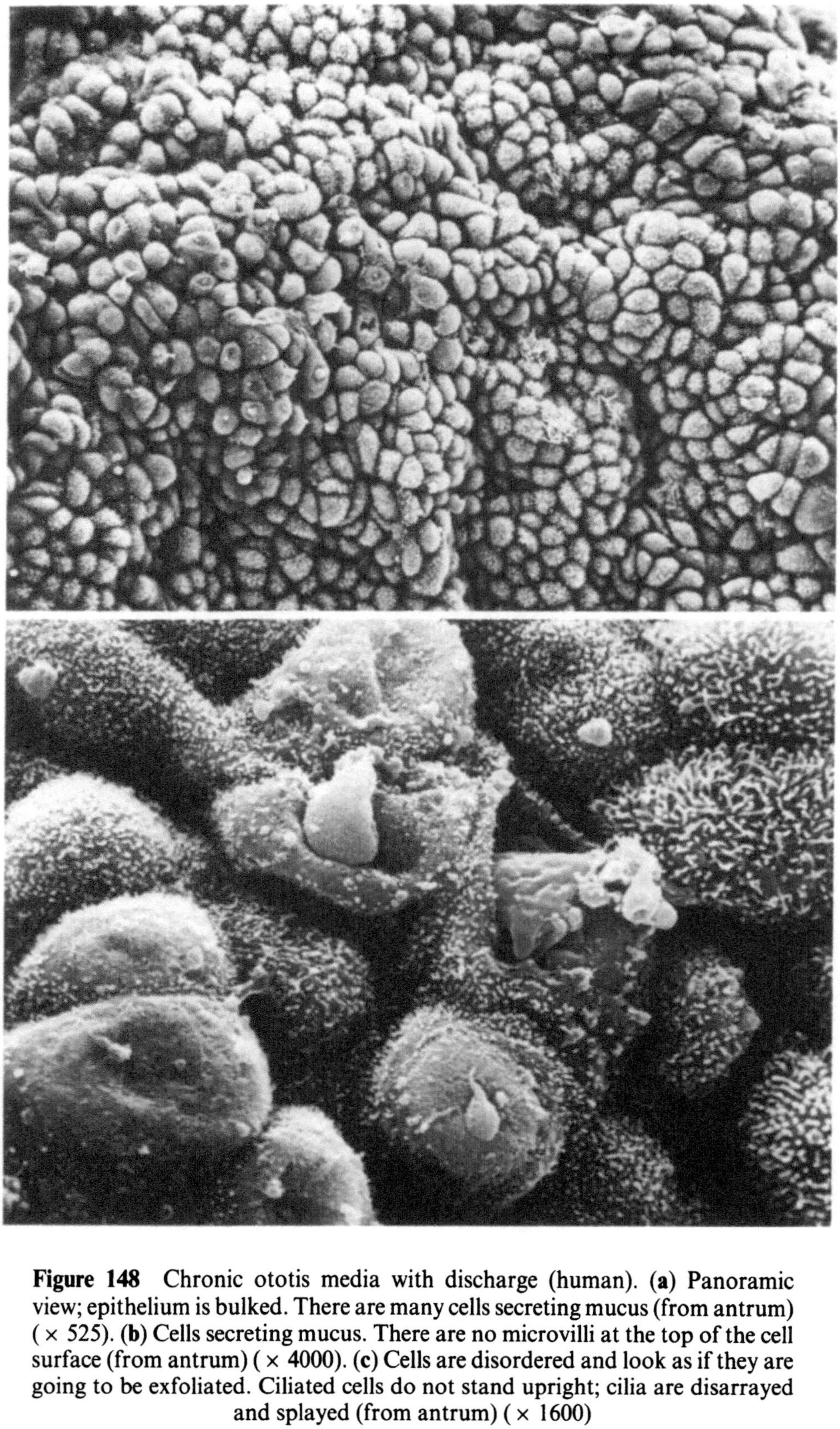

Figure 148 Chronic ototis media with discharge (human). (**a**) Panoramic view; epithelium is bulked. There are many cells secreting mucus (from antrum) (× 525). (**b**) Cells secreting mucus. There are no microvilli at the top of the cell surface (from antrum) (× 4000). (**c**) Cells are disordered and look as if they are going to be exfoliated. Ciliated cells do not stand upright; cilia are disarrayed and splayed (from antrum) (× 1600)

c

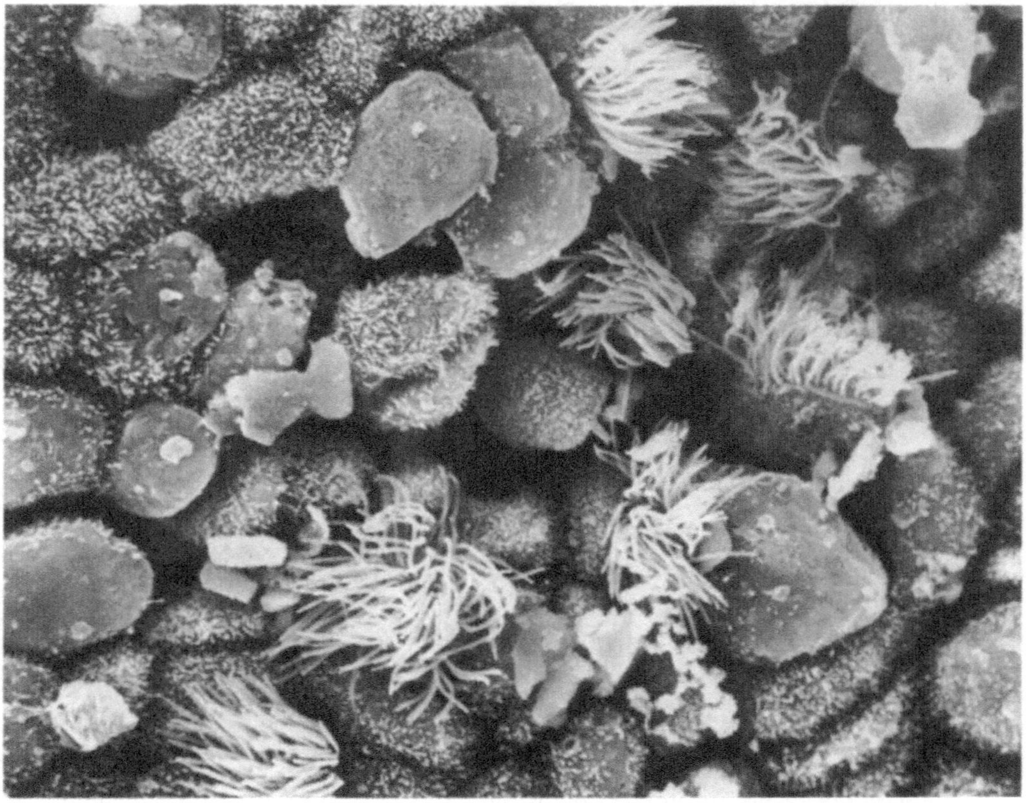

Figure 148

a

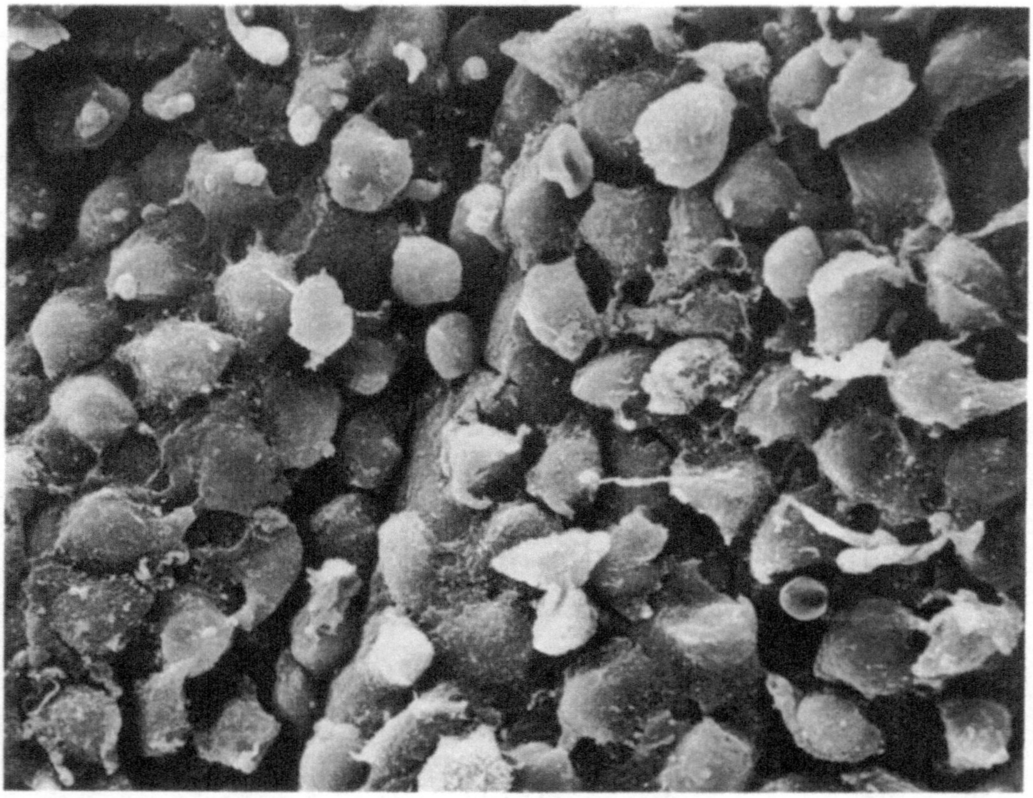

Figure 149 Chronic ototis media without discharge (human). (**a**) Epithelium has already lost its superficial layer. Underlying cells disposed in a few layers are exposed (from promontory) (× 1300). (**b**) Epithelium has lost part of its superficial layer (from promontory) (× 2600). (**c**) Basal cells, fusiform cells resting on the basal lamina (from promontory) (× 4500)

b

c

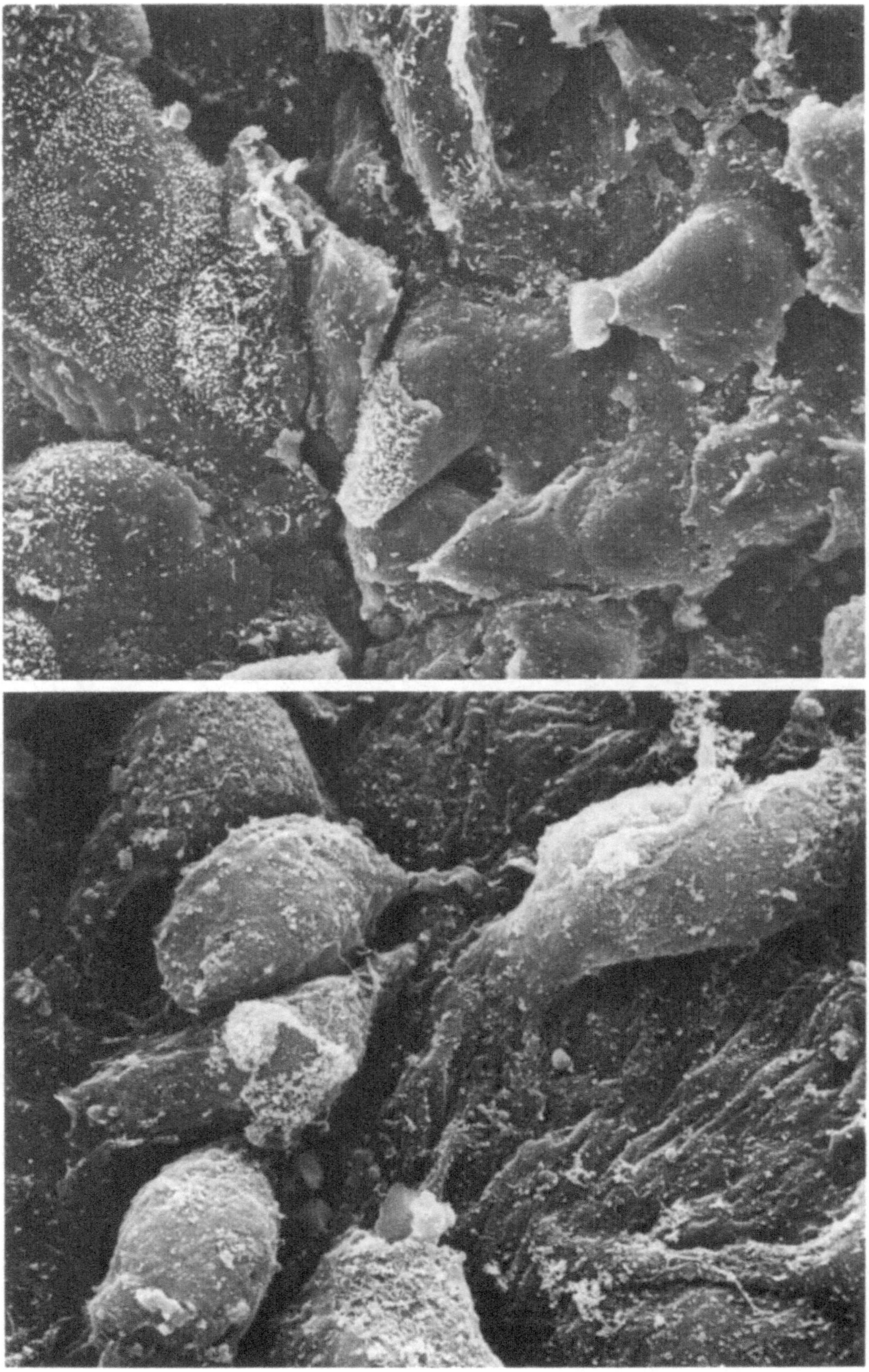

Figure 149

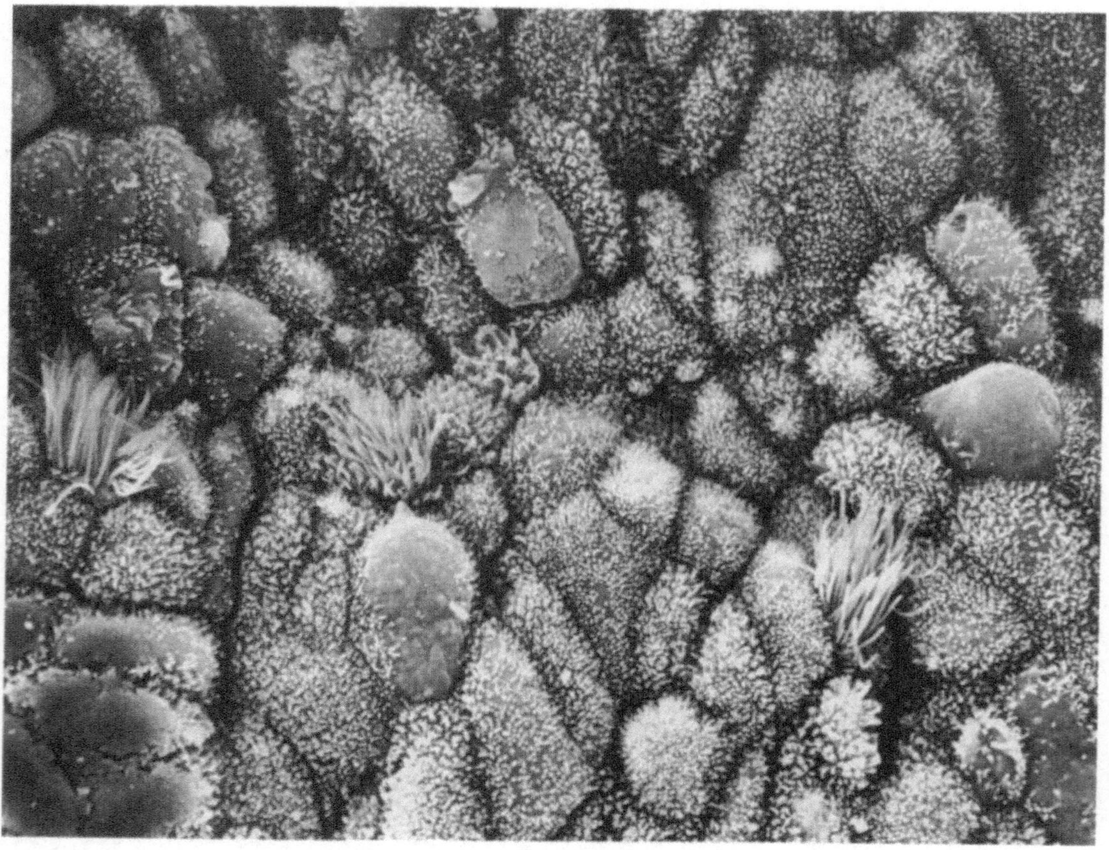

Figure 150 Epithelium appears uniform. There are a few ciliated cells. (Biopsy taken from promontory when the silicon sheet was removed in the second operation) (× 2000)

Cholesteatoma

Cholesteatoma is characterized by keratinizing stratified squamous epithelium within the middle ear cleft. This epithelial layer is continuously desquamated and the sheets of desquamated epithelium form the mass of cholesteatoma.

a

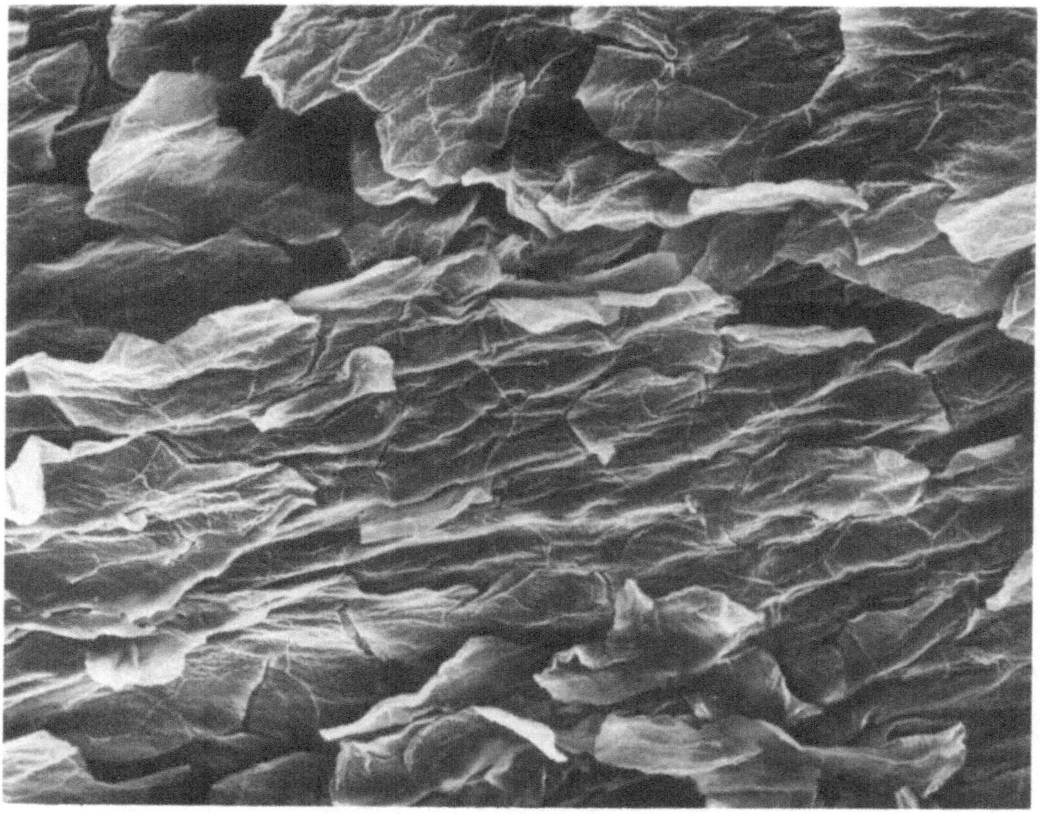

b

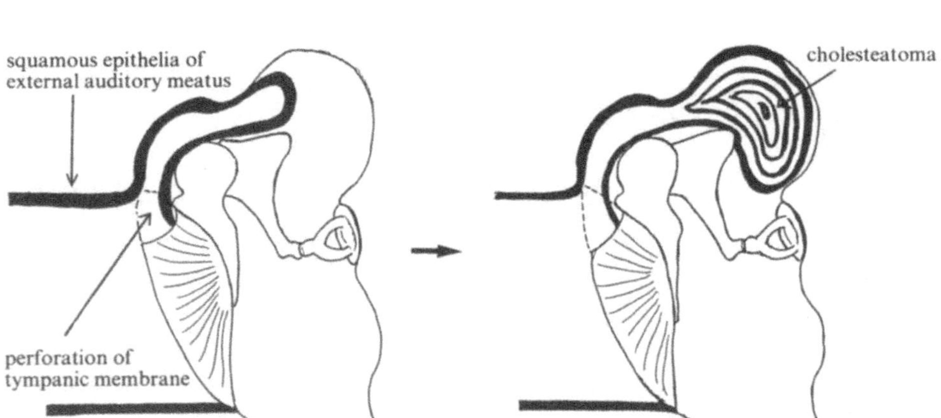

Figure 151 Cholesteatoma (human). (**a**) Squamous epithelium. There are many flat desquamated cells (from mastoid) (× 450). (**b**) Formation of cholesteatoma

Morphological changes of the organ of Corti by aminoglycosides

Some aminoglycosides, such as dihydrostreptomycin, kanamycin and gentamycin affect the organ of Corti. Severe damage is represented by fusion or loss of the sensory cilia and degeneration of the hair cell which is replaced by the supporting cell. Changes of the sensory cilia are more remarkable in the lower turn and the outer hair cell is more vulnerable. However, some studies showed that the inner hair cell is more vulnerable in the upper turn. Intracellular changes are an increase in lysozomal activity under the cuticular plate and an appearance of non-structural substance and vacuoles of various size. These are seen in the early stage, but changes of the sensory cilia develop more slowly than the changes due to acoustic trauma.

Reference

1. Nakai, Y. *et al.* (1976). Combined effect of aminoglycoside antibiotic and potent diuretics on the cochlea. *Audiology Japan*, **19**, 67

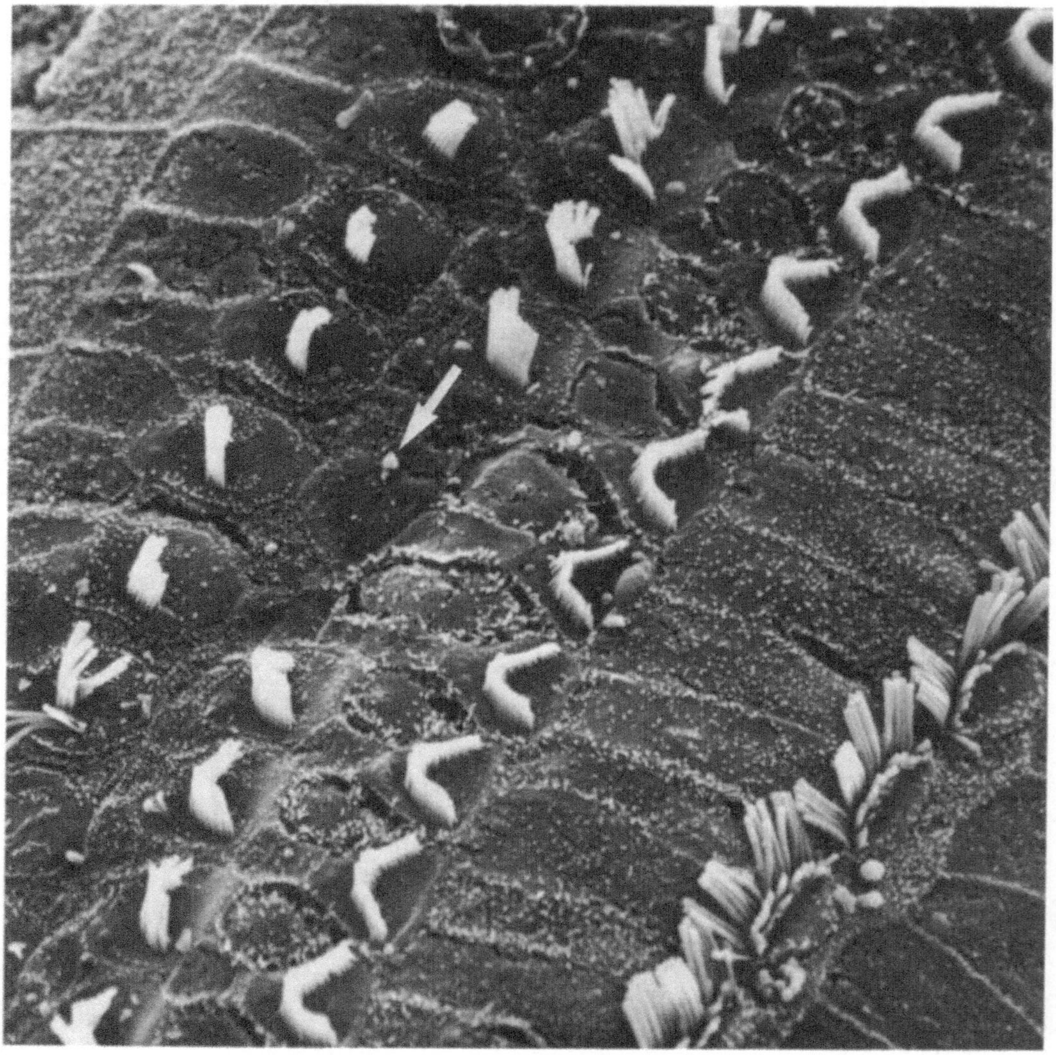

Figure 152 Damage to the organ of Corti due to streptomycin (guinea pig). Loss of a few stereocilia and a degenerated hair cell (arrow) in the second row are observed. The specimen was removed immediately after cessation of streptomycin injection (250 mg/kg) given every other day for a period of 4 weeks (× 3000)

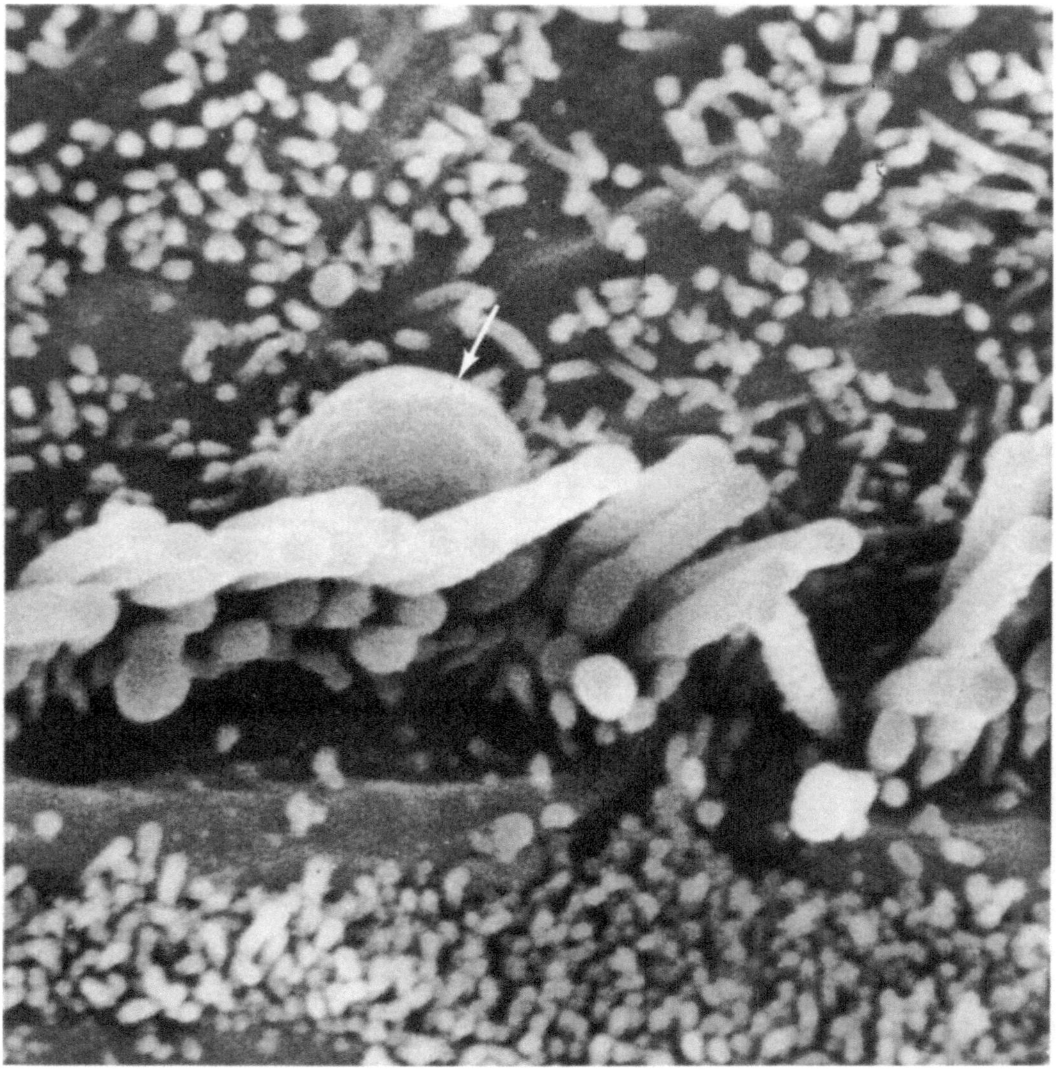

Figure 153 Surface of the third turn inner hair cell (guinea pig). Loss of some stereocilia and cytoplasmic protrusion (arrow) are observed (× 15 000)

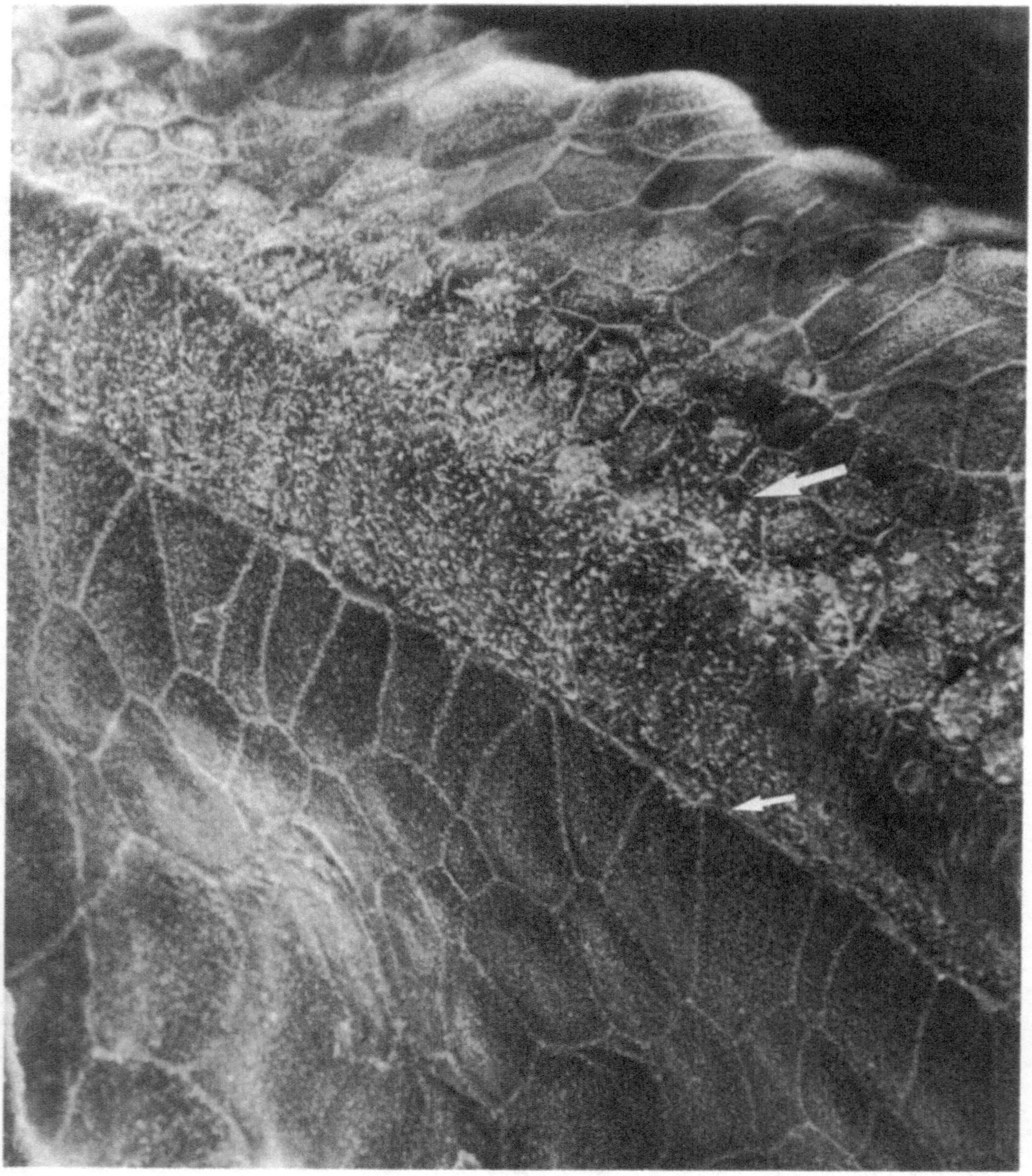

Figure 154 Second turn of the guinea pig cochlea after treatment by streptomycin injection for 8 weeks. Sterocilia are completely wiped out. Note tidy appearance of the cuticular plates after being replaced by the supporting cells in 2 months after treatment (arrow) (× 1200)

Figure 155 Change of the endolymphatic sac due to streptomycin (250 mg/kg) injection for 4 weeks (guinea pig). Examination of the rugose portion revealed some changes in the light cells. (**a**) Microvilli of the light cells appear small (× 3600), (**b**) surface of the light cell. Microvilli are short with bulging on top (× 12 000), (**c**) high magnification of the microvilli. Bulging of the tips is obvious (× 36 000)

a

b

c

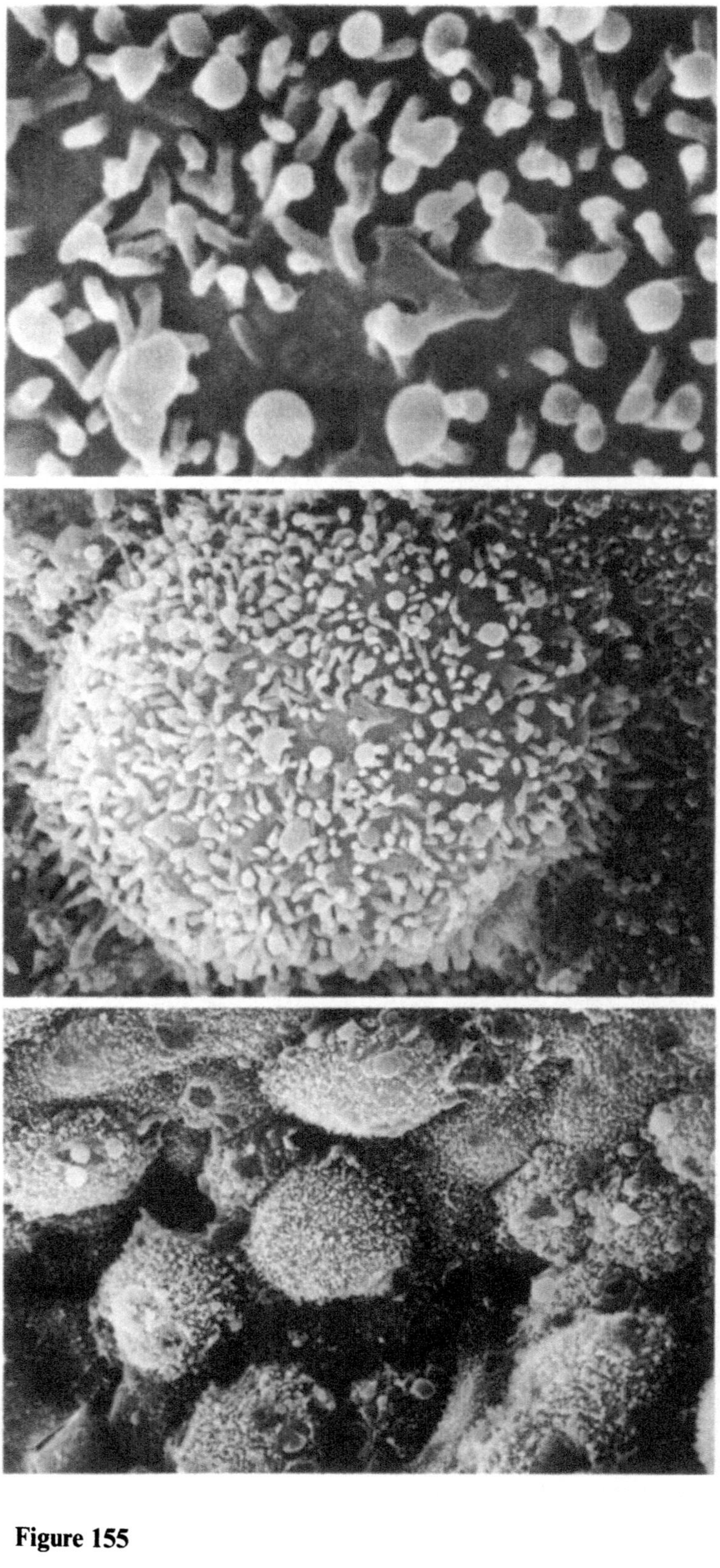

Figure 155

Acoustic damage to the organ of Corti

Acoustic damage to the organ of Corti is already well known as C^5-dip. Many studies on acoustic trauma in human cases have been done. Acoustic trauma has also studied in animals at both light and electron microscopic levels. The scanning electron-microscope enables observation of many hair cells continuously from turn to turn. Change of the hair cell is characterized by loss of the hair cell which is replaced by the supporting cells (Murakami, 1970; Melnick, 1971; Fujimoto, 1972; Duvar, 1978; Theopold, 1978). In this chapter, our guinea pig study is presented.

The animals were exposed to the white noise (100 dB/SPL) for 5 hours. In the basal turn, no remarkable change was found. In the second turn, slight disarray and shortening of the outer hair cell cilia were observed. The inner hair cell cilia remained almost intact. The third turn was most severely affected. From the lower one third of the third turn, changes of the second and third rows of the outer hair cells developed. Next, the first row of the outer hair cells was also affected. These changes were disarray and loss of the cilia. The inner hair cells showed protrusion of the cytoplasm from the basal body, fusion of the cilia and giant cilia. Further changes were degeneration and disappearance of the hair cells. In the fourth turn, however, only a few cilia were disarrayed, indicating that acoustic overstimulation selectively affects the third turn.

References

1. Duvar, H. (1978). Electron microscopic assessment of the cochlea – some technique and results. *Acta Otolaryngol.* (*Stockholm*), Suppl. 351
2. Melnick, W. (1971). Acoustic damage of the cochlea. A scanning and transmission electron microscopic observation. *Arch. Otolaryngol.*, **94**, 294
3. Theopold, H. M. (1978). Das akustische trauma im tierexperiment – Morphologische veränderung der Meerschweinchen Cochlea nach Knalltrauma (Rasterelektronen mikroskopie). *Laryngol. Rhinol.*, **57**, 706

Figure 156 Cochlear damage due to acoustic overstimulation (guinea pig). (**a**) Change in the third turn. Initial damage occurs in the outer hair cells in the 2nd and 3rd turns. Loss of the sensory cilia in the 3rd turn and cytoplasmic protrusion in the 2nd turn are observed (arrow) (× 640). (**b**) High magnification of (a). Protrusion of the cytoplasm and loss of sensory cilia in the second row are seen. Cytoplasm of the inner hair cell (arrow) (× 1600)

a

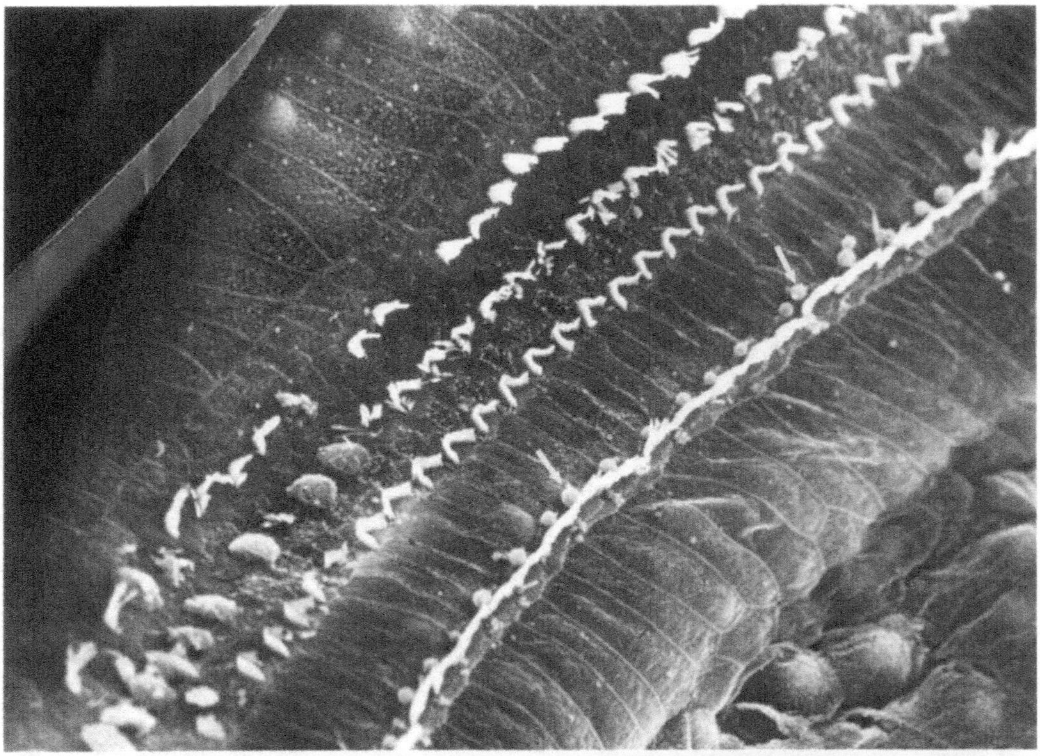

b

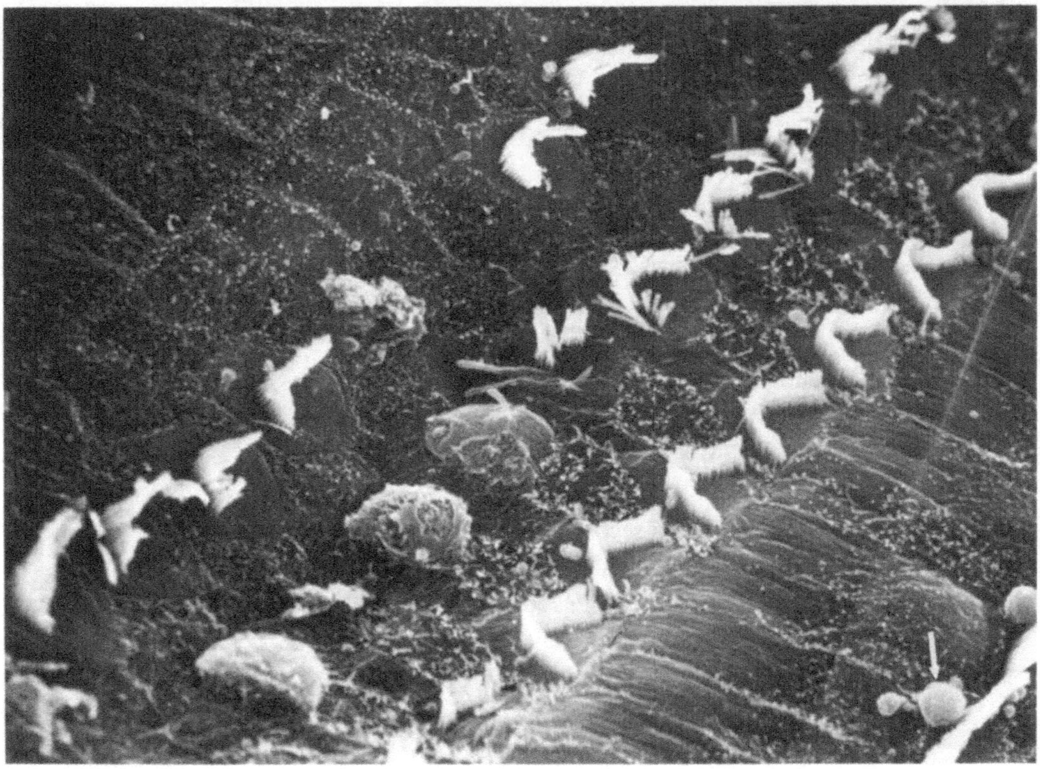

Figure 156

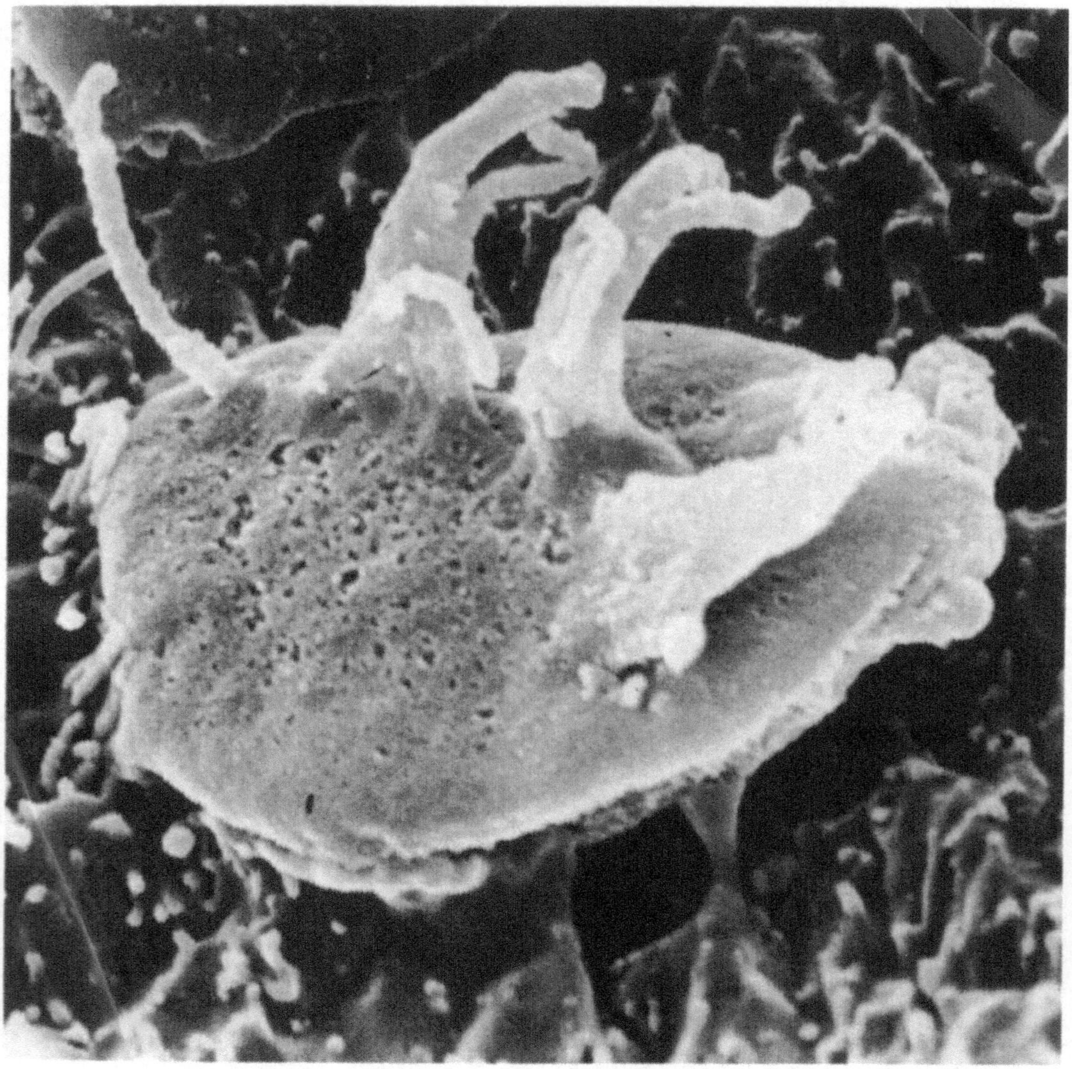

Figure 157 Degenerated second row outer hair cell (guinea pig, third turn). Loss of sensory cilia and protrusion of the cell body. Only deformed sensory cilia are left on the protruded hair cell body (× 22 500)

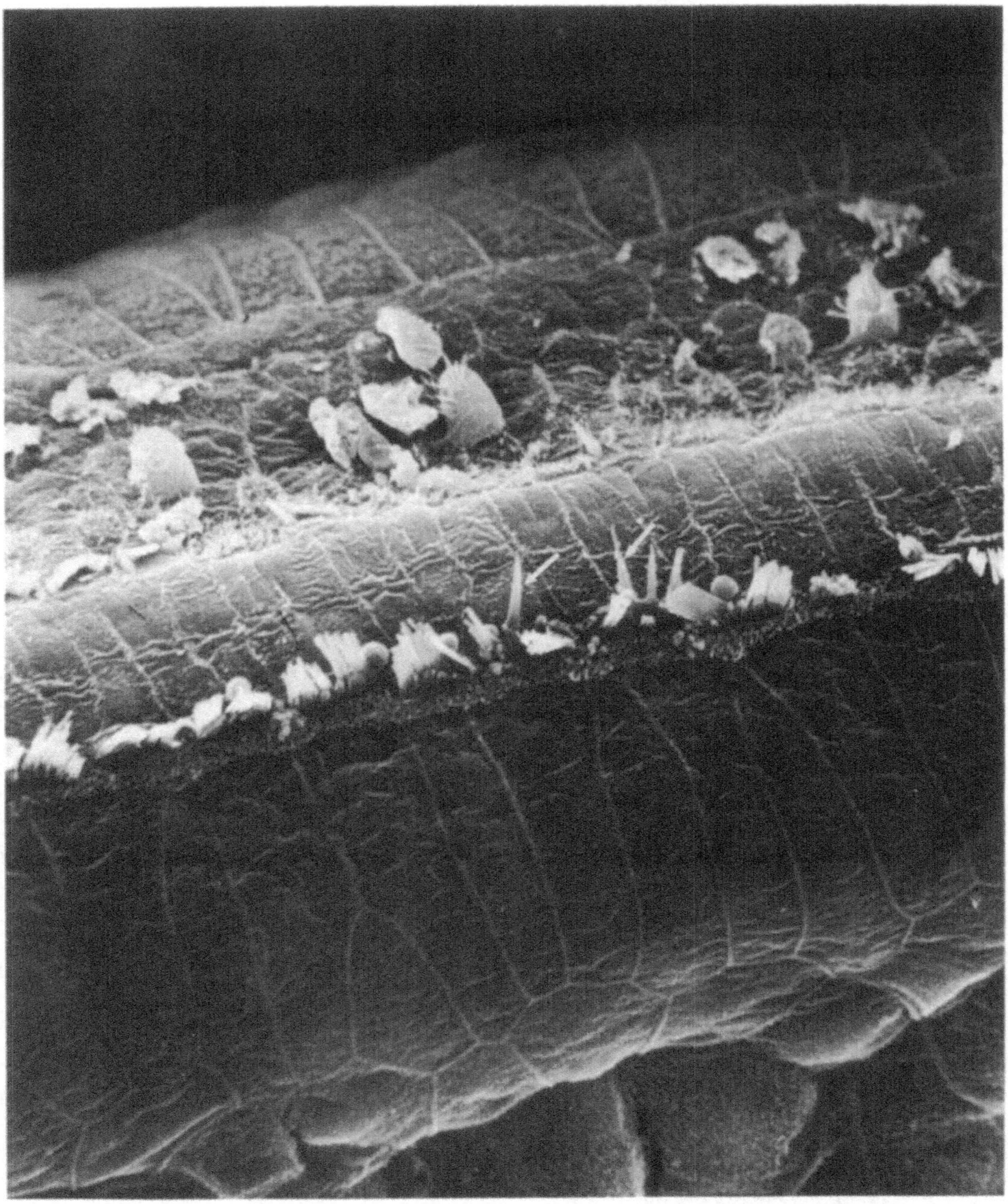

Figure 158 Severe damage of the outer hair cells (guinea pig, third turn). Outer hair cells sustained more damage than the inners. Change in the outer hair cells observed here could be described 'cell body extrusion' rather than 'cytoplasmic protrusion'. A few giant cilia (arrow) are seen in the inner hair cells (× 1100)

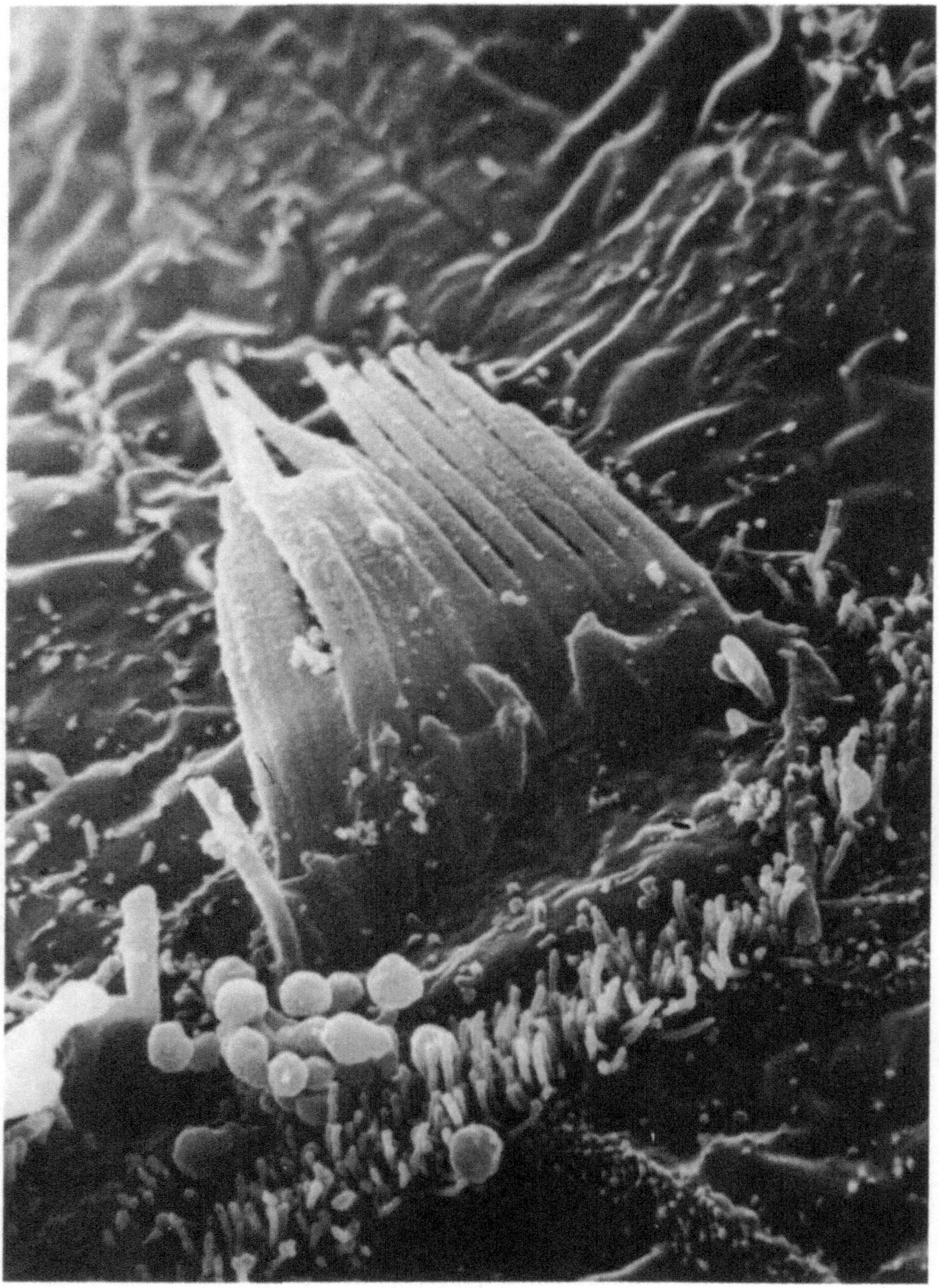

Figure 159 Fused inner hair cell cilia. Fusion of cilia is seen in the process of hair cell degeneration. Extremely tall cilia are called giant cilia. Global substance on the cell surface are swollen microvilli (× 8800)

Pathological changes of human vestibular organs

A great number of histological studies on human temporal bones have been performed. However, only a few SEM studies were found, because specimens taken from the cadaver are so frequently contaminated by artifact. In cases of acoustic neuroma and Ménière's disease, specimens were taken during labyrinthectomy. These specimens revealed a decrease in the sensory cilia and sensory cells (Harada, 1977). Loss and shortening of the cilia were observed in the lateral semicircular canal of another case of Ménière's disease (Harada, 1973). In a few cases, the otolithic organ showed some changes, such as crack formation in the otoconia which was also recognized in the animal study (Harada, 1975, 1978).

References

1. Harada, Y. (1973). Observation of morphological changes in the vestibular sensory epithelia. *Equilibrium. Res.*, **3**, 48
2. Harada, Y. *et al.* (1977). Scanning electron microscopic studies on the pathological changes of human vestibular organs. *Otologia* (*Fukuoka*), **23**, 597
3. Harada, Y. *et al.* (1978). Human otoconia in surgical specimens. *Arch. Otolaryngol.*, **104**, 371

Index